Basic and Clinical Science Course

Louis B. Cantor, MD, Indianapolis, Indiana, *Senior Secretary for Clinical Education*

Christopher J. Rapuano, MD, Philadelphia, Pennsylvania, *Secretary for Lifelong Learning and Assessment*

George A. Cioffi, MD, New York, New York, *BCSC Course Chair*

Section 11

Faculty

Sharon L. Jick, MD, *Chair*, St Louis, Missouri
Thomas L. Beardsley, MD, Asheville, North Carolina
Chadwick R. Brasington, MD, Burlington, North Carolina
Carlos Buznego, MD, Miami, Florida
Richard J. Grostern, MD, Chicago, Illinois
Lisa Park, MD, New York, New York
Timothy V. Roberts, MD, Sydney, Australia

The Academy wishes to acknowledge the *American Society of Cataract and Refractive Surgery* and the *Contact Lens Association of Ophthalmologists* for recommending faculty members to the BCSC Section 11 committee.

The Academy also wishes to acknowledge the following committees for review of this edition:

Committee on Aging: Tim Johnson, MD, Iowa City, Iowa

Vision Rehabilitation Committee: John D. Shepherd, MD, Omaha, Nebraska

Practicing Ophthalmologists Advisory Committee for Education: Edward K. Isbey III, MD, *Primary Reviewer* and *Chair*, Asheville, North Carolina; Alice Bashinsky, MD, Asheville, North Carolina; David Browning, MD, PhD, Charlotte, North Carolina; Bradley Fouraker, MD, Tampa, Florida; Dasa Gangadhar, MD, Wichita, Kansas; Steven J. Grosser, MD, Golden Valley, Minnesota; Stephen R. Klapper, MD, Carmel, Indiana; James A. Savage, MD, Memphis, Tennessee

European Board of Ophthalmology: Béatrice Cochener-Lamard, MD, PhD, *Chair*, Brest, France; Marie-José Tassignon, MD, PhD, *Liaison*, Edegem, Belgium; Roberto Bellucci, MD, Salò, Italy; Simonetta Morselli, MD, Verona, Italy; Zoltan Nagy, MD, Budapest, Hungary

Financial Disclosures

Academy staff members who contributed to the development of this product state that within the 12 months prior to their contributions to this CME activity and for the duration of development, they have had no financial interest in or other relationship with any entity discussed in this course that produces, markets, resells, or distributes ophthalmic health care goods or services consumed by or used in patients, or with any competing commercial product or service.

The authors and reviewers state that within the 12 months prior to their contributions to this CME activity and for the duration of development, they have had the following financial relationships:*

Dr Bellucci: Bausch + Lomb Surgical (C), Physiol (C), Sifi (C)

Dr Browning: Aerpio Therapeutics (S), Alimera Sciences (C), Genentech (S), Novartis Pharmaceuticals (S), Pfizer (S), Regeneron Pharmaceuticals (S)

Dr Buznego: Alcon Laboratories (C, L), Allergan (C, L), Bausch + Lomb (C, L), Calhoun Vision (O), CXL Ophthalmics (O), CXLUSA (O), Glaukos Corporation (C, L, O, S), LENSAR (C, L), Omeros (C, L), Rapid Pathogen Screening (O)

Dr Cochener-Lamard: Abbott Medical Optics (C, L), Alcon Laboratories (C, L), Bausch + Lomb (S), Horus (C, L), Physiol (C, L), ReVision Optics (C, L), Santen (C, L), Théa (C, L)

Dr Fouraker: Addition Technology (C, L), Alcon Laboratories (C, L), KeraVision (C, L), OASIS Medical (C, L)

Dr Grosser: Ivantis (O)

Dr Isbey: Alcon Laboratories (S), Bausch + Lomb (S)

Dr Nagy: Alcon Laboratories (C, L)

Dr Roberts: Abbott Medical Optics (C), Alcon Laboratories (C, L), Allergan (C), Device Technologies (C), Pfizer (C, L)

Dr Savage: Allergan (L)

Dr Tassignon: Morcher GmbH (P)

The other authors and reviewers state that within the 12 months prior to their contributions to this CME activity and for the duration of development, they have had no financial interest in or other relationship with any entity discussed in this course that produces, markets, resells, or distributes ophthalmic health care goods or services consumed by or used in patients, or with any competing commercial product or service.

*C = consultant fees, paid advisory boards, or fees for attending a meeting; L = lecture fees (honoraria), travel fees, or reimbursements when speaking at the invitation of a commercial sponsor; O = equity ownership/stock options of publicly or privately traded firms (excluding mutual funds) with manufacturers of commercial ophthalmic products or commercial ophthalmic services; P = patents and/or royalties that might be viewed as creating a potential conflict of interest; S = grant support for the past year (all sources) and all sources used for a specific talk or manuscript with no time limitation

American Academy of Ophthalmology
655 Beach Street
Box 7424
San Francisco, CA 94120-7424

Contents

General Introduction xv

Objectives 1

Introduction 3

1 Epidemiology of Cataract 5
  Introduction 5
  Rate of Cataract Surgery 5
  Distribution of Cataract Subtypes 6
  Risk Factors for the Development of Cataract 6

2 Anatomy 9
  Normal Crystalline Lens 9
    Capsule 11
    Zonular Fibers 12
    Lens Epithelium 12
    Nucleus and Cortex 13

3 Biochemistry and Physiology 15
  Molecular Biology 15
    Crystallin Proteins 15
    Membrane Structural Proteins and Cytoskeletal Proteins 16
    Increase of Water-Insoluble Proteins With Age 17
  Carbohydrate Metabolism 17
  Oxidative Damage and Protective Mechanisms 19
  Lens Physiology 20
    Maintenance of Lens Water and Cation Balance 21
  Accommodation and Presbyopia 22

4 Embryology and Developmental Defects 25
  Normal Development of the Lens 25
    Lens Placode 25
    Lens Pit 25
    Lens Vesicle 25
    Primary Lens Fibers and the Embryonic Nucleus 26
    Secondary Lens Fibers 27
    Lens Sutures and the Fetal Nucleus 28
    Tunica Vasculosa Lentis 29
    The Zonule of Zinn 29
  Congenital Anomalies and Abnormalities 30
    Congenital Aphakia 30
    Lenticonus and Lentiglobus 30

Lens Coloboma 30
Mittendorf Dot 31
Epicapsular Star 31
Peters Anomaly 31
Microspherophakia 32
Aniridia 33
Congenital Cataract 34
Developmental Defects 39
Ectopia Lentis 39
Genetic Contributions to Age-Related Cataracts 41
Ectopia Lentis et Pupillae 42
Persistent Fetal Vasculature 42

5 Pathology **43**
Age-Related Lens Changes 43
Nuclear Cataracts 43
Cortical Cataracts 45
Posterior Subcapsular Cataracts 46
Drug-Induced Lens Changes 51
Corticosteroids 51
Phenothiazines 52
Miotics 52
Amiodarone 53
Statins 53
Tamoxifen 53
Trauma 53
Contusion 53
Perforating or Penetrating Injury 55
Intraocular Procedures 55
Intralenticular Foreign Bodies 57
Radiation 57
Metallosis 58
Electrical Injury 59
Chemical Injuries 59
Metabolic Cataract 60
Diabetes Mellitus 60
Galactosemia 61
Hypocalcemia 61
Wilson Disease 62
Myotonic Dystrophy 62
Effects of Nutrition, Alcohol, and Smoking 63
Cataract Associated With Uveitis 64
Lens Changes With Hyperbaric Oxygen Therapy 65
Pseudoexfoliation Syndrome 65
Cataract and Atopic Dermatitis 66
Phacoantigenic Uveitis 66

Lens-Induced Glaucoma. 67
    Phacolytic Glaucoma 67
    Lens Particle Glaucoma 67
    Phacomorphic Glaucoma 67
    Glaukomflecken 68
Ischemia 68
Cataracts Associated With Degenerative Ocular Disorders 68

6 Evaluation and Management of Cataracts in Adults . . . 69

Clinical History: Signs and Symptoms 69
    Decreased Visual Acuity 69
    Glare and Altered Contrast Sensitivity 70
    Myopic Shift 70
    Monocular Diplopia or Polyopia 70
    Decreased Visual Function 71
Nonsurgical Management 71
Indications for Surgery 72
Preoperative Evaluation 74
    General Health of the Patient 74
    Pertinent Ocular History 75
    Social History 76
Measurements of Visual Function 76
    Visual Acuity Testing 76
    Refraction 76
    Glare Testing 77
    Contrast Sensitivity Testing 77
External Examination 77
    Motility 77
    Pupils 78
Slit-Lamp Examination 78
    Conjunctiva 78
    Cornea 78
    Anterior Chamber and Iris 79
    Crystalline Lens 79
    Limitations of Slit-Lamp Examination 80
Fundus Evaluation 80
    Ophthalmoscopy 80
    Optic Nerve 81
    Fundus Evaluation With Opaque Media 81
Special Tests 81
    Potential Acuity Estimation 81
    Visual Field Testing 82
    Objective Tests of Macular Function 82
Preoperative Measurements 82
    Biometry 82
    Corneal Topography 84
    Additional Evaluation of the Cornea 84

IOL Power Determination 84
   IOL Calculation. 85
   Preventing Errors in IOL Calculation, Selection, and Insertion 87
   Improving Outcomes 87
Patient Preparation and Informed Consent 87

7 Surgery for Cataract **89**
Historical Overview of Cataract Surgery 89
Anesthesia for Cataract Surgery. 91
Antimicrobial Prophylaxis 93
   Before Surgery 93
   In Surgery 94
   After Surgery 95
Ophthalmic Viscosurgical Devices 95
   Physical Properties 96
   Uses of Ophthalmic Viscosurgical Devices 97
Phacoemulsification: Instrumentation, Terminology,
   and Key Concepts 98
   Instrumentation 98
   Ultrasonic Technology Terminology 99
   Key Concepts and Advances in Phaco Power Delivery 100
   Irrigation 101
   Fluidics and Phacodynamics Terminology 102
   Aspiration Pumps 103
Outline of the Phacoemulsification Procedure 104
   Eye Marking and Time-Out 104
   Exposure of the Globe 105
   Paracentesis 105
   Clear Corneal Incision 106
   Scleral Tunnel Incision. 107
   Continuous Curvilinear Capsulorrhexis 108
   Hydrodissection 110
   Hydrodelineation 110
   Nucleus Rotation 111
   Nucleus Disassembly and Removal 111
   Location of Emulsification 111
   Techniques of Nucleus Disassembly 112
   Irrigation and Aspiration 115
   Insertion of the IOL 115
   After IOL Insertion 117
IOLs: Historical Perspectives and Lens Modifications 118
   Historical Perspectives. 118
   Posterior Chamber IOLs and Other Lens Modifications 119
Modification of Preexisting Astigmatism. 123
   Astigmatic Keratotomy. 123
   Limbal Relaxing Incisions 123
   Toric IOLs 124

Alternative Technologies for Cataract Extraction 125
    Laser Photolysis. 125
    Fluid-Based Phacolysis. 125
    Femtosecond Laser Cataract Extraction 125
Outcomes of Cataract Surgery 126

8   Complications of Cataract Surgery 127

Corneal Complications 128
    Corneal Edema 128
    Incision and Wound Complications 130
    Descemet Membrane Detachment. 131
    Induced Astigmatism 131
    Corneal Melting 132
Other Anterior Segment Complications 132
    Epithelial or Fibrous Ingrowth 132
    Toxic Anterior Segment Syndrome 133
    Shallow or Flat Anterior Chamber. 134
    Elevated Intraocular Pressure. 136
    Intraoperative Floppy Iris Syndrome. 136
    Lens–Iris Diaphragm Retropulsion Syndrome. 138
    Iridodialysis and Iris Trauma 138
    Cyclodialysis 139
    Ciliary Block Glaucoma 139
    Postoperative Uveitis 139
    Retained Lens Material 140
    Capsular Rupture 142
    Vitreous Prolapse in the Anterior Chamber 143
Complications of IOL Implantation 144
    Decentration and Dislocation. 144
    Pupillary Capture 148
    Capsular Block Syndrome 148
    Uveitis-Glaucoma-Hyphema Syndrome 149
    Pseudophakic Bullous Keratopathy 149
    Unexpected Refractive Results 149
    IOL Glare, Dysphotopsia, and Opacification 150
Capsular Opacification and Contraction. 152
    Posterior Capsule Opacification. 152
    Anterior Capsule Fibrosis and Phimosis 153
    Nd:YAG Laser Capsulotomy 154
Hemorrhage 157
    Systemic Anticoagulation 157
    Retrobulbar Hemorrhage 158
    Hyphema 158
    Suprachoroidal Effusion or Hemorrhage 159
    Expulsive Suprachoroidal Hemorrhage 159
    Delayed Suprachoroidal Hemorrhage 160

Endophthalmitis 160
   Diagnosis 162
   Treatment 162
Retinal Complications. 163
   Cystoid Macular Edema 163
   Retinal Light Toxicity 166
   Retinal Detachment 166

9 Preparing for Cataract Surgery in Special Situations 169

Psychosocial Considerations 169
   Claustrophobia 169
   Neurocognitive and Neurodevelopmental Disorders 169
   Patient Communication During Eye Surgery 170
Systemic Considerations. 170
   Medical Status 170
   Anticoagulation Therapy or Bleeding Disorders 171
External Ocular Abnormalities 172
   Blepharitis and Acne Rosacea. 172
   Keratoconjunctivitis Sicca 173
   Mucous Membrane Pemphigoid 173
   Exposure Keratitis and Seventh Nerve Palsy 174
Corneal Conditions. 174
   Corneal Disease 174
   Cataract and Keratoplasty 175
   Cataract Following Keratoplasty. 176
   Cataract Following Refractive Surgery 176
Compromised Visualization of the Lens 177
   Small Pupil. 177
   Poor Red Reflex. 178
Altered Lens and Zonular Anatomy 179
   Intumescent Cataract 179
   Advanced Cataract 180
   Iris Coloboma and Corectopia 180
   Posterior Polar Cataract 180
   Zonular Dehiscence With Lens Subluxation or Dislocation 181
   Pseudoexfoliation Syndrome 184
   Cataract in Aniridia. 184
Conditions Associated With Extremes in Axial Length. 184
   High Myopia 184
   High Hyperopia and Nanophthalmos 185
   Hypotony 185
Glaucoma and Cataract 186
   Assessment. 186
   Cataract Surgery in an Eye With a Functioning Filter 187
Uveitis 188

Retinal Conditions 189
    Retinal Disease 189
    Cataract Following Pars Plana Vitrectomy 190
    Cataract With Intraocular Silicone Oil 190
Ocular Trauma. 190
    Ocular Assessment 190
    Visualization During Surgery 191
    Inflammation. 191
    Retained Foreign Matter 191
    Cataract in an Eye With Damage to Other Ocular Tissues 191
    Removal of Traumatic Cataract 192
    Vision Rehabilitation 193
    IOL Selection After Trauma 193

Appendix: Surgical Procedures for Extracapsular and Intracapsular
    Cataract Extraction. 195
Basic Texts. 203
Related Academy Materials 205
Requesting Continuing Medical Education Credit. 207
Study Questions 209
Answer Sheet for Section 11 Study Questions. 215
Answers. 217
Index 223

General Introduction

The Basic and Clinical Science Course (BCSC) is designed to meet the needs of residents and practitioners for a comprehensive yet concise curriculum of the field of ophthalmology. The BCSC has developed from its original brief outline format, which relied heavily on outside readings, to a more convenient and educationally useful self-contained text. The Academy updates and revises the course annually, with the goals of integrating the basic science and clinical practice of ophthalmology and of keeping ophthalmologists current with new developments in the various subspecialties.

The BCSC incorporates the effort and expertise of more than 90 ophthalmologists, organized into 13 Section faculties, working with Academy editorial staff. In addition, the course continues to benefit from many lasting contributions made by the faculties of previous editions. Members of the Academy Practicing Ophthalmologists Advisory Committee for Education, Committee on Aging, and Vision Rehabilitation Committee review every volume before major revisions. Members of the European Board of Ophthalmology, organized into Section faculties, also review each volume before major revisions, focusing primarily on differences between American and European ophthalmology practice.

Organization of the Course

The Basic and Clinical Science Course comprises 13 volumes, incorporating fundamental ophthalmic knowledge, subspecialty areas, and special topics:

1 Update on General Medicine
2 Fundamentals and Principles of Ophthalmology
3 Clinical Optics
4 Ophthalmic Pathology and Intraocular Tumors
5 Neuro-Ophthalmology
6 Pediatric Ophthalmology and Strabismus
7 Orbit, Eyelids, and Lacrimal System
8 External Disease and Cornea
9 Intraocular Inflammation and Uveitis
10 Glaucoma
11 Lens and Cataract
12 Retina and Vitreous
13 Refractive Surgery

In addition, a comprehensive Master Index allows the reader to easily locate subjects throughout the entire series.

References

Readers who wish to explore specific topics in greater detail may consult the references cited within each chapter and listed in the Basic Texts section at the back of the book.

These references are intended to be selective rather than exhaustive, chosen by the BCSC faculty as being important, current, and readily available to residents and practitioners.

Multimedia

This edition of Section 11, *Lens and Cataract,* includes videos related to topics covered in the book. The videos were selected by members of the BCSC faculty and are available to readers of the print and electronic versions of Section 11 (www.aao.org/bcscvideo_section11). Mobile-device users can scan the QR code below (a QR-code reader must already be installed on the device) to access the video content.

Self-Assessment and CME Credit

Each volume of the BCSC is designed as an independent study activity for ophthalmology residents and practitioners. The learning objectives for this volume are given on page 1. The text, illustrations, and references provide the information necessary to achieve the objectives; the study questions allow readers to test their understanding of the material and their mastery of the objectives. Physicians who wish to claim CME credit for this educational activity may do so by following the instructions given at the end of the book.

This Section of the BCSC has been approved by the American Board of Ophthalmology as a Maintenance of Certification Part II self-assessment and CME activity.

Conclusion

The Basic and Clinical Science Course has expanded greatly over the years, with the addition of much new text, numerous illustrations, and video content. Recent editions have sought to place greater emphasis on clinical applicability while maintaining a solid foundation in basic science. As with any educational program, it reflects the experience of its authors. As its faculties change and medicine progresses, new viewpoints emerge on controversial subjects and techniques. Not all alternate approaches can be included in this series; as with any educational endeavor, the learner should seek additional sources, including Academy Preferred Practice Pattern Guidelines.

The BCSC faculty and staff continually strive to improve the educational usefulness of the course; you, the reader, can contribute to this ongoing process. If you have any suggestions or questions about the series, please do not hesitate to contact the faculty or the editors.

The authors, editors, and reviewers hope that your study of the BCSC will be of lasting value and that each Section will serve as a practical resource for quality patient care.

Objectives

Upon completion of BCSC Section 11, *Lens and Cataract,* the reader should be able to

- describe the normal anatomy, embryologic development, physiology, and biochemistry of the crystalline lens

- identify congenital anomalies of the lens

- list types of congenital and acquired cataracts

- describe the association of cataracts with aging, trauma, medications, and systemic and ocular diseases

- describe the evaluation and management of patients with cataract and other lens abnormalities

- state the principles of cataract surgery techniques and associated surgical technology

- describe an appropriate differential diagnosis and management plan for intraoperative and postoperative complications of cataract surgery

- identify special circumstances in which cataract surgery techniques should be modified, and describe appropriate treatment plans

Introduction

The ancient Greeks and Romans believed that the lens was the part of the eye responsible for the faculty of seeing. They theorized that the optic nerves were hollow channels through which "visual spirits" traveled from the brain to meet visual rays from the outside world at the lens, which they thought was located in the center of the globe. The visual information would then flow back to the brain. This concept was known as the *emanation theory of vision*. Celsus (25 BC–AD 50) drew the lens in the center of the globe, with an empty space called the *locus vacuus* anterior to it, in AD 30 (Fig I-1).

These erroneous ideas about lens position and function persisted through the Middle Ages and into the Renaissance, as shown by the drawing of the Belgian anatomist Andreas Vesalius in 1543 (Fig I-2). The true position of the crystalline lens was illustrated by the Italian anatomist Fabricius ab Aquapendente in 1600 (Fig I-3), and the Swiss physician Felix Plater (1536–1614) was the first to postulate that the retina, not the lens, was the part of the eye responsible for sight.

Today, many areas of lens physiology and biochemistry are still subjects of active research. No medical treatment, for example, can yet prevent the formation or progression of cataract in the lens of the otherwise healthy adult eye, and theories about cataract formation and innovative forms of management continue to be controversial. Although various risk factors for cataract development have been identified (discussed in Chapter 1), data to develop guidelines for reducing the risk of cataract remain inconclusive.

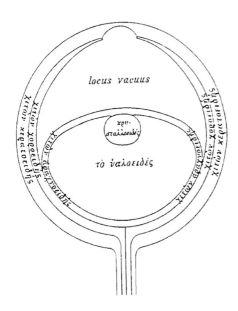

Figure I-1 The eye, after Celsus. *(From Gorin G. History of Ophthalmology. Wilmington: Publish or Perish, Inc; 1982.)*

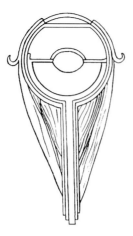

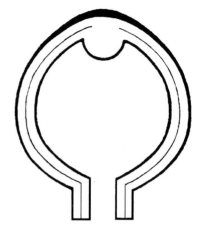

Figure I-2 Schematic eye from *De fabrica corporis humani* of Andreas Vesalius (1514–1564). *(Reproduced with permission from the Ophthalmic Publishing Company. Feigenbaum A. Early history of cataract and the ancient operation for cataract. Am J Ophthalmol. 1960;49:307.)*

Figure I-3 Sketch from *De oculo* of Fabricius ab Aquapendente (1537–1619), showing the correct position of the lens within the eyeball. *(Reproduced with permission from the Ophthalmic Publishing Company. Feigenbaum A. Early history of cataract and the ancient operation for cataract. Am J Ophthalmol. 1960;49:307.)*

The prevalence of lens disorders and continuing developments in their management make the basic and clinical science of this structure a vital component of ophthalmology training. The goal of Section 11 is to provide a curriculum for the study of the structure and function of the normal lens, the features of diseases involving the lens, and the surgical management of cataract.

CHAPTER 1

Epidemiology of Cataract

Introduction

Cataract is the leading cause of vision loss in the world. The World Health Organization (WHO) has estimated that 18 million people are bilaterally blind due to cataract and that the condition causes 48% of cases of blindness worldwide. Cataract is also a leading cause of visual impairment, with 33% of the world's population experiencing decreased vision because of this disorder; only refractive error has a greater impact in this regard. It is important to note that most cases of blindness due to cataract (up to 90%) are found in developing nations.

While the adverse impact of cataract on vision worldwide is undeniable, the lack of a widely accepted, standardized classification for lens opacities makes it difficult to precisely determine the incidence and prevalence of this condition. As discussed in Chapters 4 and 5, cataracts may be congenital, metabolic, age related, or traumatic in origin. Because of their high prevalence, age-related cataracts are presumed to have the greatest socioeconomic impact. However, most estimates of the frequency of age-related cataract are based on data from select groups rather than from the general population. Finally, in many older patients, coexisting pathology may cause vision loss that is incorrectly attributed to lens change.

The Centers for Disease Control and Prevention (CDC) Vision Health Initiative estimates that cataracts affect more than 24 million individuals in the United States and that this number will rise to 30.1 million by 2020.

Resnikoff S, Pascolini D, Etya'ale D, et al. Global data on visual impairment in the year 2002. *Bull World Health Organ.* 2004;82(11):844–851.

Rate of Cataract Surgery

Approximately 3 million cataract surgeries are performed annually in the United States, making this procedure the most common surgery performed on an outpatient basis. The direct medical cost related to the treatment of cataract in the United States, including surgery, office visits, and prescriptions, is approximately $6.8 billion annually.

The rate of cataract surgery in developed countries is up to 10,000 per million population per year. In China, the rate is 300–400 per million. In parts of the developing world, the number may be as low as 50 surgeries per million.

In 1999, the International Agency for the Prevention of Blindness (IAPB) and the WHO collaborated to launch VISION 2020: The Right to Sight, an initiative to develop the infrastructure necessary for sustainable provision of high-quality cataract surgical services throughout the developing world. The WHO determined that the number of cataract surgeries performed worldwide would have to triple to keep pace with need, with a goal of 3000 surgeries per million population annually.

Distribution of Cataract Subtypes

The Beaver Dam Eye Study, a large population-based study performed in the late 1980s, reported that 38.8% of men and 45.9% of women older than 74 years had visually significant cataracts. For this study "significance" was determined by photographic grading of lens opacities and a specified best-corrected visual acuity of 20/32 (logarithm of the minimum angle of resolution [logMAR] equivalent closest to the 20/30 Snellen fraction), excluding individuals with severe age-related maculopathy.

A follow-up to the Beaver Dam Eye Study was performed between 1993 and 1995 to estimate the incidence of nuclear, cortical, and posterior subcapsular cataracts (PSCs) in the study cohort. Incident nuclear cataract was present in 13.1% of the study cohort; cortical cataract, in 8.2%; and PSC, in 3.4%. The cumulative incidence of nuclear cataract increased from 2.9% in persons aged 43–54 years at baseline to 40% in those aged 75 years or older. For cortical cataract, the corresponding values were 1.9% and 21.8%, respectively; for PSC, 1.4% and 7.3%. Women were more likely than men to have nuclear cataracts, even after adjustments for age were made.

The Salisbury Eye Evaluation project, which reported results in 1998, was a prospective, population-based cohort study designed to identify racial differences in the prevalence of cataracts in a group of Americans older than 65 years. Nuclear cataract was noted in 50.7% of Caucasians versus 33.5% of African Americans. Conversely, cortical cataract was far more likely to be identified in African Americans than in Caucasians. PSC was found at roughly the same rate, between 5% and 10%, in both groups.

The Barbados Eye Study provided prevalence data on lens opacities in a predominantly black population. Cortical opacities were the most frequent type of cataract, and women had a higher frequency of opacification than did men.

Studies of Asian populations, including the Singapore Malay Eye Study and the Handan Eye Study, have been performed to evaluate the incidence of different cataract subtypes. These studies suggest a higher rate of cortical cataract in Asians than in Caucasians.

West SK, Muñoz B, Schein OD, Duncan DD, Rubin GS. Racial differences in lens opacities: the Salisbury Eye Evaluation (SEE) project. *Am J Epidemiol.* 1998;148(11):1033–1039.

Risk Factors for the Development of Cataract

Smoking is an established risk factor for development of nuclear sclerotic cataract and PSC. The Beaver Dam Eye Study and the Blue Mountains Eye Study, among others, concluded that there is a higher and dose-related risk of visually significant nuclear sclerosis for study participants who smoke. Some smoking-related damage to the lens may be reversible upon cessation.

Additional risk factors for cataract identified by multiple studies include UV-light exposure, diabetes mellitus, prolonged corticosteroid use (systemic, inhaled, and topical), ocular trauma (including prior ocular surgery), and high myopia. Also implicated in the development of cataract are exogenous estrogen use, alcohol consumption, and increased body mass index; however, study results regarding the impact of these factors are inconsistent.

The role of nutrition in preventing cataracts (specifically, the potential benefit of supplementation with antioxidants) has been a subject of recent interest. Some studies have shown a benefit to increased intake of vitamins C and E. However, in the Age-Related Eye Disease Study 1 (AREDS1), a formulation of vitamin C, vitamin E, beta carotene, zinc, and copper did not reduce the risk of progression to cataract surgery. In a large Italian trial, use of a multivitamin and mineral supplement benefited individuals with nuclear sclerotic cataract but increased the risk of PSC. Age-Related Eye Disease Study 2 (AREDS2), results of which were published in 2013, evaluated the effects of lutein/zeaxanthin supplementation. This study concluded that these supplements had no significant overall effect on rates of progression to cataract surgery, although patients in the lowest quintile of dietary lutein/zeaxanthin intake did have a reduced risk of cataract development following supplementation.

Age-Related Eye Disease Study (AREDS) Research Group. Risk factors associated with age-related nuclear and cortical cataract: a case-control study in the Age-Related Eye Disease Study, AREDS report no. 5. *Ophthalmology*. 2001;108(8):1400–1408.

Age-Related Eye Disease Study (AREDS) Research Group. A randomized placebo-controlled, clinical trial of high-dose supplementation with vitamins C and E and beta carotene for age-related cataract and vision loss: AREDS report no. 9. *Arch Ophthalmol*. 2001;119(10): 1439–1452.

Chew EY, SanGiovanni JP, Ferris FL, et al; Age-Related Eye Disease Study 2 (AREDS2) Research Group. Lutein/zeaxanthin for the treatment of age-related cataract: AREDS2 randomized trial report no. 4. *JAMA Ophthalmol*. 2013;131(7):843–850.

Klein R, Lee KE, Gangnon RE, Klein BEK. Relation of smoking, drinking, and physical activity to changes in vision over a 20-year period: The Beaver Dam Eye Study. *Ophthalmology*. 2014;121(6):1220–1228.

Maraini G, Williams SL, Sperduto RD, et al; Clinical Trial of Nutritional Supplements and Age-Related Cataract Study Group. A randomized, double-masked, placebo-controlled clinical trial of multivitamin supplementation for age-related lens opacities. Clinical trial of nutritional supplements and age-related cataract report no. 3. *Ophthalmology*. 2008;115(4): 599–607.

Mukesh BN, Le A, Dimitrov PN, Ahmed S, Taylor HR, McCarty CA. Development of cataract and associated risk factors: the Visual Impairment Project. *Arch Ophthalmol*. 2006;124(1): 79–85.

Tan JS, Wang JJ, Younan C, Cumming RG, Rochtchina E, Mitchell P. Smoking and the long-term incidence of cataract: the Blue Mountains Eye Study. *Ophthalmic Epidemiol*. 2008; 15(3):155–161.

CHAPTER 2

Anatomy

See BCSC Section 2, *Fundamentals and Principles of Ophthalmology,* for additional discussion and illustrations of the topics covered in this chapter.

Normal Crystalline Lens

The crystalline lens is a transparent, biconvex structure located posterior to the iris and anterior to the vitreous body (Fig 2-1). The lens is suspended in position by delicate yet strong fibers (zonular fibers, sometimes referred to as the *zonules of Zinn*) that support and attach it to the ciliary body. Components of the lens are the capsule, epithelium, cortex, and nucleus (Fig 2-2).

The anterior and posterior poles of the lens are joined by an imaginary line called the *optic axis,* which passes through them. Hypothetical lines on the lens surface passing from one pole to the other are referred to as *meridians.* The *equator* of the lens is its greatest circumference.

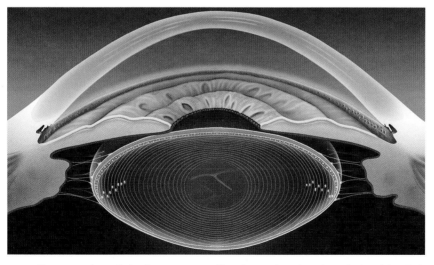

Figure 2-1 Cross section of the human crystalline lens, showing the relationship of the lens to surrounding ocular structures. *(Illustration by Christine Gralapp.)*

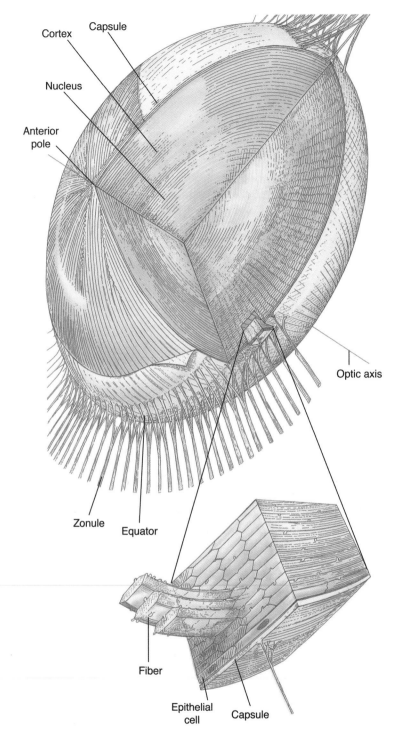

Figure 2-2 Structure of the normal human lens. *(Illustration by Carol Donner. Reproduced with permission from Koretz JF, Handelman GH. How the human eye focuses. Scientific American. July 1988:94.)*

The functions of the lens are

- to maintain its own clarity
- to refract light
- to provide accommodation, in conjunction with the zonule and ciliary body

Lacking a blood supply and innervation after fetal development, the lens depends entirely on the aqueous humor to meet its metabolic requirements and to remove its wastes.

The lens is able to refract light because its index of refraction—normally about 1.4 centrally and 1.36 peripherally—is different from that of the aqueous and vitreous surrounding it. In its nonaccommodative state, the lens contributes approximately 20.00 diopters (D) of the approximately 60.00 D of convergent refractive power of the average human eye; the air–cornea interface provides the rest, or 40.00–45.00 D.

The lens continues to grow throughout life. At birth, it measures about 6.4 mm equatorially and 3.5 mm anteroposteriorly and weighs approximately 90 mg. The adult lens typically measures 9–10 mm equatorially and about 5 mm anteroposteriorly and weighs approximately 255 mg. With age, the relative thickness of the cortex increases; the lens also adopts an increasingly curved shape so that older lenses have more refractive power. However, the index of refraction decreases with age, probably as a result of the increasing presence of insoluble protein particles. Thus, the eye may become either more hyperopic or more myopic with age, depending on the balance of these opposing changes.

Capsule

The lens capsule is an elastic, transparent basement membrane that is composed of type IV collagen and other matrix proteins and laid down by the epithelial cells. The capsule contains the lens substance and is capable of molding it during accommodative changes. The outer layer of the lens capsule, the *zonular lamella,* also serves as the point of attachment for the zonular fibers. The lens capsule is thickest in the anterior and posterior preequatorial zones and thinnest at the central posterior pole, where it may measure only 2–4 μm (Fig 2-3). The anterior lens capsule is considerably thicker than the posterior capsule at birth, and its thickness increases throughout life.

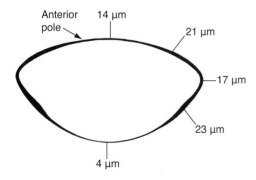

Figure 2-3 Schematic of the adult lens capsule showing the relative thickness of the capsule in different zones. *(Illustration by Christine Gralapp.)*

Zonular Fibers

The lens is supported by the system of fibers (the zonule) that originate from the basal lamina of the nonpigmented epithelium of the pars plana and pars plicata of the ciliary body. The zonular fibers consist of microfibrils composed of elastic tissue, and they insert at discrete points on the lens capsule 1.5 mm anterior to the equator and 1.25 mm posterior to the equator. With age, the equatorial zonular fibers regress, leaving separate anterior and posterior layers that appear in a triangular shape on cross section of the zonular ring. The fibers are 5–30 μm in diameter; light microscopy shows them to be eosinophilic structures that have a positive periodic acid–Schiff (PAS) reaction. Ultrastructurally, the strands, or microfibrils, composing the fibers are 8–10 nm in diameter, with 12–14 nm of banding.

Lens Epithelium

Immediately posterior to the anterior lens capsule is a single layer of epithelial cells. These cells are metabolically active and carry out all normal cell activities, including biosynthesis of DNA, RNA, protein, and lipid. They also generate adenosine triphosphate to meet the energy demands of the lens. The epithelial cells are mitotic, with the greatest activity of premitotic (replicative, or S phase) DNA synthesis occurring in a ring around the anterior lens known as the *germinative zone*. The newly formed cells migrate toward the equator, where they differentiate into fibers. As the epithelial cells migrate toward the bow region of the lens, they begin the process of terminal differentiation into lens fibers (Fig 2-4).

Perhaps the most dramatic morphologic change occurs when the epithelial cells elongate to form lens fiber cells. This change is associated with a tremendous increase in the mass of cellular proteins in the fiber cell membrane. At the same time, the cells lose organelles, including nuclei, mitochondria, and ribosomes. The loss of these organelles is optically advantageous, because light passing through the lens is no longer absorbed or

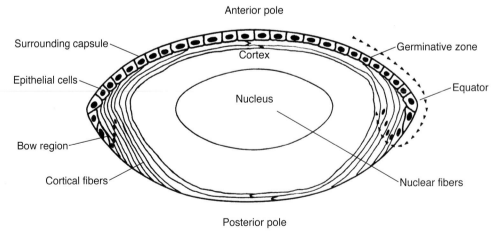

Figure 2-4 Schematic of the mammalian lens in cross section. *Arrowheads* indicate the direction of cell migration from the epithelium to the cortex. *(From Anderson RE, ed. Biochemistry of the Eye. San Francisco: American Academy of Ophthalmology; 1983;6:112.)*

scattered by these structures. However, because these new lens fiber cells lack the metabolic functions previously carried out by the organelles, they are now dependent on glycolysis for energy production (see Chapter 3).

Nucleus and Cortex

No cells are lost from the lens; as new fibers are laid down, they crowd and compact the previously formed fibers, with the older layers located toward the center. The oldest layers, the *embryonic and fetal lens nuclei,* were produced in embryonic life and persist in the center of the lens (see Chapter 4, Fig 4-1). The outermost fibers are the most recently formed and make up the cortex of the lens.

Lens sutures (see Chapter 4, Fig 4-1) are formed by the interdigitation of the anterior and posterior tips of the spindle-shaped fibers. Multiple optical zones, as well as Y-shaped sutures located within the lens nucleus, are visible by slit-lamp biomicroscopy. (See Chapter 4 for further discussion of the embryonic nucleus and lens sutures.) These zones of demarcation occur because strata of epithelial cells with differing optical densities are laid down throughout life. There is no morphologic distinction between the cortex and the nucleus; rather, the transition between these regions is gradual. Although some surgical texts and this volume make distinctions between the nucleus, epinucleus, endonucleus, and cortex, these terms relate only to potential differences in the behavior and appearance of the material during surgical procedures.

Kuszak JR, Clark JI, Cooper KE, et al. Biology of the lens: lens transparency as a function of embryology, anatomy and physiology. In: Albert DM, Jakobiec FA, eds. *Principles and Practice of Ophthalmology.* 3rd ed. Philadelphia: Saunders; 2008: vol 1, chapter 104.

Snell RS, Lemp MA. *Clinical Anatomy of the Eye.* 2nd ed. Boston: Blackwell; 1998:197–204.

CHAPTER 3

Biochemistry and Physiology

See BCSC Section 2, *Fundamentals and Principles of Ophthalmology*, for additional discussion of several of the topics discussed in this chapter.

Molecular Biology

Crystallin Proteins

The human lens has a protein concentration of 33% of its wet weight, which is at least twice that of most tissues. Lens proteins are commonly divided into 2 groups, based on water solubility (Fig 3-1). The water-soluble fraction of the young lens accounts for approximately 80% of lens proteins; aging-related changes result in an increase in the percentage of water-insoluble protein. The water-soluble portion consists mainly of a group of proteins called *crystallins*. The crystallins can be divided into 2 major groups, α-crystallins and β,γ-crystallins.

α-Crystallins represent about one-third of the lens proteins by mass. In their native state, they are the largest of the crystallins, with a molecular mass ranging between 600 and 800 kDa. In addition, they may associate with other crystallins, yielding complexes greater than 2×10^6. There are 2 α-crystallin subunits, αA and αB, each with a molecular mass of

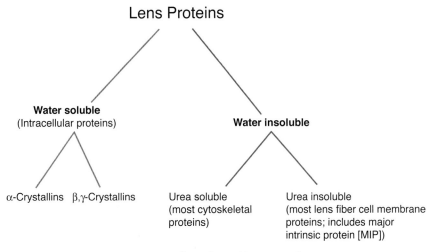

Figure 3-1 Overview of lens proteins.

approximately 20 kDa, which form heteromeric complexes containing about 30 subunits. The sequence of the α-crystallins identifies them as members of the family of small heat-shock proteins. α-Crystallin complexes bind to partially denatured proteins and prevent them from aggregating. Their primary function in lens fiber cells appears to be to inhibit the complete denaturation and insolubilization of the other crystallins.

β,γ-Crystallins are subdivided into 2 groups, based on molecular mass and isoelectric points. The β-crystallins, a complex group of oligomers composed of polypeptides, are encoded by 7 genes. These crystallins have molecular masses ranging from 23 to 32 kDa. The individual polypeptides associate with each other, forming dimers and higher-order complexes in their native state. By gel chromatography, the β-crystallins can be separated into βH (β high-molecular-mass) and βL (β low-molecular-mass) fractions.

The γ-crystallins are the smallest of the crystallins, with a molecular mass in the range of 20 kDa or less. The native γ-crystallins do not associate with each other or with other proteins and, therefore, have the lowest molecular mass of the crystallin fractions. In humans, the gamma family is encoded by 4 genes. X-ray crystallographic studies have determined the 3-dimensional structure of the γ-crystallins to high resolution. Fourfold repetition of a core 3-dimensional structural motif suggests that the β,γ-crystallins might have arisen from double duplication and fusion of a gene for a 40-residue polypeptide. The basic structure of the β-crystallins and γ-crystallins has been maintained through hundreds of millions of years of vertebrate evolution.

Bloemendal H, de Jong W, Jaenicke R, Lubsen NH, Slingsby C, Tardieu A. Aging and vision: structure, stability and function of lens crystallins. *Prog Biophys Mol Biol.* 2004;86(3): 407–485.

Membrane Structural Proteins and Cytoskeletal Proteins

The water-insoluble fraction of lens proteins can be further divided into 2 fractions, 1 soluble and 1 insoluble in 8 M urea. The *urea-soluble fraction* of the young lens contains cytoskeletal proteins that provide the structural framework of the lens cells. Microfilaments and microtubules found in lens cells are similar to those found in other cell types. However, the lens contains 2 types of intermediate filaments that are unusual: one class is made from the protein *vimentin,* which is not usually found in epithelial cells; the other class, the *beaded filaments,* is composed of the proteins phakinin and filensin, which are specific to the lens. Genetic disruption of the structure of the beaded filaments leads to disruption of the structure of the lens fiber cells and formation of a cataract.

The *urea-insoluble fraction* of the young lens contains the plasma membranes of the lens fiber cells. Several proteins are associated with these fiber cell plasma membranes. One makes up nearly 50% of the membrane proteins and is known as the *major intrinsic protein (MIP; also known as aquaporin 0)*, a member of a class of proteins called *aquaporins.* Other members of the aquaporin family are found throughout the body, where they serve predominantly as water channels. MIP first appears in the lens just as the fibers begin to elongate. With age, this protein, which has a molecular mass of 28 kDa, undergoes proteolytic cleavage, forming a protein fragment with a molecular mass of 22 kDa. The relative proportions of these 2 proteins become about equal at 20–30 years of age. Over time, the protein with molecular mass of 22 kDa predominates in the lens nucleus.

Hejtmancik JF, Piatigorsky J. Lens proteins and their molecular biology. In: Albert DM, Jakobiec FA, eds. *Principles and Practice of Ophthalmology.* 3rd ed. Philadelphia: Saunders; 2008: vol 1, chapter 105.

Increase of Water-Insoluble Proteins With Age

As the lens ages, its proteins aggregate to form very large particles. These particles become water-insoluble and scatter light, increasing the opacity of the lens. Of note, the water-insoluble protein fraction increases with age, even if the lens remains relatively transparent. Conversion of the water-soluble proteins into water-insoluble proteins appears to be a natural process in lens fiber maturation, but it may occur more quickly in cataractous lenses.

In cataracts with significant browning of the lens nucleus *(brunescent cataracts),* the increase in the amount of water-insoluble protein correlates well with the degree of opacification. In markedly brunescent cataracts, as much as 90% of the nuclear proteins may be in the insoluble fraction. Associated oxidative changes occur, including protein-to-protein and protein-to-glutathione disulfide bond formation. These changes result in decreased levels of the reduced form of glutathione and increased levels of glutathione disulfide (oxidized glutathione) in the cytoplasm of the nuclear fiber cells. It is the general view that glutathione is essential to maintain a reducing environment in the lens cytoplasm. Depletion of the reduced form of glutathione accelerates protein crosslinking, protein aggregation, and light scattering. In addition to the increased formation of disulfide bonds, nuclear proteins are highly crosslinked by nondisulfide bonds. This insoluble protein fraction contains yellow-to-brown pigments that are found in higher concentration in nuclear cataracts. Increased fluorescence is generated by the nondisulfide crosslinks that form in brunescent nuclear cataracts.

Carbohydrate Metabolism

The goal of lens metabolism is the maintenance of lens transparency. In the lens, energy production largely depends on glucose metabolism. Glucose enters the lens from the aqueous humor both by *simple diffusion* and by a mediated transfer process called *facilitated diffusion.* Most of the glucose transported into the lens is phosphorylated to glucose-6-phosphate (G6P) by the enzyme hexokinase. This reaction is 70–100 times slower than that of other enzymes involved in lens glycolysis and is, therefore, rate-limited in the lens. Once formed, G6P enters 1 of 2 metabolic pathways: anaerobic glycolysis or the hexose monophosphate (HMP) shunt (Fig 3-2).

The more active of these 2 pathways is *anaerobic glycolysis,* which provides most of the high-energy phosphate bonds required for lens metabolism. Substrate-linked phosphorylation of adenosine diphosphate (ADP) to adenosine triphosphate (ATP) occurs at 2 steps along the pathway from glucose metabolism to lactate. The rate-limiting step in the glycolytic pathway itself is at the level of the enzyme phosphofructokinase, which is regulated through feedback control by metabolic products of the glycolytic pathway. This

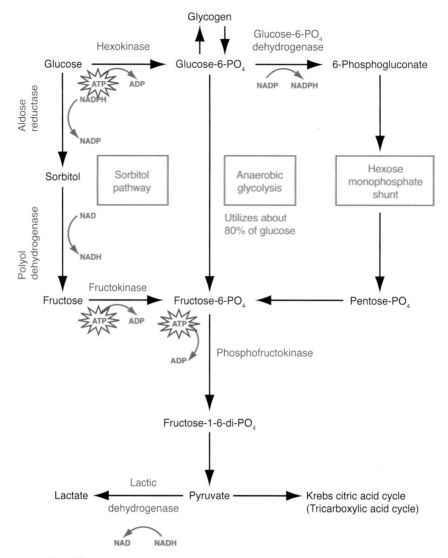

Figure 3-2 Simplified scheme of glucose metabolism in the lens. *(Adapted with permission from Hart WM Jr, ed. Adler's Physiology of the Eye: Clinical Application. 9th ed. St Louis: Mosby; 1992:362.)*

pathway is much less efficient than aerobic glycolysis, because only 2 net molecules of ATP are produced for each glucose molecule utilized, whereas aerobic glycolysis produces an additional 36 molecules of ATP from each glucose molecule metabolized in the citric acid cycle (oxidative metabolism). Because of the low oxygen tension in the lens, only about 3% of the lens glucose passes through the citric acid cycle (also called the tricarboxylic acid cycle or the Krebs cycle) to produce ATP; however, even this low level of aerobic metabolism produces approximately 25% of the lens ATP.

That the lens is not dependent on oxygen is demonstrated by its ability to sustain normal metabolism in a nitrogen environment. Provided with ample glucose, the anoxic in vitro lens remains completely transparent, has normal levels of ATP, and maintains its ion and amino acid pump activities. However, when deprived of glucose, the lens cannot maintain these functions and becomes hazy after several hours, even in the presence of oxygen.

The less active pathway for utilization of G6P in the lens is the HMP shunt, also known as the *pentose phosphate pathway.* While on average, less than 5% of lens glucose is metabolized by this route, the pathway is stimulated in the presence of elevated levels of glucose.

The glucose that is not phosphorylated to G6P enters the *sorbitol pathway,* which is yet another pathway for lens glucose metabolism, or it is converted into gluconic acid. Aldose reductase is the key enzyme in this pathway and has been found to play a pivotal role in the development of "sugar" cataracts. In comparison with hexokinase, aldose reductase has a very low affinity for glucose. Less than 4% of lens glucose is normally converted to sorbitol.

As previously noted, the hexokinase reaction is rate-limited in phosphorylating glucose in the lens and is inhibited by the feedback mechanisms of the products of glycolysis. Therefore, when the amount of glucose increases in the lens (as occurs in hyperglycemic states), the sorbitol pathway is activated relatively more than the glycolytic pathway, and sorbitol accumulates. Sorbitol is metabolized to fructose by the enzyme polyol dehydrogenase. Unfortunately, this enzyme has a relatively low affinity (high K_m [apparent affinity constant]), meaning that considerable sorbitol will accumulate before being further metabolized. This characteristic, combined with the poor permeability of the lens to sorbitol, results in retention of sorbitol in the lens.

A high ratio of NADPH/NADH drives the reaction in the direction of sorbitol accumulation. The accumulation of NADP that occurs as a consequence of activation of the sorbitol pathway may cause the HMP shunt stimulation that is observed in the presence of an elevated lens glucose level. In addition to sorbitol, fructose levels increase in a lens incubated in a high-glucose environment. Together, the 2 sugars increase the osmotic pressure within the lens, drawing in water. At first, the energy-dependent pumps of the lens are able to compensate, but ultimately they are overwhelmed. The result is swelling of the fibers, disruption of the normal cytoskeletal architecture, and opacification of the lens.

The pivotal role of aldose reductase in cataractogenesis in animals is apparent from studies of cataract development in various hyperglycemic animal species. Those species that have high aldose reductase activities develop lens opacities, whereas those lacking aldose reductase do not. In addition, specific inhibitors of this enzymatic activity, applied either systemically or topically to 1 eye, decrease the rate of onset and the severity of glucose cataracts in experimental studies.

Oxidative Damage and Protective Mechanisms

Free radicals are generated in the course of normal cellular metabolic activities and may also be produced by external agents such as radiant energy. These free radicals are highly reactive and can damage lens fibers. Peroxidation of lens fiber plasma or plasma membrane lipids has been suggested as a factor contributing to lens opacification.

Because oxygen tension in and around the lens is normally low, free radical reactions may not involve molecular oxygen; instead, the free radicals may react directly with molecules. DNA is easily damaged by free radicals. Although some of the damage to the lens is reparable, some of it may be permanent. Free radicals can also attack the proteins or membrane lipids in the lens cortex. No repair mechanisms are known to ameliorate such damage. In lens fibers, where protein synthesis no longer takes place, free radical damage may lead to polymerization and crosslinking of lipids and proteins, resulting in an increase in the water-insoluble protein content.

The lens is equipped with several enzymes that protect against free radical or oxidative damage, including superoxide dismutase, catalase, and glutathione peroxidase. Superoxide dismutase catalyzes the destruction of the superoxide anion, O_2^-, and produces hydrogen peroxide, which is broken down by catalase. Next, glutathione peroxidase catalyzes a reaction resulting in the formation of glutathione disulfide (GSSG), which is then reconverted to glutathione (GSH) by glutathione reductase, using the pyridine nucleotide NADPH. The primary source of erythrocyte NADPH, the HMP shunt provides NADPH as the reducing agent. Thus, glutathione acts indirectly as a major free radical scavenger in the lens. In addition, both vitamin E and ascorbic acid are present in the lens. Each of these substances can act as a free radical scavenger and thus protect against oxidative damage.

Increasing oxygen levels within the eye may have a role in cataract formation. For example, exposure of the lens to an increased level of oxygen during long-term hyperbaric oxygen therapy leads to a myopic shift, increased opacification of the lens nucleus, and, in many cases, the formation of nuclear cataracts. The lens is also exposed to increased levels of oxygen acutely during retinal surgery and chronically following vitrectomy. Because vitrectomy is associated with very high rates of nuclear cataract formation, it has been suggested that the low oxygen level existing around the lens protects it from oxidative damage and that loss of the gel structure of the vitreous body increases exposure of the lens to oxygen and the risk of nuclear cataracts.

Beebe DC. The lens. In: Kaufman PL, Alm A, eds. *Adler's Physiology of the Eye: Clinical Application.* 11th ed. St Louis: Mosby; 2009:131–163.

Boulton ME, Rozanowska M, Wride M. Biophysics and age changes of the crystalline lens. In: Albert DM, Jakobiec FA, eds. *Principles and Practice of Ophthalmology.* 3rd ed. Philadelphia: Saunders; 2008: vol 1, chapter 106.

Lens Physiology

Throughout life, lens epithelial cells at the equator divide and develop into lens fibers, resulting in continual growth of the lens (see Chapter 2, Figs 2-2 and 2-4). The lens cells with the highest metabolic rate are found in the epithelium and outer cortex. These superficial cells utilize oxygen and glucose for the active transport of electrolytes, carbohydrates, and amino acids into the lens. Because the lens is avascular, the task of maintaining transparency poses several challenges. The older cells, found toward the center of the lens, must be able to communicate with the superficial cells and the environment outside the lens. This communication is accomplished through low-resistance gap junctions that facilitate the exchange of small molecules from cell to cell. Lens fiber cells also have abundant water channels in their membranes, made from MIP. It is not yet certain whether MIP serves primarily as a water channel, as an adhesion molecule that minimizes the extracellular space between fiber cells, or as both in the lens. Minimizing the extracellular space between fiber cells is important to reduce the scattering of light as it passes through the lens.

Maintenance of Lens Water and Cation Balance

The normal human lens contains approximately 66% water and 33% protein, and this proportion changes very little with aging. The lens cortex is more hydrated than the lens nucleus. About 5% of the lens volume is the water found between the lens fibers in the extracellular spaces. Within the lens, sodium and potassium concentrations are maintained at 20 mM and 120 mM, respectively.

Perhaps the most important aspect of lens physiology is the mechanism that controls water and electrolyte balance, which is critical to lens transparency. Because transparency is highly dependent on the structural and macromolecular components of the lens, perturbation of cellular hydration can readily lead to opacification. It is noteworthy that disruption of water and electrolyte balance is not a feature of nuclear cataracts. In cortical cataracts, however, the water content rises significantly.

Lens epithelium: site of active transport

The lens is less hydrated and has higher levels of potassium ions (K^+) and amino acids than the surrounding aqueous and vitreous. Conversely, the lens contains lower levels of sodium ions (Na^+), chloride ions (Cl^-), and water than the surrounding environment. The cation balance between the inside and outside of the lens is the result both of the permeability properties of the lens cell membranes and of the activity of the sodium-potassium pumps, which reside within the cell membranes of the lens epithelium and each lens fiber. The sodium-potassium pumps function by pumping sodium ions out while taking potassium ions in. This mechanism depends on the breakdown of ATP and is regulated by the enzyme Na^+,K^+-ATPase. Inhibition of Na^+,K^+-ATPase leads to loss of cation balance and elevated water content in the lens.

Pump–leak theory

The combination of active transport and membrane permeability is often referred to as the pump–leak system of the lens (Fig 3-3). According to the *pump–leak theory*, potassium and various other molecules, such as amino acids, are actively transported into the lens via the epithelium anteriorly. They then diffuse out with the concentration gradient through the back of the lens, where there are no active-transport mechanisms. Conversely, sodium flows in through the back of the lens with the concentration gradient and then is actively exchanged for potassium by the epithelium. In support of this theory, an anteroposterior gradient was found for both ions: potassium was concentrated in the anterior lens; sodium, in the posterior lens. Most of the Na^+,K^+-ATPase activity is found in the lens epithelium and the superficial cortical fiber cells. The active-transport mechanisms are lost if the capsule and attached epithelium are removed from the lens but not if the capsule alone is removed by enzymatic degradation with collagenase. These findings support the hypothesis that the epithelium is the primary site for active transport in the lens.

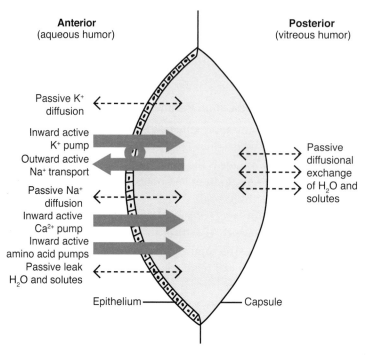

Anterior
(aqueous humor)

Posterior
(vitreous humor)

Passive K⁺ diffusion

Inward active K⁺ pump
Outward active Na⁺ transport

Passive Na⁺ diffusion
Inward active Ca²⁺ pump
Inward active amino acid pumps
Passive leak H₂O and solutes

Passive diffusional exchange of H_2O and solutes

Epithelium — Capsule

Figure 3-3 The pump–leak hypothesis of pathways of solute movement in the lens. The major site of active-transport mechanisms is the anterior epithelium, whereas passive diffusion occurs over both surfaces of the lens. *(Modified with permission from Paterson CA, Delamere NA. The lens. In: Hart WM Jr, ed.* Adler's Physiology of the Eye. *9th ed. St Louis: Mosby; 1992:365.)*

Accommodation and Presbyopia

Accommodation, the mechanism by which the eye changes focus from distant to near images, occurs through a change in lens shape resulting from the action of the ciliary muscle on the zonular fibers. The lens substance is most malleable during childhood and the young-adult years, progressively losing its ability to change shape with age.

According to the Helmholtz theory of accommodation, most of the accommodative change in lens shape occurs at the central anterior lens surface. The central anterior capsule is thinner than the peripheral capsule (see Chapter 2, Fig 2-3), and the anterior zonular fibers insert slightly closer to the visual axis than do the posterior zonular fibers, resulting in a central anterior bulge with accommodation. The curvature of the posterior lens surface changes minimally with accommodation. The central posterior capsule, which is the thinnest area of the capsule, maintains the same curvature regardless of zonular tension.

The ciliary muscle is a ring-shaped muscle that, on contraction, has the opposite effect from what one intuitively expects of a sphincter. When a sphincter muscle contracts, it usually tightens its grip. However, when the ciliary muscle contracts, the diameter of the muscle ring is reduced, thereby relaxing the tension on the zonular fibers and allowing the lens to become more spherical. Thus, when the ciliary muscle contracts, the axial thickness of the lens increases, the equatorial diameter of the lens decreases, and

Table 3-1 Changes With Accommodation

	With Accommodation	Without Accommodation
Ciliary muscle action	Contraction	Relaxation
Ciliary ring diameter	Decreases	Increases
Zonular tension	Decreases	Increases
Lens shape	More spherical	Flatter
Lens equatorial diameter	Decreases	Increases
Axial lens thickness	Increases	Decreases
Central anterior lens capsule curvature	Steepens	Flattens
Central posterior lens capsule curvature	Minimal change	Minimal change
Lens dioptric power	Increases	Decreases

the dioptric power of the lens increases, resulting in accommodation. When the ciliary muscle relaxes, the zonular tension increases, the lens flattens, and the dioptric power of the eye decreases (Table 3-1).

The accommodative response may be stimulated by the known or apparent size and distance of an object or by blur, chromatic aberration, or a continual oscillation of ciliary tone. Accommodation is mediated by the parasympathetic fibers of cranial nerve III (oculomotor). Parasympathomimetic drugs (eg, pilocarpine) induce accommodation, whereas parasympatholytic medications (eg, atropine) block accommodation. Drugs that relax the ciliary muscle are called *cycloplegics*.

The *amplitude of accommodation* is the amount of change in the eye's refractive power that is produced by accommodation. It diminishes with age and may be affected by some medications and diseases. Adolescents generally have 12.00–16.00 D of accommodation, whereas adults at age 40 years have 4.00–8.00 D. After age 50 years, accommodation decreases to less than 2.00 D.

Presbyopia is the gradual loss of accommodative response, resulting from reduced elasticity of the crystalline lens. Once an individual is approximately 40 years of age or older, the rigidity of the lens nucleus reduces accommodation, as contraction of the ciliary muscle no longer results in increased convexity and dioptric power of the anterior surface of the lens. This decreased accommodation then becomes clinically significant. Studies have shown that, throughout life, the hardness or stiffness of the human lens increases more than 1000-fold. (See also BCSC Section 3, *Clinical Optics.*) Researchers continue to explore other factors that may contribute to presbyopia, such as changes in lens dimensions, in the elasticity of the lens capsule, and in the geometry of zonular attachments with age.

Glasser A. Accommodation. In: Kaufman PL, Alm A, eds. *Adler's Physiology of the Eye: Clinical Application.* 11th ed. St Louis: Mosby; 2009:40–69.

Heys KR, Cram SL, Truscott RJ. Massive increase in the stiffness of the human lens nucleus with age: the basis for presbyopia? *Mol Vis.* 2004;10:956–963.

This chapter was prepared with the assistance of David Beebe, PhD.

CHAPTER 4

Embryology and Developmental Defects

Normal Development of the Lens

The formation of the human crystalline lens begins very early in embryogenesis (Fig 4-1). At approximately 25 days of gestation, 2 lateral evaginations, called the *optic vesicles,* form from the forebrain, or diencephalon. As the optic vesicles enlarge and extend laterally, they become closely apposed and adherent to the *surface ectoderm,* a single layer of cuboidal cells, in 2 patches on either side of the head. (See BCSC Section 2, *Fundamentals and Principles of Ophthalmology,* for additional discussion and illustrations of ocular development.)

Lens Placode

The ectoderm cells that overlie the optic vesicles become columnar at approximately 27 days of gestation. This area of thickened cells is called the *lens placode.* Growth factors of the *bone morphogenetic protein (BMP)* family are required for formation of the lens placode and, subsequently, the lens.

Lens Pit

The lens pit appears at 29 days of gestation as an indentation (infolding) of the lens placode. The lens pit deepens and invaginates to form the lens vesicle.

Lens Vesicle

As the lens pit continues to invaginate, the stalk of cells connecting it to the surface ectoderm degenerates by programmed cell death (apoptosis), thereby separating the lens cells from the surface ectoderm. The resultant sphere, a single layer of cuboidal cells encased in a basement membrane (the *lens capsule*), is called the *lens vesicle.* At the time of its formation at 30 days of gestation, the lens vesicle is approximately 0.2 mm in diameter.

Because the lens vesicle was formed through a process of invagination of the surface ectoderm, the apices of the cuboidal cells are oriented toward the lumen of the lens vesicle, with the base of each cell attached to the capsule around the periphery of the vesicle. At the same time that the lens vesicle is forming, the optic vesicle is invaginating to form the 2-layered *optic cup.*

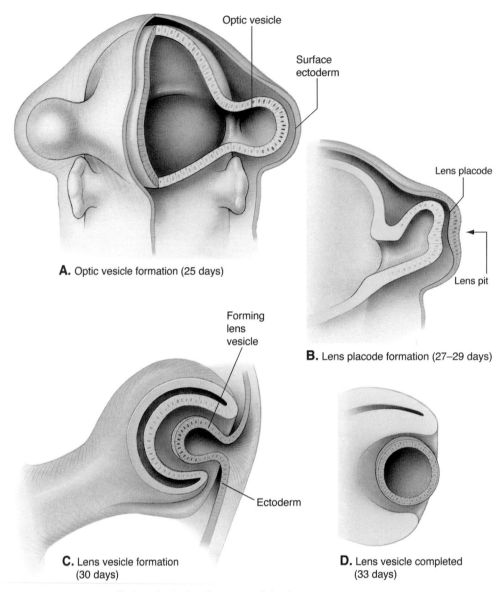

Figure 4-1 Embryologic development of the lens. *(Illustration by Christine Gralapp.)*

(Continued)

Primary Lens Fibers and the Embryonic Nucleus

The cells in the posterior layer of the lens vesicle stop dividing and begin to elongate. As they elongate, they begin to fill the lumen of the lens vesicle. At approximately 40 days of gestation, the lumen of the lens vesicle is obliterated. The elongated cells are called the *primary lens fibers.* As the fiber cells mature, their nuclei and other membrane-bound organelles undergo degradation, a process that reduces light scattering. The primary lens fibers make up the embryonic nucleus that will ultimately occupy the central area of the adult lens.

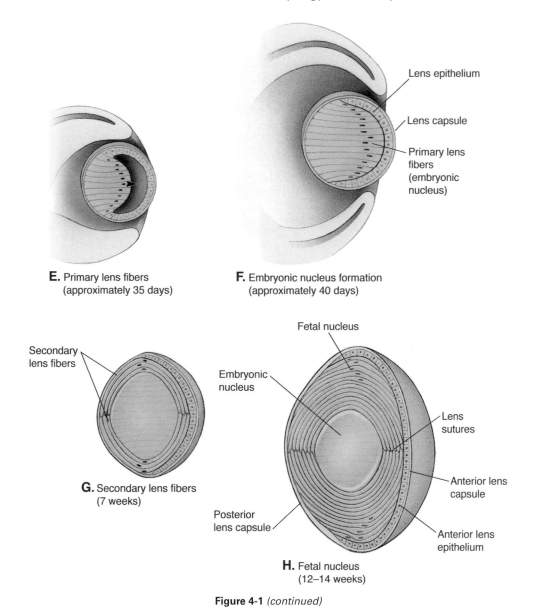

E. Primary lens fibers
(approximately 35 days)

F. Embryonic nucleus formation
(approximately 40 days)

G. Secondary lens fibers
(7 weeks)

H. Fetal nucleus
(12–14 weeks)

Figure 4-1 *(continued)*

The cells of the anterior lens vesicle remain as a monolayer of cuboidal cells, the *lens epithelium.* Subsequent growth of the lens is due to proliferation within the epithelium. The *lens capsule* develops as a basement membrane elaborated by the lens epithelium anteriorly and by lens fibers posteriorly.

Secondary Lens Fibers

After they proliferate, the epithelial cells near the lens equator elongate to form secondary lens fibers. The anterior aspect of each developing lens fiber extends anteriorly beneath the lens epithelium, toward the anterior pole of the lens. The posterior aspect of each developing lens fiber extends posteriorly along the capsule, toward the posterior pole of the lens. In this manner, new lens fibers are continually formed, layer upon layer. As each secondary fiber cell detaches from the capsule, it loses its nucleus and membrane-bound organelles. The secondary lens fibers formed between 2 and 8 months of gestation make up the *fetal nucleus.*

Lens Sutures and the Fetal Nucleus

As lens fibers grow anteriorly and posteriorly, a pattern emerges where the ends of the fibers meet and interdigitate with the ends of fibers arising on the opposite side of the lens, near the anterior and posterior poles. These patterns of cell association are known as *sutures.* Y-shaped sutures are recognizable at approximately 8 weeks of gestation, with an erect Y-suture appearing anteriorly and an inverted Y-suture posteriorly (Fig 4-2). As the lens fibers continue to form and the lens continues to grow, the pattern of lens sutures becomes increasingly complex, resulting in 12 or more suture branches in the adult eye. The mechanisms responsible for the precise formation and changing organization of the suture pattern remain obscure.

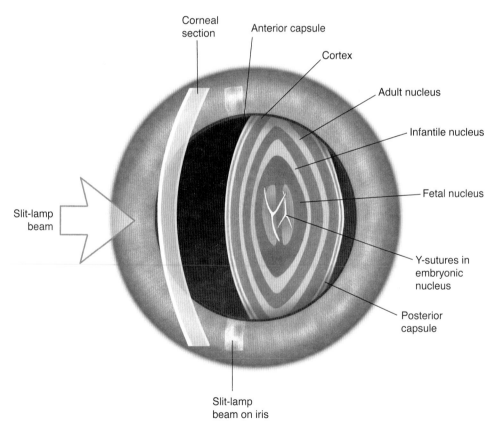

Figure 4-2 Y-shaped sutures, formed during embryogenesis, are visible within the adult lens with the use of the slit lamp. *(Illustration by Christine Gralapp.)*

The human lens weighs approximately 90 mg at birth, and it increases in mass by approximately 2 mg per year as new fibers form throughout life. The central, or oldest, lens fibers gradually become less malleable, and the lens nucleus becomes more rigid. This process progressively reduces the amplitude of accommodation.

Tunica Vasculosa Lentis

Around 1 month of gestation, the hyaloid artery, which enters the eye at the optic nerve head (also called the optic disc), branches to form a network of capillaries, the tunica vasculosa lentis, on the posterior surface of the lens capsule (Fig 4-3). These capillaries grow toward the equator of the lens, where they anastomose with a second network of capillaries, called the *anterior pupillary membrane.* This membrane derives from the ciliary veins and covers the anterior surface of the lens. At approximately 9 weeks of gestation, the capillary network surrounding the lens is fully developed; it disappears by an orderly process of programmed cell death shortly before birth. Sometimes a remnant of the tunica vasculosa lentis persists as a small opacity or strand, called a *Mittendorf dot* (discussed later in this chapter), on the posterior aspect of the lens. In other eyes, remnants of the pupillary membrane are often visible as pupillary strands.

The Zonule of Zinn

Experimental evidence suggests that the zonular fibers are secreted by the ciliary epithelium, although how these fibers insert into the lens capsule is not known. The zonular fibers begin to develop at the end of the third month of gestation.

Duke-Elder S, ed. *System of Ophthalmology.* St Louis: Mosby; 1973:127–137.

Kuszak JR, Clark JI, Cooper KE, Rae JL. Biology of the lens: lens transparency as a function of embryology, anatomy, and physiology. In: Albert DM, Jakobiec FA, eds. *Principles and Practice of Ophthalmology.* 3rd ed. Philadelphia: Saunders; 2008:1291–1339.

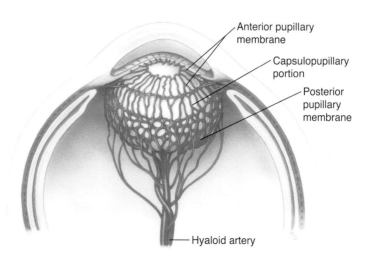

Anterior pupillary membrane

Capsulopupillary portion

Posterior pupillary membrane

Hyaloid artery

Figure 4-3 Components of the tunica vasculosa lentis. *(Illustration by Christine Gralapp.)*

Congenital Anomalies and Abnormalities

Most significant congenital anomalies of the eye and orbit are apparent on ultrasonography before birth. As a rule, the more profound the abnormality, the earlier in development it occurred. Disorders of the lens include abnormalities in lens shape, size, location, and development, as well as cataract.

Congenital Aphakia

The lens is absent in congenital aphakia, a very rare anomaly. Two forms of congenital aphakia have been described. In *primary aphakia,* the lens placode fails to form from the surface ectoderm in the developing embryo. In *secondary aphakia,* the more common type, the developing lens is spontaneously absorbed. Both forms of aphakia are usually associated with other malformations of the eye.

Lenticonus and Lentiglobus

Lenticonus is a localized, cone-shaped deformation of the anterior or posterior lens surface (Fig 4-4). Posterior lenticonus is more common than anterior lenticonus and is usually unilateral and axial in location. Anterior lenticonus is often bilateral and may be associated with Alport syndrome.

In lentiglobus, the localized deformation of the lens surface is spherical. Posterior lentiglobus is more common than anterior lentiglobus and is often associated with posterior polar opacities that vary in density.

Retinoscopy through the center of the lens reveals a distorted and myopic reflex in both lenticonus and lentiglobus. These deformations can also be seen in the red reflex, where, by retroillumination, they appear as an "oil droplet." (This condition should not be confused with the "oil droplet" cataract of galactosemia, which is discussed in Chapter 5.) The posterior bulging may progress with initial worsening of the myopia, followed by opacification of the defect. Surrounding cortical lamellae may also opacify.

Lens Coloboma

A lens coloboma is an anomaly of lens shape (Fig 4-5). *Primary coloboma* is a wedge-shaped defect or indentation of the lens periphery that occurs as an isolated anomaly.

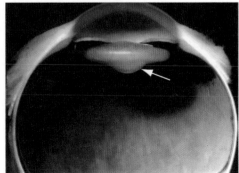

Figure 4-4 Posterior lenticonus *(arrow). (Courtesy of Mission for Vision.)*

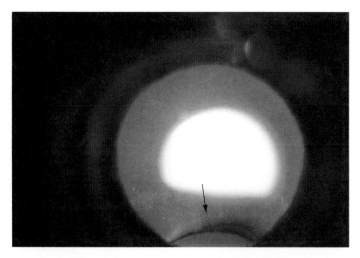

Figure 4-5 Coloboma of the lens *(arrow)* as viewed by retroillumination.

Secondary coloboma is a flattening or indentation of the lens periphery caused by the lack of ciliary body or zonular development. Lens colobomas are typically located inferonasally and may be associated with colobomas of the iris, optic nerve, or retina. Cortical lens opacification or thickening of the lens capsule may appear adjacent to the coloboma. The zonular attachments in the region of the coloboma are usually weakened or absent.

Mittendorf Dot

Mittendorf dot, mentioned earlier in this chapter, is a common anomaly observed in many healthy eyes. A small, dense white spot generally located inferonasal to the posterior pole of the lens, a Mittendorf dot is a remnant of the posterior pupillary membrane of the tunica vasculosa lentis (Fig 4-6). It marks the place where the hyaloid artery came into contact with the posterior surface of the lens in utero. Sometimes a Mittendorf dot is associated with a fibrous tail or remnant of the hyaloid artery projecting into the vitreous body.

Epicapsular Star

Another very common remnant of the tunica vasculosa lentis is an epicapsular star (Fig 4-7). As its name suggests, this anomaly is a star-shaped distribution of tiny brown or golden flecks on the central anterior lens capsule. It may be unilateral or bilateral.

Peters Anomaly

Peters anomaly is part of a spectrum of disorders known as *anterior segment dysgenesis syndrome,* also referred to as *neurocristopathy* or *mesodermal dysgenesis.* (See also BCSC Section 6, *Pediatric Ophthalmology and Strabismus.*) Peters anomaly is characterized by a central or paracentral corneal opacity (leukoma) associated with thinning or absence of adjacent endothelium and Descemet membrane. In Peters anomaly type 1, iris strands adherent to the cornea are often present. In Peters anomaly type 2, the lens is adherent to the posterior cornea. In normal ocular development, the lens vesicle separates from the

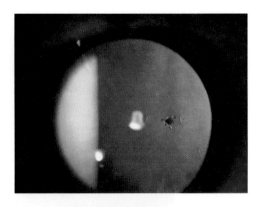

Figure 4-6 Mittendorf dot, as viewed by retroillumination. *(Courtesy of Matt Weed, MD. Photograph by D. Brice Critser, CRA. Used with permission from the University of Iowa and EyeRounds.org.)*

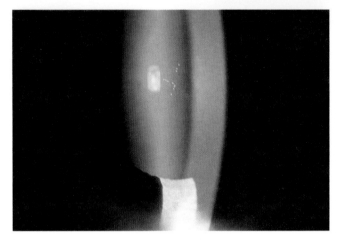

Figure 4-7 Epicapsular star.

surface ectoderm (the future corneal epithelium) at approximately 33 days of gestation. Peters anomaly is typically linked with the absence of this separation. It is often associated with mutations in or deletion of 1 allele of the genes normally involved in anterior segment development, including the transcription factors *PAX6*, *PITX2*, and *FOXC1*. Patients with Peters anomaly type 2 may also display the following lens anomalies:

- anterior cortical or polar cataract
- a misshapen lens displaced anteriorly into the pupillary space and the anterior chamber
- microspherophakia

Microspherophakia

Microspherophakia is a developmental abnormality in which the lens is small in diameter and spherical. The entire lens equator can be visualized at the slit lamp when the pupil is widely dilated (Fig 4-8). The spherical shape of the lens results in increased refractive power, which causes the eye to be highly myopic.

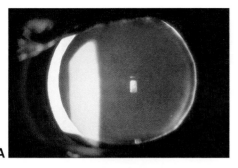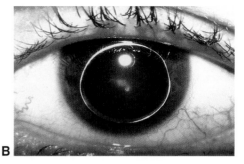

A   **B**

Figure 4-8 Microspherophakia. **A,** When the pupil is dilated, the entire lens equator can be seen at the slit lamp. **B,** Anterior dislocation of a microspherophakic lens. *(Part A courtesy of Karla J. Johns, MD.)*

Faulty development of the secondary lens fibers during embryogenesis is believed to be the cause of microspherophakia. Microspherophakia is most often seen as a part of Weill-Marchesani syndrome, but it may also occur as an isolated hereditary abnormality or, occasionally, in association with Peters anomaly, Marfan syndrome, Alport syndrome, Lowe syndrome, or congenital rubella. Individuals with Weill-Marchesani syndrome commonly have small stature, short and stubby fingers, and broad hands with reduced joint mobility. Weill-Marchesani syndrome is usually inherited as an autosomal recessive trait.

The spherical lens can block the pupil, causing secondary angle-closure glaucoma. Use of miotics aggravates this condition by increasing pupillary block and allowing additional forward lens displacement. Cycloplegics are the medical treatment of choice to break an attack of angle-closure glaucoma in patients with microspherophakia, because they decrease pupillary block by tightening the zonular fibers, decreasing the anteroposterior lens diameter, and pulling the lens posteriorly. A laser iridotomy may also be useful in relieving angle closure in patients with microspherophakia. (See also BCSC Section 10, *Glaucoma.*)

Aniridia

Aniridia is an uncommon panocular syndrome in which the most dramatic manifestation is partial or nearly complete absence of the iris (Fig 4-9). Aniridia has been linked to the loss of 1 allele of the *PAX6* gene, a transcription factor that is important for the development and function of the cornea, lens, and retina. Associated findings include corneal pannus and epitheliopathy, glaucoma, foveal and optic nerve hypoplasia, and nystagmus. Aniridia is almost always bilateral. Two-thirds of cases are familial; one-third of cases are sporadic. Sporadic cases of aniridia are associated with a high incidence of Wilms tumor and the WAGR complex (*W*ilms tumor, *a*niridia, *g*enitourinary malformations, and mental *r*etardation).

Anterior or posterior polar lens opacities may be present at birth in patients with aniridia. Cortical, subcapsular, or lamellar opacities develop in 50%–85% of patients within the first 2 decades of life. The lens opacities may progress, further impairing vision. Poor zonular integrity and ectopia lentis have also been reported in patients with aniridia.

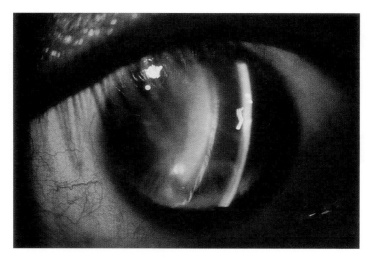

Figure 4-9 Cataract in a patient with aniridia.

Congenital Cataract

Cataracts that are present at birth or that develop within the first year of life are called *congenital* or *infantile* cataracts. Because some lens opacities escape detection at birth and are noted only on later examination, these terms are used interchangeably by many physicians. In this book, the term *congenital cataract* is used for both categories of lens opacities. These cataracts are fairly common, occurring in 1 of every 2000 live births, and cover a broad spectrum of severity. While some lens opacities do not progress and are visually insignificant, others can cause profound visual impairment.

Congenital cataracts may be unilateral or bilateral. They can be classified by morphology, presumed or defined genetic etiology, presence of specific metabolic disorders, or associated ocular anomalies or systemic findings (Table 4-1). In general, approximately one-third of congenital cataracts are a component of a more extensive syndrome or disease (eg, cataract resulting from congenital rubella syndrome), one-third occur as an isolated inherited trait, and one-third result from undetermined causes. Metabolic diseases tend to be more commonly associated with bilateral cataracts. (For a discussion of the evaluation of pediatric patients with congenital cataracts, see BCSC Section 6, *Pediatric Ophthalmology and Strabismus.*) Congenital cataracts occur in a variety of morphologic configurations, including lamellar, polar, sutural, coronary, cerulean, nuclear, capsular, complete, and membranous.

Lamellar

Of the congenital cataracts, lamellar, or *zonular,* cataracts are the most common type (Fig 4-10). They are characteristically bilateral and symmetric, and their effect on vision varies with the size and density of the opacity. Lamellar cataracts may be inherited as an autosomal dominant trait. In some cases, they may occur as a result of a transient toxic influence during embryonic lens development. The earlier this toxic influence occurs, the smaller and deeper is the resulting lamellar cataract.

Table 4-1 Etiology of Pediatric Cataracts

Type	Causes
Bilateral	Idiopathic
	Heredity*
	Genetic and metabolic diseases
	Down syndrome
	Hallermann-Streiff syndrome
	Lowe syndrome
	Galactosemia
	Marfan syndrome
	Trisomy 13–15
	Hypoglycemia
	Alport syndrome
	Myotonic dystrophy
	Fabry disease
	Hypoparathyroidism
	Conradi-Hünermann syndrome
	Maternal infections
	Cytomegalovirus
	Rubella
	Syphilis
	Toxoplasmosis
	Varicella
	Ocular anomalies
	Aniridia
	Anterior segment dysgenesis syndrome
	Toxicity
	Corticosteroids
	Radiation (may be unilateral or bilateral)
Unilateral	Idiopathic
	Ocular anomalies
	Persistent fetal vasculature
	Anterior segment dysgenesis
	Posterior lenticonus
	Posterior lentiglobus
	Posterior pole tumors
	Trauma (rule out child abuse)
	Rubella
	Masked bilateral cataract
	Radiation (may be unilateral or bilateral)

*Autosomal dominant most common; also autosomal recessive or X-linked.

Lamellar cataracts are opacifications of specific layers or zones of the lens. Clinically, the cataract is visible as an opacified layer that surrounds a clearer center and is itself surrounded by a layer of clear cortex. Viewed from the front, the lamellar cataract has a disc-shaped configuration. Often, additional arcuate opacities within the cortex straddle the equator of the lamellar cataract; these horseshoe-shaped opacities are called *riders.*

Polar

Polar cataracts are lens opacities that involve the subcapsular cortex and capsule of the anterior or posterior pole of the lens. *Anterior polar cataracts* are usually small,

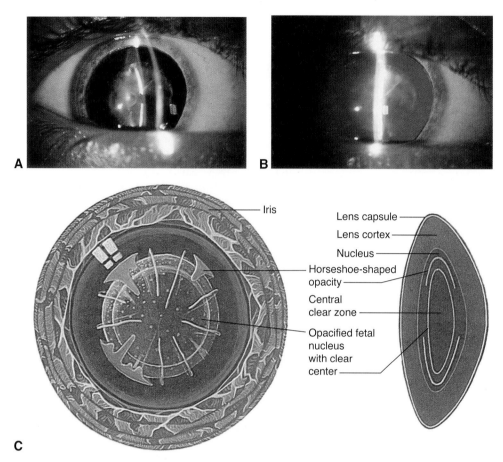

Figure 4-10 A, Lamellar cataract. **B,** Lamellar cataract viewed by retroillumination. **C,** Schematic of lamellar cataract. *(Part C courtesy of Alcon. Illustration by John A. Craig.)*

bilateral, symmetric, nonprogressive opacities that do not impair vision (Fig 4-11). Most commonly, they are congenital and sporadic, but they may be inherited in an autosomal dominant pattern. Anterior polar cataracts are sometimes seen in association with other ocular abnormalities, including microphthalmos, persistent pupillary membrane, and anterior lenticonus. They usually do not require treatment but often cause anisometropia.

Posterior polar cataracts are generally associated with more profound decrease in vision than anterior polar cataracts, because they tend to be larger and are positioned closer to the nodal point of the eye. Capsular fragility has been reported in association with these cataracts, which are usually stable but occasionally progress. They may be familial or sporadic. Familial posterior polar cataracts are usually bilateral and inherited in an autosomal dominant pattern. Sporadic posterior polar cataracts are often unilateral and may be associated with remnants of the tunica vasculosa lentis or with an abnormality of the posterior lens surface such as lenticonus or lentiglobus.

Sutural

The sutural, or stellate, cataract is an opacification of the Y-sutures of the fetal nucleus (Fig 4-12). It usually does not impair vision. These opacities often have branches or knobs projecting from them. Sutural cataracts are bilateral and symmetric and are frequently inherited in an autosomal dominant pattern.

Coronary

Coronary cataracts are so named because they consist of a group of club-shaped cortical opacities that are arranged around the equator of the lens like a crown, or corona. They cannot be seen unless the pupil is dilated, and they usually do not affect visual acuity. Coronary cataracts are often inherited in an autosomal dominant pattern.

Cerulean

Also known as *blue-dot cataracts*, cerulean cataracts are small bluish opacities located in the lens cortex (Fig 4-13). They are nonprogressive and usually do not cause visual symptoms.

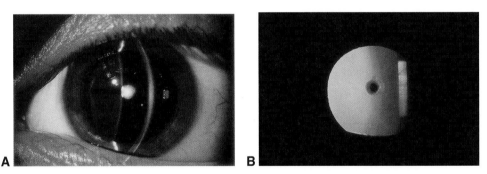

Figure 4-11   **A,** Anterior polar cataract. **B,** Anterior polar cataract viewed by retroillumination.

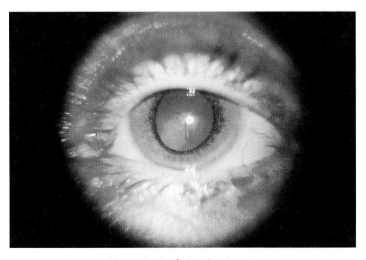

Figure 4-12   Sutural cataract.

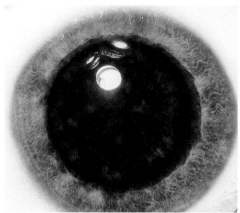

Figure 4-13 Cerulean cataract. *(Courtesy of Karla J. Johns, MD.)*

Nuclear

Congenital nuclear cataracts are opacities of the embryonic nucleus alone or of both embryonic and fetal nuclei (Fig 4-14). They are usually bilateral, with a wide spectrum of severity. Lens opacification may involve the complete nucleus, or it may be limited to discrete layers within the nucleus. Eyes with congenital nuclear cataracts tend to be microphthalmic, and they are at increased risk of developing aphakic glaucoma.

Capsular

Capsular cataracts are small opacifications of the lens epithelium and anterior lens capsule that spare the cortex. They are differentiated from anterior polar cataracts by their protrusion into the anterior chamber. Capsular cataracts generally do not adversely affect vision.

Complete

With complete, or total, cataract, all of the lens fibers are opacified. The red reflex is completely obscured, and the retina cannot be seen with either direct or indirect ophthalmoscopy. Some cataracts may be subtotal at birth and progress rapidly to become complete cataracts. Complete cataracts may be unilateral or bilateral, and they cause profound visual impairment.

Membranous

Membranous cataracts occur when lens proteins are resorbed from either an intact or a traumatized lens, allowing the anterior and posterior lens capsules to fuse into a dense white membrane (Fig 4-15). The resulting opacity and lens distortion generally cause significant visual disability.

Rubella

Maternal infection with the rubella virus, an RNA togavirus, can cause fetal damage, especially if the infection occurs during the first trimester of pregnancy. Cataracts resulting from *congenital rubella syndrome* are characterized by pearly white nuclear opacifications. Sometimes the entire lens is opacified (complete cataract), and the cortex may liquefy. Histologically, lens-fiber nuclei are retained deep within the lens substance. Live virus particles may be recovered from the lens as late as 3 years after the patient's birth. Cataract

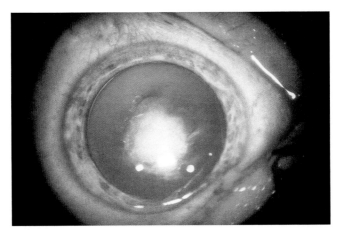

Figure 4-14 Congenital nuclear cataract. *(Reproduced from Day SH.* Understanding and Preventing Amblyopia: Slide & Script Presentation. *Eye Care Skills for the Primary Care Physician Series. San Francisco: American Academy of Ophthalmology; 1987.)*

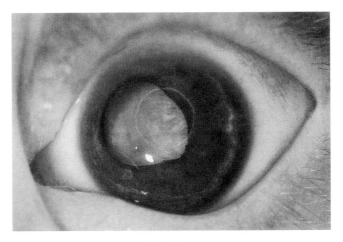

Figure 4-15 Membranous cataract.

removal may be complicated by excessive postoperative inflammation caused by release of these particles. (See also BCSC Section 6, *Pediatric Ophthalmology and Strabismus.*) Other ocular manifestations of congenital rubella syndrome include diffuse pigmentary retinopathy, microphthalmos, glaucoma, and transient or permanent corneal clouding. Although congenital rubella syndrome may cause cataract or glaucoma, both conditions are usually not present simultaneously in the same eye.

Developmental Defects

Ectopia Lentis

Ectopia lentis is a displacement of the lens that may be congenital, developmental, or acquired. A *subluxated* lens is partially displaced from its normal position but remains in the pupillary area. A *luxated,* or *dislocated,* lens is completely displaced from the pupil, implying separation of all zonular attachments. Findings associated with lens subluxation include decreased vision, marked astigmatism, monocular diplopia, and iridodonesis (tremulous iris). Potential complications of ectopia lentis include cataract and displacement of the lens into the anterior chamber or the vitreous space. Dislocation into the anterior chamber or pupil may cause pupillary block and angle-closure glaucoma. Dislocation of the lens posteriorly into the vitreous cavity often has no adverse sequelae aside from a profound change in refractive error.

Trauma is the most common cause of acquired lens displacement. Nontraumatic ectopia lentis is commonly associated with Marfan syndrome, homocystinuria, aniridia, and congenital glaucoma. Less frequently, it appears with Ehlers-Danlos syndrome, hyperlysinemia, Weill-Marchesani syndrome, and sulfite oxidase deficiency. Ectopia lentis may occur as an isolated anomaly (simple ectopia lentis), usually inherited as an autosomal dominant trait. Ectopia lentis can also be associated with pupillary abnormalities in the ocular syndrome ectopia lentis et pupillae (discussed later in this chapter).

Marfan syndrome

Marfan syndrome is a heritable disorder with ocular, cardiovascular, and skeletal manifestations. Though usually inherited as an autosomal dominant trait, the disorder appears with no family history in approximately 15% of cases. Marfan syndrome is caused by mutations in the fibrillin gene on chromosome 15. Affected individuals are tall, with arachnodactyly (Fig 4-16A) and chest wall deformities. Associated cardiovascular abnormalities include dilated aortic root and mitral valve prolapse.

Between 50% and 80% of patients with Marfan syndrome exhibit ectopia lentis (Fig 4-16B). The lens subluxation tends to be bilateral and symmetric (usually superior and temporal), but variations do occur. The zonular attachments commonly remain intact but become stretched and elongated. Ectopia lentis in Marfan syndrome is probably congenital in most cases. Progression of lens subluxation occurs in some patients over time, but in many patients the lens position remains stable.

Other ocular abnormalities associated with Marfan syndrome include axial myopia and an increased risk of retinal detachment. Patients with Marfan syndrome may develop

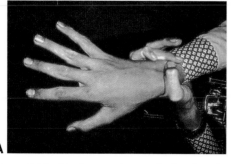 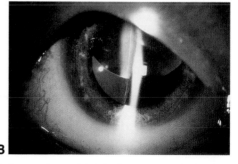

A   B

Figure 4-16 Marfan syndrome. **A,** Arachnodactyly in a patient with Marfan syndrome. **B,** Subluxated lens in Marfan syndrome. *(Part A courtesy of Karla J. Johns, MD.)*

pupillary block glaucoma if the lens dislocates into the pupil or anterior chamber. Open-angle glaucoma may also occur. Amblyopia may develop in children with lens subluxation if their refractive error shows significant asymmetry or remains uncorrected in early childhood. Spectacle or contact lens correction of the refractive error provides satisfactory vision in most cases. Pupillary dilation is sometimes helpful. The clinician may refract both the phakic and the aphakic portions of the pupil to determine the optimum visual acuity. A reading add is often necessary because the subluxated lens lacks sufficient accommodation.

In some cases, adequate visual acuity cannot be obtained with spectacle or contact lens correction, and removal of the lens may be indicated. Lens extraction—either extra-capsular or intracapsular—in patients with Marfan syndrome is associated with a high rate of complications such as vitreous loss and complex retinal detachment. Advanced surgical techniques, including the use of capsular tension rings and capsular tension segments, are increasingly being used to improve outcomes in these cases (see Chapter 9).

Homocystinuria

Homocystinuria is an inborn error of methionine metabolism that is transmitted in an autosomal recessive pattern. Serum levels of homocysteine and methionine are elevated. Affected individuals are healthy at birth; however, seizures and osteoporosis develop, and cognitive impairment soon becomes apparent. These patients are usually tall and have light-colored hair. Patients with homocystinuria are prone to thromboembolic episodes, and surgery and general anesthesia are thought to increase the risk of thromboembolism.

Lens dislocation in homocystinuria tends to be bilateral and symmetric. The dislocation appears in infancy in approximately 30% of affected individuals, and by the age of 15 years, it appears in 80% of those affected. The lenses are usually subluxated inferiorly and nasally, but variations have been reported. Because zonular fibers of the lens are known to have a high concentration of cysteine, deficiency of cysteine is thought to disturb normal zonular development; affected fibers tend to be brittle and easily disrupted. Studies of infants with homocystinuria treated with a low-methionine, high-cysteine diet and vitamin supplementation with the coenzyme pyridoxine (vitamin B_6) have shown that this therapy may reduce the incidence of sequelae, including ectopia lentis, in some patients. (See also BCSC Section 6, *Pediatric Ophthalmology and Strabismus*.)

Hyperlysinemia

Hyperlysinemia, an inborn error of metabolism of the amino acid lysine, is associated with ectopia lentis. Affected individuals also show cognitive impairment and muscular hypotony.

Genetic Contributions to Age-Related Cataracts

Studies of identical and fraternal twins and of familial associations suggest that a large proportion of the risk of age-related cataracts is inherited. It is estimated that inheritance accounts for more than 50% of the risk of cortical cataracts. Recent studies have identified mutations in the gene associated with congenital and age-related cortical cataracts, *EPHA2*, which has been mapped to 1p36. This is the first gene known to cause hereditary, nonsyndromic age-related cortical cataracts, although mutations at this locus account for only a small fraction of cortical opacities. Similarly, 35%–50% of the risk of nuclear cataracts can be traced to inheritance. Identification of the genes associated with increased risk of cortical and nuclear cataracts is important, because understanding the biochemical pathways in which they function may suggest ways to slow the progression or prevent the development of age-related cataracts in a large number of cases.

Jun G, Guo H, Klein BEK, et al. *EPHA2* is associated with age-related cortical cataract in mice and humans. *PLoS Genet.* 5(7):e1000584.

Shiels A, Bennett TM, Knopf HLS, et al. The *EPHA2* gene is associated with cataracts linked to chromosome 1p. *Mol Vis.* 2008;14:2042–2055.

Ectopia Lentis et Pupillae

In the autosomal recessive disorder ectopia lentis et pupillae, the lens and the pupil are displaced in opposite directions. The pupil is irregular, usually slit shaped, and displaced from the normal position. The dislocated lens may bisect the pupil or may be completely absent from the pupillary space. This disorder is usually bilateral but not symmetric. Characteristically, the iris dilates poorly. Associated ocular anomalies include severe axial myopia, retinal detachment, enlarged corneal diameter, cataract, and abnormal iris transillumination.

Persistent Fetal Vasculature

Persistent fetal vasculature (PFV), also known as *persistent hyperplastic primary vitreous (PHPV),* is a congenital, nonhereditary ocular malformation that frequently involves the lens. In 90% of patients, it is unilateral. A white, fibrous retrolental tissue is present, often in association with posterior cortical opacification. Progressive cataract formation often occurs, sometimes leading to a complete cataract. Other abnormalities associated with PFV include elongated ciliary processes, prominent radial iris vessels, and persistent hyaloid artery. (See BCSC Section 6, *Pediatric Ophthalmology and Strabismus,* and Section 12, *Retina and Vitreous,* for additional discussion.)

Beebe DC. The lens. In: Kaufman PL, Alm A, eds. *Adler's Physiology of the Eye: Clinical Application.* 11th ed. St Louis: Mosby; 2011:131–163.

Congdon NG, Chang MA, Botelho P, Stark WJ, Datiles MB III. Cataract: clinical types. In: Tasman W, Jaeger EA, eds. *Duane's Clinical Ophthalmology.* Philadelphia: Lippincott Williams & Wilkins; 2006; vol 1, chapter 73.

Hiles DA, Kilty LA. Disorders of the lens. In: Isenberg SJ, ed. *The Eye in Infancy.* 2nd ed. St Louis: Mosby; 1994:336–373.

Streeten BW. Pathology of the lens. In: Albert DM, Jakobiec FA, eds. *Principles and Practice of Ophthalmology.* 2nd ed. Philadelphia: Saunders; 2000:3685–3749.

CHAPTER 5

Pathology

Age-Related Lens Changes

As the lens ages, it increases in mass and thickness and decreases in accommodative power. As new layers of cortical fibers form concentrically, the lens nucleus compresses and hardens (a process known as nuclear sclerosis). Chemical modification and proteolytic cleavage of crystallins (lens proteins) result in the formation of high-molecular-mass protein aggregates. These aggregates may become large enough to cause abrupt fluctuations in the local refractive index of the lens, thereby scattering light and reducing transparency. Chemical modification of lens nuclear proteins also increases opacity, such that the lens becomes increasingly yellow or brown with advancing age (Fig 5-1). Other age-related changes include decreased concentrations of glutathione and potassium and increased concentrations of sodium and calcium in the lens cell cytoplasm.

A frequent cause of visual impairment in older adults is *age-related cataract,* the pathogenesis of which is multifactorial and not completely understood. There are 3 main types of age-related cataracts: nuclear, cortical, and posterior subcapsular. In many patients, components of more than 1 type are present. (See also BCSC Section 4, *Ophthalmic Pathology and Intraocular Tumors.*)

Nuclear Cataracts

Some degree of nuclear sclerosis and yellowing is normal in patients older than 50 years. In general, this condition interferes only minimally with visual function. In eyes with nuclear cataracts, the central opacity causes an increased amount of light scattering, which the ophthalmologist observes as a yellow-brown central lens nucleus. A nuclear cataract (Fig 5-2) is best evaluated by using a slit-lamp biomicroscope with off-axis illumination through a dilated pupil.

Nuclear cataracts tend to progress slowly. They are usually bilateral but may be asymmetric. Nuclear cataracts typically cause greater impairment of distance vision than of near vision. In the early stages of cataract development, the progressive hardening of the lens nucleus frequently causes an increase in the refractive index of the lens and thus a myopic shift in refraction *(lenticular myopia).* In hyperopic or emmetropic eyes, the myopic shift enables otherwise presbyopic individuals to read without spectacles, a condition referred to as "second sight." A change in astigmatism and, in rare instances, a hyperopic shift can occur as the nucleus matures. Occasionally, the abrupt change in refractive index between the sclerotic nucleus (or other lens opacities) and the lens cortex can cause monocular

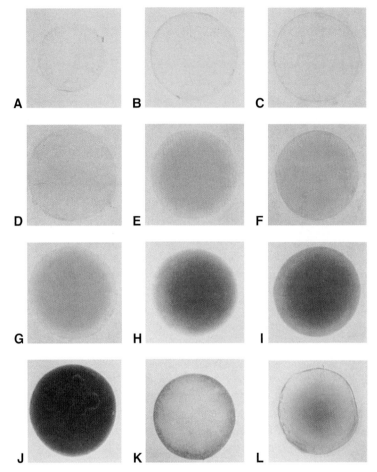

Figure 5-1 Increasing yellow-to-brown coloration of the human lens from age 6 months **(A)** to 8 years **(B)**, 12 years **(C)**, 25 years **(D)**, 47 years **(E)**, 60 years **(F)**, 70 years **(G)**, 82 years **(H)**, and 91 years **(I)**. **J,** Brown nuclear cataract in a 70-year-old patient. **K,** Cortical cataract in a 68-year-old patient. **L,** Mixed nuclear and cortical cataract in a 74-year-old patient. *(Reproduced with permission from Lerman S. Phototoxicity: clinical considerations. Focal Points: Clinical Modules for Ophthalmologists. San Francisco: American Academy of Ophthalmology; 1987, module 8.)*

diplopia. Progressive yellowing or browning of the lens causes patients to have poor color discrimination, especially at the blue end of the visible-light spectrum. In bilateral cases, patients are frequently unaware of their altered color discrimination.

Visual dysfunction in low light often occurs with advancing nuclear cataract. In the most advanced cases, the lens nucleus becomes increasingly opaque and brown and is called a *brunescent nuclear cataract.* The term *oil droplet cataract* is sometimes used to describe a cataract in which nuclear sclerosis is most pronounced in the central nucleus. Such cataracts are best evaluated on retinoscopy.

Histologically, the nucleus in a nuclear cataract is difficult to distinguish from the nucleus of a normal, aged lens. Investigations by electron microscopy have identified an

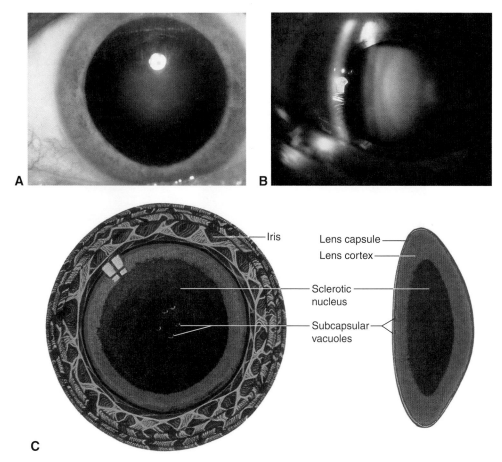

Figure 5-2 Nuclear cataract viewed with diffuse illumination **(A)** and with a slit beam **(B)**. **C,** Schematic of nuclear cataract. *(Part C courtesy of Alcon. Illustration by John A. Craig.)*

increased number of lamellar membrane whorls in some nuclear cataracts. The degree to which protein aggregates or these membrane modifications contribute to the increased light scattering of nuclear cataracts is unclear.

Cortical Cataracts

In contrast to nuclear cataracts, cortical cataracts are associated with the local disruption of the structure of mature lens fiber cells. Once membrane integrity is compromised, essential metabolites are lost from the affected cells. This loss leads to extensive protein oxidation and precipitation. Like nuclear cataracts, cortical cataracts are usually bilateral but are often asymmetric. Their effect on visual function varies greatly, depending on the location of the opacity relative to the visual axis. A common symptom of cortical cataracts is glare from intense focal light sources, such as car headlights. Monocular diplopia may also result. Cortical cataracts vary greatly in their rate of progression, with some

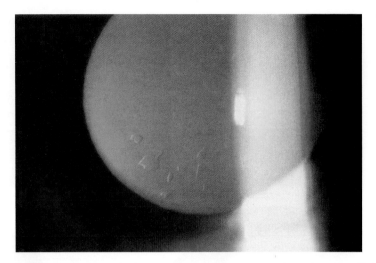

Figure 5-3 Vacuoles in early cortical cataract development, as viewed at the slit lamp using retroillumination.

cortical opacities remaining unchanged for prolonged periods and others progressing rapidly.

The first signs of cortical cataract formation visible with the slit-lamp biomicroscope are vacuoles (Fig 5-3) and water clefts in the anterior or posterior cortex. The cortical lamellae may be separated by fluid. Wedge-shaped opacities (often called *cortical spokes* or *cuneiform opacities*) form near the periphery of the lens, with the pointed end of the opacities oriented toward the center (Fig 5-4). The cortical spokes appear as white opacities when viewed with the slit-lamp biomicroscope and as dark shadows when viewed by retroillumination. The wedge-shaped opacities may spread to adjacent fiber cells and along the length of affected fibers, causing the degree of opacity to increase and extend toward the visual axis. When the entire cortex from the capsule to the nucleus becomes white and opaque, the cataract is said to be *mature* (Fig 5-5). In mature opacities, the lens absorbs water, becoming swollen and enlarged (termed *intumescent* cortical cataract); such cataracts may lead to angle-closure glaucoma.

When degenerated cortical material leaks through the lens capsule, leaving the capsule wrinkled and shrunken, the cataract is referred to as *hypermature* (Fig 5-6). When further liquefaction of the cortex allows free movement of the nucleus within the capsular bag, the cataract is described as *morgagnian* (Fig 5-7).

Histologically, cortical cataracts are characterized by local swelling and disruption of the lens fiber cells. Globules of eosinophilic material (morgagnian globules) are observed in slitlike spaces between lens fibers.

Posterior Subcapsular Cataracts

Patients with posterior subcapsular cataracts (PSCs) are often younger than those presenting with nuclear or cortical cataracts. PSCs are located in the posterior cortical layer and

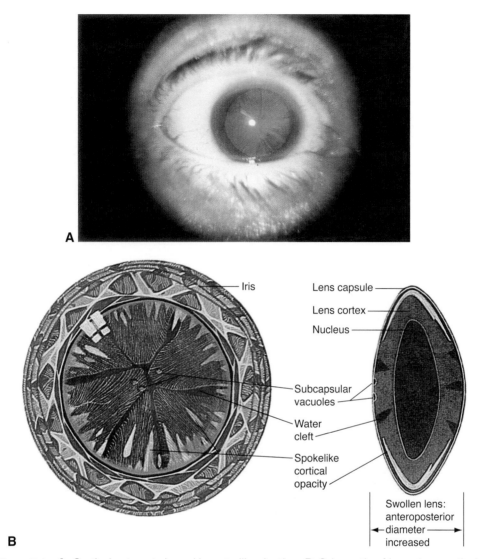

Figure 5-4 **A,** Cortical cataract viewed by retroillumination. **B,** Schematic of immature cortical cataract. *(Part B courtesy of Alcon. Illustration by John A. Craig.)*

are visually significant only when they become axial (Fig 5-8). The first indication of PSC formation is a subtle iridescent sheen in the posterior cortical layers that is visible with the slit lamp. At later stages, granular opacities and a plaquelike opacity of the posterior subcapsular cortex appear.

The patient often reports symptoms of glare and poor vision under bright-light conditions because a central PSC obscures more of the pupillary aperture when miosis is induced by bright lights, accommodation, or miotics. Near vision tends to be reduced more than distance vision. Some patients experience monocular diplopia. Slit-lamp detection of PSCs can best be accomplished through a dilated pupil. Retroillumination is also helpful.

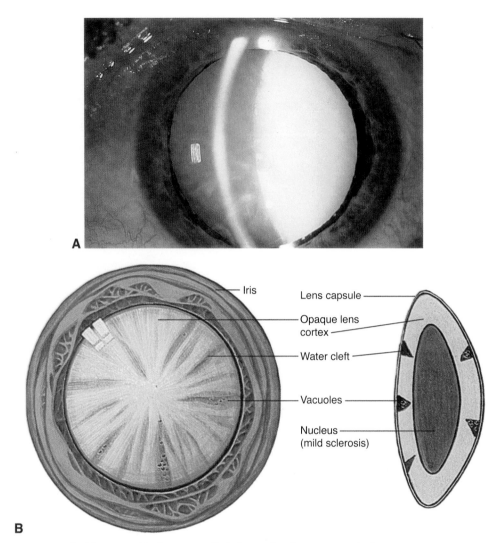

Figure 5-5 **A,** Mature cortical cataract. **B,** Schematic of mature cortical cataract. *(Part B courtesy of Alcon. Illustration by John A. Craig.)*

As stated earlier, PSCs are one of the main types of cataract related to aging. However, they can also occur as a result of trauma; systemic, topical, or intraocular corticosteroid use; inflammation; exposure to ionizing radiation; and prolonged alcohol abuse.

Histologically, PSCs are associated with posterior migration of the lens epithelial cells from the lens equator to the visual axis on the inner surface of the posterior capsule. During their migration to or after their arrival at the posterior axis, the cells undergo aberrant enlargement. These swollen cells are called *Wedl* (or *bladder*) cells.

Hammond CJ, Duncan DD, Snieder H, et al. The heritability of age-related cortical cataract: the twin eye study. *Invest Ophthalmol Vis Sci.* 2001;42(3):601–605.

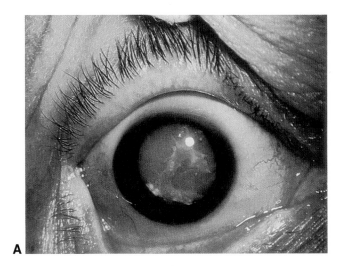

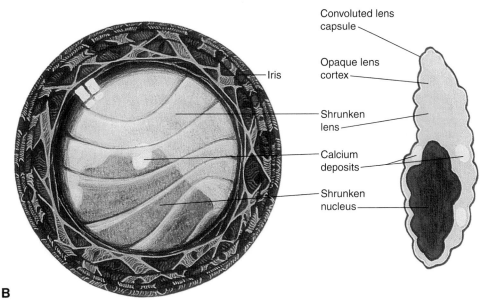

Figure 5-6 **A,** Hypermature cortical cataract. **B,** Schematic of hypermature cortical cataract. *(Part B courtesy of Alcon. Illustration by John A. Craig.)*

Hammond CJ, Snieder H, Spector TD, Gilbert CE. Genetic and environmental factors in age-related nuclear cataracts in monozygotic and dizygotic twins. *N Engl J Med.* 2000;342(24):1786–1790.

Heiba IM, Elston RC, Klein BE, Klein R. Genetic etiology of nuclear cataract: evidence for a major gene. *Am J Med Genet.* 1993;47(8):1208–1214.

Iyengar SK, Klein BE, Klein R, et al. Identification of a major locus for age-related cortical cataract on chromosome 6p12-q12 in the Beaver Dam Eye Study. *Proc Natl Acad Sci USA.* 2004;101(40):14485–14490.

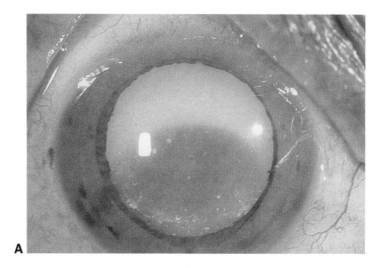

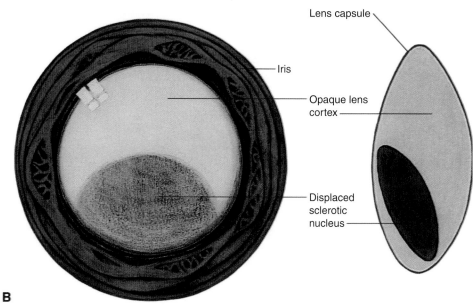

Figure 5-7 **A,** Morgagnian cataract. **B,** Schematic of morgagnian cataract. *(Part B courtesy of Alcon. Illustration by John A. Craig.)*

Kuszak JR, Deutsch TA, Brown HG. Anatomy of aged and senile cataractous lenses. In: Albert DM, Jakobiec FA, eds. *Principles and Practice of Ophthalmology.* Philadelphia: Saunders; 1994:564–575.

Pesudovs K, Elliott DB. Refractive error changes in cortical, nuclear, and posterior subcapsular cataracts. *Br J Ophthalmol.* 2003;87(8):964–967.

West SK, Valmadrid CT. Epidemiology of risk factors for age-related cataract. *Surv Ophthalmol.* 1995;39(4):323–334.

Young RW. *Age-Related Cataract.* New York: Oxford University Press; 1991.

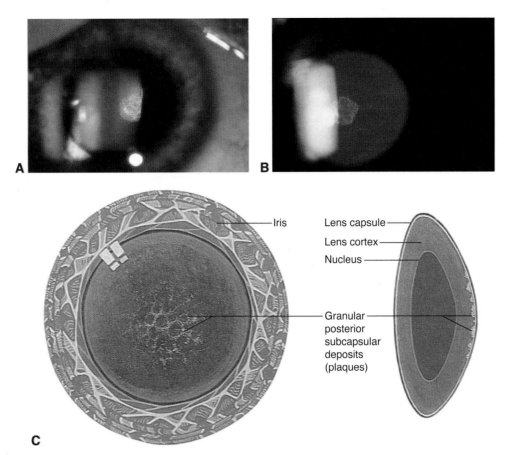

Figure 5-8 Posterior subcapsular cataract (PSC) viewed at the slit lamp **(A)** and with indirect illumination **(B). C,** Schematic of PSC. *(Part C courtesy of Alcon. Illustration by John A. Craig.)*

Drug-Induced Lens Changes

Corticosteroids

As mentioned earlier, long-term use of corticosteroids may cause PSCs. The development of corticosteroid-induced PSCs is related to the dose and treatment duration. Cataract formation can occur following administration of corticosteroids orally, topically, or by inhalation. The use of high-dose intraocular steroids to treat retinal neovascularization and inflammation also results in the development of PSCs and ocular hypertension. The advent of slow-release steroid repositories, including subconjunctival and intravitreal implants, has not altered the adverse ocular effects (intraocular pressure elevation and PSC development) of these medications.

Histologically and clinically, PSC formation occurring subsequent to corticosteroid use cannot be distinguished from senescent PSC formation. Some steroid-induced PSCs in children may resolve with cessation of the drug.

Fraunfelder FT, Fraunfelder FW. *Drug-Induced Ocular Side Effects.* 7th ed. Boston: Butterworth-Heinemann; 2014.

Jaffe GJ, Martin D, Callanan D, et al; Fluocinolone Acetonide Uveitis Study Group. Fluocinolone acetonide implant (Retisert) for noninfectious posterior uveitis: thirty-four-week results of a multicenter randomized clinical study. *Ophthalmology.* 2006;113(6):1020–1027.

Kiernan DF, Mieler WF. The use of intraocular corticosteroids. *Expert Opin Pharmacother.* 2009;10(15):2511–2525.

Phenothiazines

Phenothiazines, a major group of psychotropic medications, can cause pigmented deposits in the anterior lens epithelium in an axial configuration (Fig 5-9). The occurrence of these deposits appears to depend on both drug dose and treatment duration. In addition, they are more likely to occur with the use of some phenothiazines, notably chlorpromazine and thioridazine, than with others. The vision changes associated with phenothiazine use are generally insignificant.

Miotics

Topical anticholinesterases, which have been used in the treatment of glaucoma, can cause cataract formation. This type of cataract is increasingly uncommon, however, as these medications are now rarely used. The incidence of cataracts has been reported to be as high as 20% in patients after 55 months of pilocarpine use and 60% in patients after echothiophate iodide use.

Usually, this type of cataract first appears as small vacuoles within and posterior to the anterior lens capsule and epithelium. The cataract may progress to posterior cortical and nuclear lens changes. Cataract formation is more likely in patients receiving anticholinesterase therapy over a long period and in those receiving more frequent dosing.

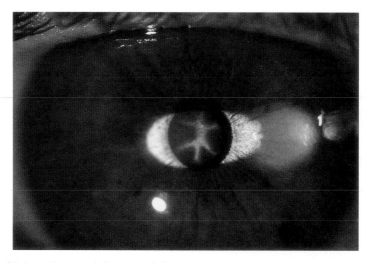

Figure 5-9 Slit-lamp image of pigmented deposits on anterior lens capsule in a patient treated with phenothiazines.

Amiodarone

Amiodarone, an antiarrhythmia medication, has been reported to cause stellate pigment deposition in the anterior cortical axis. Only very rarely is this condition visually significant. Amiodarone is also deposited in the corneal epithelium (cornea verticillata) and can cause a rare optic neuropathy.

Statins

Studies performed in dogs have shown that some 3-hydroxy-3-methylglutaryl coenzyme A (HMG-CoA) reductase inhibitors, known as *statins,* are associated with cataract when taken in excessive doses. Conflicting human studies have indicated that statins are both a risk factor for development of nuclear sclerotic cataracts and protective against them. However, concomitant use of simvastatin and erythromycin, which increases circulating statin levels, may be associated with approximately a twofold-increased risk of cataract.

Klein BE, Klein R, Lee KE, Grady LM. Statin use and incident nuclear cataract. *JAMA.* 2006; 295(23):2752–2758.

Leuschen J, Mortensen EM, Frei CR, Mansi EA, Panday V, Mansi I. Association of statin use with cataracts: a propensity score-matched analysis. *JAMA Ophthalmol.* 2013;131(11): 1427–1434.

Schlienger RG, Haefeli WE, Jick H, Meier CR. Risk of cataract in patients treated with statins. *Arch Intern Med.* 2001;161(16):2021–2026.

Tamoxifen

Cataract development and tamoxifen use were once thought to be linked; this suggested association has not been substantiated. Crystalline maculopathy has been reported in patients receiving high-dose tamoxifen therapy.

Bradbury BD, Lash TL, Kaye JA, Jick SS. Tamoxifen and cataracts: a null association. *Breast Cancer Res Treat.* 2004;87(2):189–196.

Callanan D, Williams PD. Retinal toxicity of systemic medications. In: Albert DM, Miller JW, Azar DT, Blodi BA, eds. *Albert & Jakobiec's Principles and Practice of Ophthalmology.* 3rd ed. Philadelphia: Saunders; 2008: chap 176.

Trauma

Traumatic lens damage may be caused by mechanical injury and by physical forces such as radiation, chemicals, and electrical current.

Contusion

Vossius ring

Blunt injury to the eye can sometimes cause a ring of pigment (known as a *Vossius ring*) from the pupillary ruff to be imprinted on the anterior surface of the lens. Although a Vossius ring is visually insignificant and gradually resolves with time, its presence indicates prior blunt trauma.

Traumatic cataract

A blunt, nonperforating injury may cause lens opacification either as an acute event or as a late sequela. A contusion cataract may involve only a portion of the lens or the entire lens. Often, the initial manifestation of a contusion cataract is a stellate or rosette-shaped opacification *(rosette cataract)*, usually axial in location, that involves the posterior lens capsule (Fig 5-10). In some cases, blunt trauma causes both dislocation and cataract formation (Fig 5-11). In rare cases, mild contusion cataracts can improve spontaneously.

Dislocation and subluxation

During a blunt injury to the eye, rapid expansion of the globe in an equatorial plane immediately follows compression. This rapid equatorial expansion can disrupt the zonular fibers, causing dislocation or subluxation of the lens. The lens may be dislocated in any direction, including posteriorly into the vitreous cavity or anteriorly into the anterior chamber.

Symptoms and signs of traumatic lens subluxation include fluctuation of vision, impaired accommodation, monocular diplopia, and high astigmatism. Often, iridodonesis

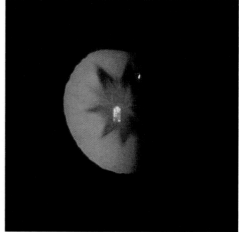

Figure 5-10 Slit-lamp retroillumination of a stellate lens opacity following contusion.

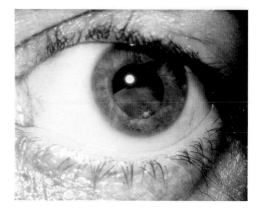

Figure 5-11 Dislocated cataractous lens following blunt trauma. *(Courtesy of Karla J. Johns, MD.)*

or phacodonesis is present. Retroillumination of the lens at the slit lamp through a dilated pupil may reveal the zonular disruption. In some cases, blunt trauma causes both dislocation and cataract formation.

Irvine JA, Smith RE. Lens injuries. In: Shingleton BJ, Hersh PS, Kenyon KR, eds. *Eye Trauma.* St Louis: Mosby; 1991:126–135.

Perforating or Penetrating Injury

A perforating or penetrating injury of the lens often causes opacification of the cortex at the site of the rupture, usually progressing rapidly to complete opacification (Fig 5-12). Occasionally, a small perforating injury of the lens capsule heals, resulting in a stationary focal cortical cataract (Fig 5-13).

Intraocular Procedures

Virtually any intraocular procedure may be associated with cataract formation, either soon after surgery or following a longer period of healing. Trans pars plana vitrectomy, especially with gas tamponade of the retina, is strongly associated with nuclear sclerotic cataract formation. A visually significant nuclear sclerotic cataract develops in up to 90% of phakic eyes within 2 years of undergoing vitrectomy.

Postvitrectomy cataracts are less common in patients younger than 50 years. The formation of nuclear cataracts after vitrectomy is associated with increases in oxygen tension in the vitreous intraoperatively and postoperatively. (See Chapter 3 for a discussion of oxygen tension in the lens.) Retinal surgery performed without vitrectomy is not associated with increased nuclear sclerosis, but any disturbance of the capsule during a vitreous cavity procedure may precipitate a PSC.

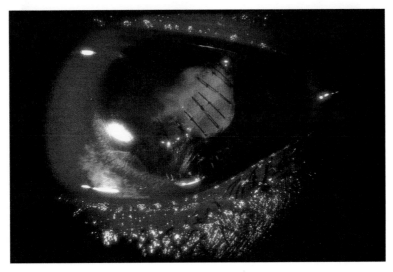

Figure 5-12 Complete cortical opacification after perforating injury, with disruption of the lens capsule.

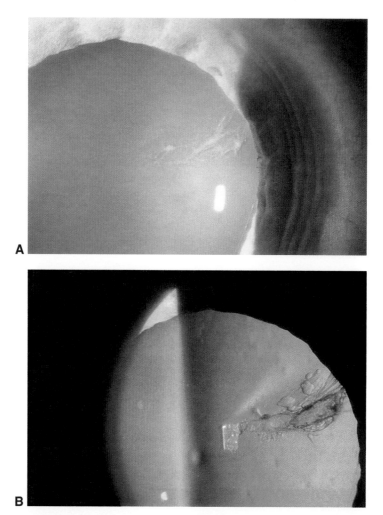

Figure 5-13 **A,** Focal cortical cataract from a small perforating injury to the lens capsule as viewed by direct illumination. **B,** Focal cortical cataract viewed by retroillumination.

Intravitreal injections may be associated with cataract formation either as a result of direct trauma to the lens or as an adverse effect of specific medications injected into the vitreous space.

Trabeculectomy is a known risk factor for development of visually significant cataract. The Collaborative Initial Glaucoma Treatment Study found that glaucoma patients' risk of needing early cataract surgery was 8 times higher in those whose initial treatment was trabeculectomy than in those whose initial treatment was with medications. This risk decreased to 3 times higher at 5 years following trabeculectomy.

Nuclear sclerotic cataract formation also occurs at significantly higher rates after penetrating keratoplasty and Descemet stripping endothelial keratoplasty.

Feng H, Adelman R. Cataract formation following vitreoretinal procedures. *Clin Ophthalmol.* 2014;8:1957–1965.

Musch DC, Gillespie BW, Niziol LM, et al; Collaborative Initial Glaucoma Treatment Study Group. Cataract extraction in the Collaborative Initial Glaucoma Treatment Study: incidence, risk factors, and the effect of cataract progression and extraction on clinical and quality-of-life outcomes. *Arch Ophthalmol.* 2006;124(12):1694–1700.

Price MO, Price DA, Fairchild KM, Price FW Jr. Rate and risk factors for cataract formation and extraction after Descemet stripping endothelial keratoplasty. *Br J Ophthalmol.* 2010; 94(11):1468–1471.

Intralenticular Foreign Bodies

In rare instances, a small foreign body can perforate the cornea and the anterior lens capsule and become lodged within the lens. If the foreign body is not composed of a ferric or cupric material and the anterior lens capsule seals the perforation site, the foreign body may be retained within the lens without significant complication. Intralenticular foreign bodies may cause cataract formation in some cases but do not always lead to lens opacification.

Radiation

Ionizing radiation

The lens is extremely sensitive to ionizing radiation; however, up to 20 years may pass after exposure before a cataract becomes clinically apparent. This period of latency is related to the dose of radiation and to the patient's age; younger patients are more susceptible because they have more lens cells that are actively growing. Ionizing radiation in the x-ray range (0.001–10.0-nm wavelength) can cause cataracts in some individuals in doses as low as 2 Gy in one fraction. (A routine chest x-ray equals 0.01-Gy exposure to the thorax.) A single computed tomography (CT) scan of the brain may expose the lens to as much as 2.5–5 cGy (100 cGy = 1 Gy).

The first clinical signs of radiation-induced cataract are often punctate opacities within the posterior capsule and feathery anterior subcapsular opacities that radiate toward the equator of the lens. These opacities may progress to complete opacification of the lens.

Infrared radiation

Exposure of the eye to infrared (IR) radiation and intense heat over time can cause the outer layers of the anterior lens capsule to peel off as a single layer. Such true exfoliation of the lens capsule, in which the exfoliated outer lamella tends to scroll up on itself, is rarely seen today. Cortical cataract may be associated with this condition, in which case it is known as *glassblower's cataract*. (See the section Pseudoexfoliation Syndrome, later in this chapter.)

Ultraviolet radiation

Experimental evidence suggests that the lens is susceptible to damage from ultraviolet (UV) radiation. Epidemiologic evidence suggests that long-term exposure to sunlight is associated with an increased risk of cortical cataracts, perhaps more frequently in men than women. Although sunlight exposure accounts for only approximately 10% of the total risk of cortical cataract in the general population in temperate climates, this risk is avoidable. Because exposure to UV radiation can lead to other morbidity, clinicians should encourage their patients to avoid excessive sunlight exposure. Lenses sold in the United States must conform to the American National Standards Institute (ANSI) requirements aimed at reducing UV transmission. Using prescription corrective lenses and non-prescription sunglasses decreases UV exposure by more than 80%, and wearing a hat with a brim decreases ocular sun exposure by 30%–50%.

Cruickshanks KJ, Klein BE, Klein R. Ultraviolet light exposure and lens opacities: the Beaver Dam Eye Study. *Am J Public Health.* 1992;82(12):1658–1662.

Klein BE, Lee KE, Danforth LG, Schaich TM, Cruickshanks KJ, Klein R. Selected sun-sensitizing medications and incident cataract. *Arch Ophthalmol.* 2010;128(8):959–963.

Metallosis

Siderosis bulbi

Intraocular iron-containing foreign bodies can cause siderosis bulbi, a condition characterized by deposition of iron molecules in the trabecular meshwork, lens epithelium, iris, and retina (Fig 5-14A). The epithelium and cortical fibers of the affected lens at first show a yellowish tinge, followed by a rusty brown discoloration (Fig 5-14B). Lens involvement

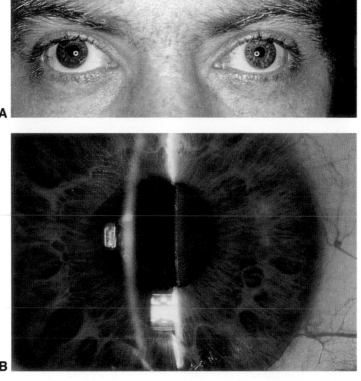

Figure 5-14 Siderosis bulbi. **A,** Heterochromia iridis caused by siderosis bulbi. **B,** Discoloration of the lens capsule and cortex.

occurs more rapidly if the retained foreign body is embedded close to the lens. Later manifestations of siderosis bulbi are complete cortical cataract formation and retinal dysfunction. (See also BCSC Section 12, *Retina and Vitreous.*)

Chalcosis

Chalcosis occurs when an intraocular foreign body deposits copper in the Descemet membrane, anterior lens capsule, or other intraocular basement membranes. The resulting *"sunflower" cataract* is a petal-shaped deposition of yellow or brown pigment in the lens capsule that radiates from the anterior axial pole of the lens to the equator. Usually, this cataract causes no significant loss of vision. However, intraocular foreign bodies containing almost pure copper (more than 90%) can cause a severe inflammatory reaction and intraocular necrosis.

Electrical Injury

Electrical shock can cause protein coagulation and cataract formation. Lens manifestations are more likely when the transmission of current involves the patient's head. Initially, lens vacuoles appear in the anterior midperiphery of the lens, followed by linear opacities in the anterior subcapsular cortex. A cataract induced by an electrical injury may regress, remain stationary, or mature to complete cataract over months or years (Fig 5-15).

Portellos M, Orlin SE, Kozart DM. Electric cataracts. *Arch Ophthalmol.* 1996;114(8): 1022–1023.

Chemical Injuries

Alkali injuries to the ocular surface often result in cataract, in addition to damaging the cornea, conjunctiva, and iris. Alkali compounds penetrate the eye readily, causing an increase in aqueous pH and a decrease in the level of aqueous glucose and ascorbate. Cortical cataract formation may occur acutely or as a delayed effect of chemical injury. Because acid tends to penetrate the eye less easily than does alkali, acid injuries are less likely to result in cataract formation.

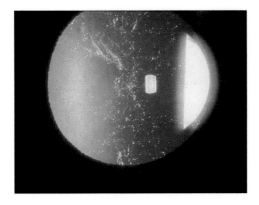

Figure 5-15 Cataract induced by electrical injury. *(Courtesy of Karla J. Johns, MD.)*

Metabolic Cataract

Diabetes Mellitus

Diabetes mellitus can affect lens clarity as well as the refractive index and accommodative amplitude of the lens. As the blood glucose level increases, so, too, does the glucose content in the aqueous humor. (See Chapter 3 for a discussion of glucose-induced lens changes.) Acute myopic shifts may indicate undiagnosed or poorly controlled diabetes mellitus. Patients with type 1 diabetes have a decreased amplitude of accommodation compared with age-matched controls, and presbyopia may present at a younger age in these patients. (See also Chapter 9.)

Cataract is a common cause of visual impairment in patients with diabetes mellitus. Acute *diabetic cataract,* or *"snowflake" cataract,* refers to bilateral, widespread subcapsular lens changes of abrupt onset and typically occurs in young individuals with uncontrolled diabetes mellitus (Fig 5-16). Multiple gray-white subcapsular opacities that have a snowflake appearance are seen initially in the superficial anterior and posterior lens cortex. Vacuoles and clefts form in the underlying cortex. Intumescence and maturity of the cortical cataract follow shortly thereafter. Although acute diabetic cataracts are rarely encountered in clinical practice today, rapidly maturing bilateral cortical cataracts in a child or young adult should alert the clinician to the possibility of diabetes mellitus.

Patients with diabetes mellitus develop age-related lens changes that are indistinguishable from nondiabetic age-related cataracts, except that these lens changes tend to occur at a younger age than in those without the disease. The increased risk or earlier onset of age-related cataracts in diabetic patients may be a result of the accumulation of sorbitol within the lens and accompanying changes in hydration, increased nonenzymatic glycosylation (glycation) of lens proteins, or greater oxidative stress from alterations in lens metabolism. These stressors may promote an increase in nuclear sclerotic cataract, cortical cataract, and PSC formation.

Flynn HW Jr, Smiddy WE, eds. *Diabetes and Ocular Disease: Past, Present, and Future Therapies.* Ophthalmology Monograph 14. San Francisco: American Academy of Ophthalmology; 2000:49–53, 226.

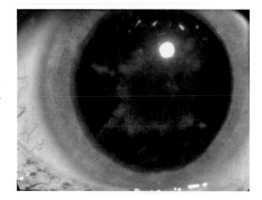

Figure 5-16 Diabetic cataract, or "snowflake" cataract, consists of gray-white subcapsular opacities. *(Courtesy of Karla J. Johns, MD.)*

Johns KJ. Diabetes and the lens. In: Feman SS, ed. *Ocular Problems in Diabetes Mellitus.* Boston: Blackwell; 1992:221–244.

Klein BE, Klein R, Wang Q, Moss SE. Older-onset diabetes and lens opacities. The Beaver Dam Eye Study. *Ophthalmic Epidemiol.* 1995;2(1):49–55.

Li L, Wan XH, Zhao GH. Meta-analysis of the risk of cataract in type 2 diabetes. *BMC Ophthalmol.* 2014;14:94.

Galactosemia

Galactosemia is an inherited autosomal recessive inability to convert galactose to glucose. As a consequence of this inability, excessive galactose accumulates in body tissues, with further metabolic conversion of galactose to galactitol (dulcitol), the sugar alcohol of galactose. Galactosemia can result from defects in 1 of 3 enzymes involved in the metabolism of galactose: (1) galactose-1-phosphate uridyltransferase (Gal-1-PUT), (2) galactokinase, or (3) uridine diphosphate galactose 4-epimerase (UDP-galactose 4-epimerase). The most common and the severest form, known as *classic galactosemia,* is caused by a defect in Gal-1-PUT.

In classic galactosemia, symptoms of malnutrition, hepatomegaly, jaundice, and intellectual deficiency present within the first few weeks of life. The disease is fatal if undiagnosed and untreated. The diagnosis of classic galactosemia can be confirmed by demonstration of galactose in the urine.

Typically, the nucleus and deep cortex become increasingly opacified, causing an "oil droplet" appearance on retroillumination (Fig 5-17). The cataracts can progress to total opacification.

Treatment of galactosemia includes elimination of milk and milk products from the diet. In some cases, early cataract formation can be reversed by timely diagnosis and dietary intervention. This oil droplet appearance is similar to the oil droplet cataract of central nuclear sclerosis but differs markedly from the oil droplet cataract of posterior lenticonus. In posterior lenticonus, a bulge in the posterior capsule causes the oil droplet appearance on red reflex examination.

Burke JP, O'Keefe M, Bowell R, Naughten ER. Ophthalmic findings in classical galactosemia—a screened population. *J Pediatr Ophthalmol Strabismus.* 1989;26(4):165–168.

Hypocalcemia

Cataracts may develop in association with any condition that results in hypocalcemia. Hypocalcemia may be idiopathic, or it may occur as a result of unintended destruction

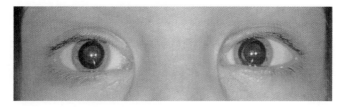

Figure 5-17 "Oil droplet" bilateral cataracts in a patient with galactosemia.

of the parathyroid glands during thyroid surgery. Usually bilateral, hypocalcemic (tetanic) cataracts are punctate iridescent opacities in the anterior and posterior cortex. They lie beneath the lens capsule and are usually separated from it by a zone of clear lens. These discrete opacities may remain stable or may mature into complete cortical cataracts.

Wilson Disease

Wilson disease (hepatolenticular degeneration) is an inherited autosomal recessive disorder of copper metabolism. The characteristic ocular manifestation of Wilson disease is the Kayser-Fleischer ring, a golden-brown discoloration of the Descemet membrane around the periphery of the cornea. In addition, a characteristic sunflower cataract often develops. Reddish-brown pigment (cuprous oxide) is deposited in the anterior lens capsule and subcapsular cortex in a stellate shape that resembles the petals of a sunflower. In most cases, the sunflower cataract does not cause serious visual impairment.

Myotonic Dystrophy

Myotonic dystrophy is an inherited autosomal dominant condition characterized by delayed relaxation of contracted muscles, ptosis, weakness of the facial musculature, cardiac conduction defects, and prominent frontal balding in affected male patients. Patients with this disorder typically develop polychromatic iridescent crystals in the lens cortex (Fig 5-18), with sequential PSC progressing to complete cortical opacification. Ultrastructurally, polychromatic iridescent crystals are composed of whorls of plasmalemma from the lens fibers. The crystals are occasionally seen in the lens cortex of patients who do not have myotonic dystrophy; these crystals are thought to be caused by cholesterol crystal deposition in the lens.

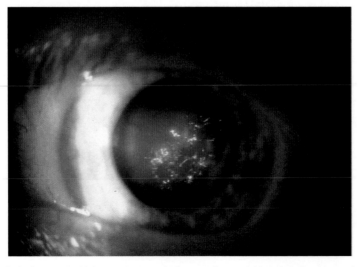

Figure 5-18 Polychromatic iridescent crystals in a patient with myotonic dystrophy. *(Courtesy of Karla J. Johns, MD.)*

Effects of Nutrition, Alcohol, and Smoking

Although nutritional deficiencies have been demonstrated to cause cataracts in animal models, this etiology has been difficult to confirm in humans. Numerous population-based studies have found that lower socioeconomic status, lower education level, and poorer overall nutrition are associated with increased prevalence of age-related cataracts. Severe episodes of dehydration caused by diarrhea may be linked to an increased risk of cataract formation.

The identification of specific dietary deficiencies that lead to cataract formation and of supplements that protect against it has been more challenging. Some studies have suggested that taking multivitamin supplements, vitamin A, vitamin C, vitamin E, niacin, thiamine, riboflavin, or beta carotene or increasing protein intake may protect against cataract development. Several studies have suggested that the antioxidants lutein and zeaxanthin provide some protection against nuclear and cortical cataracts.

The Age-Related Eye Disease Study (AREDS1) showed that, over 7 years, increased intake of vitamins C and E and beta carotene did not decrease the development or progression of cataract. Likewise, the subsequent study (Age-Related Eye Disease Study 2 [AREDS2]) showed no difference in the rates of cataract surgery among patients who took lutein and zeaxanthin supplements and those who did not.

It is important to remember that high-dose vitamin use may pose risks. Smokers taking high doses of beta carotene have an increased risk of lung cancer, death from lung cancer, and death from cardiovascular disease. In addition, women taking supplemental doses of vitamin A have an increased risk of hip fracture.

Smoking, the use of smokeless tobacco products, and excessive alcohol consumption are significant, avoidable risk factors for cataract. In numerous studies performed worldwide, these practices have consistently been associated with an increase in the frequency of nuclear opacities. Although patients may know the general health risks of smoking and excessive alcohol consumption, they may not know about the risks of ocular conditions such as macular degeneration and cataract that are related to these practices. Ophthalmologists can inform their patients about these risks, and they are in a strong position to encourage individuals to stop smoking and reduce alcohol consumption.

Age-Related Eye Disease Study Research Group (AREDS). A randomized, placebo-controlled, clinical trial of high-dose supplementation with vitamins C and E and beta carotene for age-related cataract and vision loss: AREDS report no. 9. *Arch Ophthalmol.* 2001;119(10): 1439–1452.

Berendschot TT, Broekmans WM, Klöpping-Ketalaars IA, Kardinaal AF, Van Poppel G, Van Norren D. Lens aging in relation to nutritional determinants and possible risk factors for age-related cataract. *Arch Ophthalmol.* 2002;120(12):1732–1737.

Chew EY, SanGiovanni JP, Ferris FL et al; Age-Related Eye Disease Study 2 (AREDS2) Research Group. Lutein/zeaxanthin for the treatment of age-related cataract: AREDS2 randomized trial report no. 4. *JAMA Ophthalmol.* 2013;131(7):843–850.

Cumming RG, Mitchell P, Smith W. Diet and cataract: the Blue Mountains Eye Study. *Ophthalmology.* 2000;107(3):450–456.

Kanthan GL, Mitchell P, Burlutsky G, Wang JJ. Alcohol consumption and the long-term incidence of cataract and cataract surgery: the Blue Mountains Eye Study. *Am J Ophthalmol.* 2010;150(3):434–440.

Lyle BJ, Mares-Perlman JA, Klein BE, Klein R, Greger JL. Antioxidant intake and risk of incident age-related nuclear cataracts in the Beaver Dam Eye Study. *Am J Epidemiol.* 1999; 149(9):801–809.

Milton RC, Sperduto RD, Clemons TE, Ferris FL 3rd; Age-Related Eye Disease Study Research Group (AREDS). Centrum use and progression of age-related cataract in the Age-Related Eye Disease Study: a propensity score approach. AREDS report no. 21. *Ophthalmology.* 2006;113(8):1264–1270.

Raju P, George R, Ve Ramesh S, Arvind H, Baskaran M, Vijaya L. Influence of tobacco use on cataract development. *Br J Ophthalmol.* 2006;90(11):1374–1377.

Weikel KA, Garber C, Baburins A, Taylor A. Nutritional modulation of cataract. *Nutr Rev.* 2014;72(1):30–47.

Cataract Associated With Uveitis

Lens changes often occur as a result of chronic uveitis or associated corticosteroid therapy. Typically, a PSC develops; anterior lens changes may also occur. The formation of posterior synechiae is common in uveitis, often with thickening of the anterior lens capsule, which may have an associated fibrous pupillary membrane. Lens changes in cataract secondary to uveitis may progress to a mature cataract. Calcium deposits may be observed on the anterior capsule or within the lens substance.

Cortical cataract formation occurs in up to 70% of cases of Fuchs heterochromic uveitis (Fig 5-19). Because posterior synechiae are uncommon in this syndrome, formation of pupillary membranes is unlikely, and long-term corticosteroid therapy is not indicated. Cataract extraction in patients with Fuchs heterochromic uveitis generally has a favorable

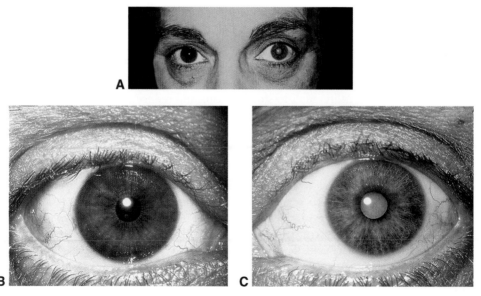

Figure 5-19 Clinical photographs from a patient with Fuchs heterochromic uveitis. **A,** The affected eye is lighter. **B,** Normal right eye. **C,** Cataract formation in the affected left eye. *(Courtesy of Karla J. Johns, MD.)*

prognosis. Intraoperative anterior chamber hemorrhage at the time of cataract surgery has been reported in approximately 25% of cases.

Lens Changes With Hyperbaric Oxygen Therapy

The lens may also undergo changes after hyperbaric oxygen (HBO) therapy. A myopic shift commonly occurs during the course of treatment with HBO. This change, thought to be due to a refractive change in the crystalline lens, usually reverses after cessation of HBO treatment. However, several reports have documented subsequent development of nuclear cataract.

> Gesell LB, Trott A. De novo cataract development following a standard course of hyperbaric oxygen therapy. *Undersea Hyperb Med.* 2007;34(6):389–392.

Pseudoexfoliation Syndrome

Pseudoexfoliation syndrome is a systemic disease in which a matrix of fibrotic material is deposited in many bodily organs. In the eye, a basement membrane–like fibrillogranular white material is deposited on the cornea, iris, lens, anterior hyaloid face, ciliary processes, zonular fibers, and trabecular meshwork. These deposits, believed to comprise elastic microfibrils, appear as grayish-white flecks that are prominent at the pupillary margin and on the lens capsule (Fig 5-20). Associated with this condition are atrophy of the iris at the pupillary margin, deposition of pigment on the anterior surface of the iris, poorly dilating pupil, increased pigmentation of the trabecular meshwork, capsular fragility, zonular weakness, and open-angle glaucoma. Pseudoexfoliation syndrome is a unilateral or bilateral disorder that becomes more apparent with increasing age. An association between lifetime UV-light exposure and the development of pseudoexfoliation syndrome has recently been documented.

Increased oxidative stress caused by abnormalities in transforming growth factor β (TGF-β) contributes to the formation of cataracts. Patients with this syndrome may also experience weakness of the zonular fibers and spontaneous lens subluxation and

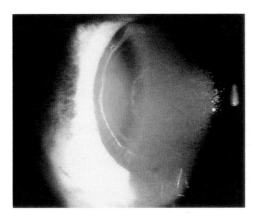

Figure 5-20 In pseudoexfoliation syndrome, deposits appear as grayish-white flecks that are prominent at the pupillary margin and on the lens capsule.

phacodonesis. Poor zonular integrity may affect cataract surgery technique and intraocular lens implantation. (See Chapter 9 for a discussion of cataract surgery in special situations.) The exfoliative material may be produced even after the crystalline lens is removed.

Pasquale LR, Jiwani AZ, Zehavi-Dorin T, et al. Solar exposure and residential geographic history in relation to exfoliation syndrome in the United States and Israel. *JAMA Ophthalmol.* 2014;132(12):1439–1445.

Schlötzer-Schrehardt U, Naumann GO. Ocular and systemic pseudoexfoliation syndrome. *Am J Ophthalmol.* 2006;141(5):921–937.

Zenkel M, Lewczuk P, Jünemann A, Kruse FE, Naumann GO, Schlötzer-Schrehardt U. Proinflammatory cytokines are involved in the initiation of the abnormal matrix process in pseudoexfoliation syndrome/glaucoma. *Am J Pathol.* 2010;176(6):2868–2879.

Cataract and Atopic Dermatitis

Atopic dermatitis is a chronic, erythematous dermatitis, accompanied by itching and often seen in conjunction with increased levels of immunoglobulin E (IgE) and a history of multiple allergies or asthma. Cataract formation has been reported in up to 25% of patients with atopic dermatitis. The cataracts are usually bilateral, and onset occurs in the second to third decade of life. Typically, these cataracts are anterior subcapsular opacities in the pupillary area that resemble shieldlike plaques.

Mannis MJ, Macsai MS, Huntley AC, eds. *Eye and Skin Disease.* Philadelphia: Lippincott-Raven; 1996.

Phacoantigenic Uveitis

In the normal eye, minute quantities of lens proteins leak out through the lens capsule. The eye appears to have immunologic tolerance to these small numbers of lens antigens. However, the release of a large quantity of lens proteins into the anterior chamber disrupts this immunologic tolerance and may trigger a severe inflammatory reaction. Phacoantigenic uveitis, previously termed *phacoanaphylactic endophthalmitis,* is an immune-mediated granulomatous inflammation initiated by lens proteins released through a ruptured lens capsule. This condition usually occurs following traumatic rupture of the lens capsule or following cataract surgery when cortical material is retained within the eye. Onset occurs days to weeks after the injury or surgery.

This disease is characterized by a red, painful eye with injection, chemosis, and anterior chamber inflammation with cells, flare, and keratic precipitates. Occasionally, glaucoma develops due to obstruction of the trabecular meshwork and formation of synechiae. Late complications include cyclitic membrane, hypotony, and phthisis bulbi. In rare instances, phacoantigenic uveitis can give rise to an inflammatory reaction in the fellow eye. Histologic examination shows a zonal granulomatous inflammation surrounding a breach of the lens capsule. Lens extraction is the definitive therapy for this condition. See also BCSC Section 4, *Ophthalmic Pathology and Intraocular Tumors,* and Section 9, *Intraocular Inflammation and Uveitis.*

Lens-Induced Glaucoma

See BCSC Section 10, *Glaucoma,* for additional discussion, including images.

Phacolytic Glaucoma

Phacolytic glaucoma is a complication of a mature or hypermature cataract. Denatured, liquefied high-molecular-mass lens proteins leak through an intact but permeable lens capsule. An immune response is not elicited; rather, macrophages ingest these lens proteins. The trabecular meshwork becomes clogged with both the lens proteins and the engorged macrophages. The usual clinical presentation of phacolytic glaucoma consists of abrupt onset of pain and redness in a cataractous eye that has had poor vision for some time. The cornea may be edematous, and significant flare reaction occurs in the anterior chamber. The lack of keratic precipitates helps distinguish phacolytic glaucoma from phacoantigenic glaucoma. White flocculent material appears in the anterior chamber and often adheres to the lens capsule as well. IOP is markedly elevated, and the anterior chamber angle is open, although the same material may be seen in the trabecular meshwork. Initial treatment of phacolytic glaucoma consists of controlling the IOP with ocular hypotensive medications and managing the inflammation with topical corticosteroids. Surgical removal of the lens is the definitive treatment.

Lens Particle Glaucoma

Following a penetrating lens injury or surgical procedure (ie, extracapsular cataract extraction, phacoemulsification with retained cortical material, or in rare instances, Nd:YAG laser capsulotomy), particles of lens cortex may migrate into the anterior chamber, where they obstruct aqueous outflow through the trabecular meshwork. In most instances, glaucoma occurs within weeks of the initial surgery or trauma, but it may occur months or years later. Gonioscopy shows that the angle is open, and cortical material can often be seen deposited along the trabecular meshwork. Medical therapy to lower IOP and to reduce intraocular inflammation is indicated. If the IOP and inflammation do not respond quickly to this treatment, surgical removal of the retained lens material may be required.

Phacomorphic Glaucoma

As the lens grows in the anterior–posterior dimension it can cause pupillary block and induce secondary angle-closure glaucoma, or it can physically push the iris forward and thus cause shallowing of the anterior chamber. Often, the patient presents with a red, painful eye and a history of vision changes as a result of cataract formation prior to the acute event (Fig 5-21). The cornea may be edematous, and gonioscopy reveals a closed anterior chamber angle. Initial management includes medical treatment to lower the IOP. The condition responds to laser iridotomy, but definitive treatment consists of cataract extraction.

Liebmann JM, Ritch R. Glaucoma secondary to lens intumescence and dislocation. In: Ritch R, Shields MB, Krupin T, eds. *The Glaucomas.* 2nd ed. St Louis: Mosby; 1996.

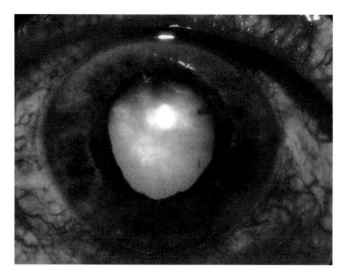

Figure 5-21 Phacomorphic glaucoma.

Glaukomflecken

Glaukomflecken are gray-white epithelial and anterior cortical lens opacities that occur following an episode of markedly elevated IOP, as in acute angle-closure glaucoma. Histologically, glaukomflecken are composed of necrotic lens epithelial cells and degenerated subepithelial cortex.

Ischemia

Ischemic ocular conditions, such as pulseless disease (Takayasu arteritis), thromboangiitis obliterans (Buerger disease), and anterior segment necrosis, can cause PSC. The cataract may progress rapidly to total opacification of the lens.

Cataracts Associated With Degenerative Ocular Disorders

Cataracts can occur in association with many degenerative ocular disorders, such as retinitis pigmentosa, essential iris atrophy, and chronic hypotony. These secondary cataracts usually begin as PSCs and may progress to total lens opacification. The mechanisms responsible for cataractogenesis in degenerative ocular disorders are not well understood.

CHAPTER 6

Evaluation and Management of Cataracts in Adults

An ophthalmologist evaluating a patient with cataracts must assess the degree to which the lens opacity affects vision and determine whether surgery will improve the patient's quality of life. The following questions should be considered in the evaluation and management of cataract:

- What is the functional impact of the cataract?
- What are the morphological characteristics of the cataract?
- Is surgery indicated either to improve the patient's quality of life or to aid in the management of other ocular conditions?
- What are the patient's expectations regarding the refractive results of surgery?
- Does the patient have ocular or systemic comorbidities that might affect the decision to proceed with surgery or alter the management plan?
- What are the possible barriers to obtaining informed consent or to ensuring good postoperative care?

In most cases, cataract surgery is an elective procedure. Thus, in addition to answering the preceding questions, the ophthalmologist should inform the patient about the impact of the cataract, the risks and benefits of surgical management, the alternatives to surgery, and the options regarding the intraocular lens (IOL) to be used if surgery takes place. Ultimately, it is important that both patient and physician be satisfied that surgery is the appropriate choice for improving vision.

Clinical History: Signs and Symptoms

Decreased Visual Acuity

Often, the clinical history of a patient with decreased vision and function due to cataract is straightforward, and the patient tells the ophthalmologist which activities have been curtailed or abandoned. Some patients, however, learn of their decline in visual acuity only after being examined. Others deny that they are having any problems until their limitations are demonstrated or privileges are withdrawn because they are no longer visually competent.

Different types of cataract may have different effects on visual acuity, depending on incident light, pupil size, and refractive error (Table 6-1). The presence of even small posterior subcapsular cataracts (PSCs) can greatly disturb near visual acuity (reading vision) without necessarily affecting distance vision. Color vision disturbances may be noted by the patient, especially with unilateral or asymmetric cataract.

Glare and Altered Contrast Sensitivity

Cataract patients often report an increase in glare, which may vary from increased photosensitivity in brightly lit environments to disabling glare in the daytime or with headlights from oncoming cars. Shorter wavelengths of light cause the most scatter; the color, intensity, and direction of lighting also affect glare. This increased sensitivity is particularly prominent with PSCs and, occasionally, with anterior cortical lens changes.

Contrast sensitivity is the ability to detect subtle variations in shading. Because patients with ocular abnormalities have altered contrast sensitivity in low light, measurement of contrast sensitivity may provide a more comprehensive estimate of the visual resolution of the eye. A significant loss in contrast sensitivity may occur without a similar loss in Snellen acuity. However, abnormal contrast sensitivity is not a specific indicator of vision loss due to cataract.

Myopic Shift

The development of cataract may increase the dioptric power of the lens, commonly causing a mild to moderate degree of myopic shift. Hyperopic and emmetropic patients find that their need for distance or reading spectacles diminishes as they experience this "second sight." This phenomenon is encountered with nuclear sclerotic cataracts and disappears when the optical clarity of the crystalline lens further deteriorates. Less commonly, hyperopic or astigmatic refractive errors can be induced by cataractous lens changes. Asymmetric development of lens-induced myopia may produce intolerable anisometropia.

Monocular Diplopia or Polyopia

Occasionally in cataractous eyes, nuclear changes are localized to the inner layers of the lens nucleus, resulting in multiple refractile areas at the center of the lens. Such areas may best be seen as irregularities in the red reflex on retinoscopy or direct ophthalmoscopy. This type of cataract can result in monocular diplopia or polyopia, including

Table 6-1 Characteristics and Effects of the Most Common Cataracts in Adults

Type	Growth Rate	Glare	Effect on Distance	Effect on Near	Induced Myopia
Cortical	Moderate	Moderate	Mild	Mild	None
Nuclear	Slow	Mild	Moderate	None	Moderate
Posterior subcapsular	Rapid	Marked	Mild	Marked	None

ghost images and occasionally a true second image. Monocular diplopia can also occur with other ocular media opacities or other disorders of the eye (see BCSC Section 5, *Neuro-Ophthalmology*).

Decreased Visual Function

Assessing the overall effect of the cataract on visual function is almost certainly a more appropriate way to determine visual disability than is acuity testing alone. Patients should be asked whether their vision (at near, at distance, and under different lighting conditions) is adequate to allow them to perform relevant activities of daily living and participate in any hobbies. While no one test can comprehensively assess the effects of a cataract, questionnaires for measuring visual function may be useful. These include the Activities of Daily Vision Scale (ADVS), the Visual Function Index (VF-14), the National Eye Institute Visual Function Questionnaire (NEI-VFQ), and the Visual Disability Assessment (VDA).

Mangione CM, Lee PP, Gutierrez PR, Spritzer K, Berry S, Hays RD; National Eye Institute Visual Function Questionnaire Field Test Investigators. Development of the 25-item National Eye Institute Visual Function Questionnaire. *Arch Ophthalmol.* 2001;119(7): 1050–1058.

Mangione CM, Phillips RS, Seddon JM, et al. Development of the 'Activities of Daily Vision Scale'. A measure of visual functional status. *Med Care.* 1992;30(12):1111–1126.

Pesudovs K, Wright TA, Gothwal VK. Visual disability assessment: valid measurement of activity limitation and mobility in cataract patients. *Br J Ophthalmol.* 2010;94(6):777–781.

Steinberg EP, Tielsch JM, Schein OD, et al. The VF-14. An index of functional impairment in patients with cataract. *Arch Ophthalmol.* 1994;112(5):630–638.

Nonsurgical Management

Nonsurgical approaches may be attempted to improve visual function in cataract patients who do not desire surgery and in those for whom surgical management is not feasible. Careful refraction may improve spectacle correction for distance and near vision. For example, patients who have experienced a myopic shift secondary to cataract may hold reading material closer and may not report symptoms until a change in their glasses is made; a corresponding increase in the power added for near vision is necessary. Use of specialized tints may reduce glare, and brighter illumination can improve the contrast of reading material. Handheld monoculars may facilitate spotting objects at a distance; high-plus spectacles, magnifiers, closed-circuit televisions, and telescopic loupes may be used for reading and close work.

Referral to low vision services may be appropriate. To learn about the American Academy of Ophthalmology's Initiative in Vision Rehabilitation and obtain a patient handout, visit the Low Vision and Vision Rehabilitation page on the ONE Network at https://www.aao.org/low-vision-and-vision-rehab.

In patients with small axial cataracts, pupillary dilation, achieved either pharmacologically or by laser pupilloplasty, may improve visual function by allowing more light to pass through peripheral portions of the lens. However, there is a risk of inducing additional glare with this approach.

Pharmacologic reversal of cataracts is a subject of ongoing research. No commercially available medication has been proven to delay or reverse cataract formation in humans. Aldose reductase inhibitors, which block the conversion of glucose to sorbitol, have been shown to prevent cataracts in animals with experimentally induced diabetes mellitus. However, studies in humans show no such effect. Antioxidants such as zinc and beta carotene and vitamins E and C do not slow cataract progression.

American Academy of Ophthalmology Cataract and Anterior Segment Panel. Preferred Practice Pattern Guidelines. *Cataract in the Adult Eye*. San Francisco: American Academy of Ophthalmology; 2011. Available at www.aao.org/ppp.

Kanthan GL, Wang JJ, Rochtchina E, Mitchell P. Use of antihypertensive medications and topical beta-blockers and the long-term incidence of cataract and cataract surgery. *Br J Ophthalmol*. 2009;93(9):1210–1214.

Indications for Surgery

The most common indication for cataract surgery is the patient's desire for improved vision. The decision to operate is not based solely on a specific level of reduced acuity. Key to the decision is determining whether the patient's visual function would improve enough to warrant cataract surgery. Some governmental agencies and industries have minimum standards of visual function for their workers for tasks such as driving, flying, and operating complex equipment. A patient whose best-corrected visual acuity (BCVA) does not meet these visual requisites may need to consider cataract surgery. The ophthalmic surgeon must determine, through discussion with the patient and family and analysis of the results of subjective and objective testing, whether cataract surgery is advisable.

To approve reimbursement for cataract surgery, some third-party payers require that patients have a certain level of vision loss; in such cases, glare testing may be useful for documenting loss of visual function beyond that measured by Snellen acuity. In some cases, patients have lens changes that cause unwanted refractive errors or symptoms but do not meet criteria for third-party reimbursement. After a careful discussion of the risks, benefits, alternatives, and costs, surgery may be offered to patients who would benefit from the procedure.

Medical indications for cataract surgery include phacolytic glaucoma, phacomorphic glaucoma, phacoantigenic uveitis, and dislocation of the lens. An additional indication for surgery is the presence of a cataract sufficiently opaque to obscure the view of the fundus and impair the diagnosis or management of other ocular diseases, such as diabetic retinopathy, macular degeneration, or glaucoma.

Cataract in elderly persons, especially those with significant deafness or early dementia, may lead to isolation. The quality of life of such patients may be greatly improved with spectacle independence following cataract surgery. Also, cataract extraction has been shown to decrease the frequency of falls and hip fractures and to reduce morbidity and mortality.

Common indications for surgery in a patient with a monocular cataract include loss of stereopsis, diminished peripheral vision, disabling glare, and symptomatic anisometropia. The presence of cataract in one eye has a negative effect on driving performance and accident avoidance.

When a patient has bilateral, visually significant cataracts, surgery is usually performed first in the eye with the more advanced cataract. In patients with active or severe systemic illness, or in those with other ocular diseases contributing to decreased vision, it may be appropriate to operate first on the eye with better visual potential, should only one surgical procedure be anticipated. Other strategies to facilitate patient adaptation include operating on the dominant eye or the more ametropic eye first.

After undergoing second-eye cataract surgery, patients have been shown to experience significant improvements not only in acuity and satisfaction with their vision but also measures of bilateral visual function, such as stereopsis and contrast sensitivity. But the decision of whether to proceed with cataract surgery on the second eye must be individualized to the patient's needs and visual potential, just as it was for the first eye. One consideration is the development of symptomatic anisometropia, which may occur as a result of the initial cataract surgery. The anisometropia may be unsatisfactorily addressed by nonsurgical treatment, and the patient may find it disabling enough to justify surgery on the second eye, even if the cataract is at an early stage of development.

Before proceeding with the second surgery, the physician and the patient traditionally allow sufficient time to confirm the success and safety of the first operation and to assess the refractive outcome. Interest has recently increased in immediate sequential (same-day) bilateral cataract surgery. Most ophthalmologists do not use this approach because of the potential for bilateral complications and the inability to incorporate information regarding refractive outcome into planning for the second eye. However, it may be a viable option for patients who are unable to return for second-eye surgery and for those who have limited access to surgical resources. Some patients with high refractive errors may voice a preference for immediate sequential bilateral cataract surgery to avoid functional impairment due to anisometropia between procedures. If same-day surgery is performed, the surgeon should treat each eye as an entirely separate case by using new gloves, draping, instruments, and equipment.

Arshinoff SA, Odorcic S. Same-day sequential cataract surgery. *Curr Opin Ophthalmol.* 2009; 20(1):3–12.

Bohigian GM, Kamenetzky SA. Risk management in cataract surgery. *Focal Points: Clinical Modules for Ophthalmologists.* San Francisco: American Academy of Ophthalmology; 2007, module 8.

Brown GC, Brown MM, Menezes A, Busbee BG, Lieske HB, Lieske PA. Cataract surgery cost utility revisited in 2012. *Ophthalmology.* 2013;120(12):2367–2376.

Castells X, Alonso J, Ribó C, et al. Comparison of the results of first and second cataract eye surgery. *Ophthalmology.* 1999;106(4):676–682.

Castells X, Comas M, Alonso J, et al. In a randomized controlled trial, cataract surgery in both eyes increased benefits compared to surgery in one eye only. *J Clin Epidemiol.* 2006; 59(2):201–207.

Ishii K, Kabata T, Oshika T. The impact of cataract surgery on cognitive impairment and depressive mental status in elderly patients. *Am J Ophthalmol.* 2008;146(3):404–409.

Ivers RQ, Cumming RG, Mitchell P, Attebo K. Visual impairment and falls in older adults: the Blue Mountains Eye Study. *J Am Geriatr Soc.* 1998;46(1):58–64.

Preoperative Evaluation

The clinician should obtain the following information to determine whether cataract surgery is advisable. The parameters suggested should be tailored to the individual patient.

General Health of the Patient

A complete medical history is the starting point for the preoperative evaluation. The ophthalmologist should work with the patient's primary care physician to achieve optimal management of all medical problems, especially diabetes mellitus, ischemic heart disease, chronic obstructive pulmonary disease, bleeding disorders, or adrenal suppression caused by systemic corticosteroid use. The ophthalmologist should be aware of the patient's drug sensitivities and use of medications that might alter the outcome of surgery, such as immunosuppressants and anticoagulants. Given the low risk of hemorrhage with topical anesthesia and clear corneal incisions, anticoagulant medications do not need to be discontinued prior to cataract surgery. Any alteration in the patient's use of these medications is ideally done in consultation with the prescribing physician.

The ophthalmologist should specifically ask about the use of systemic α_1-adrenergic antagonist medications (including prazosin, terazosin, doxazosin, silodosin, alfuzosin, and tamsulosin, as well as herbal supplements, such as saw palmetto) for the treatment of benign prostatic hyperplasia, urinary incontinence, urolithiasis, and hypertension. These medications are strongly associated with intraoperative floppy iris syndrome (IFIS) and fluctuations in pupil size. All α_1-blockers can bind to postsynaptic nerve endings of the iris dilator muscle for a prolonged period, causing excessive iris mobility. This effect may occur after only 1 dose of the medication and may persist indefinitely, even after discontinuation of the drug. Anecdotal reports document potential α_1-antagonist properties and potential associations with IFIS in other medications, including certain antipsychotic and antihypertensive medications. See Chapter 8 for further discussion of IFIS.

The ophthalmologist should inquire about and document any allergies, adverse reactions, and sensitivities to sedatives, narcotics, anesthetics, povidone-iodine, and latex. Factors limiting the patient's ability to cooperate in the operating room or to lie comfortably on the operating room table (eg, deafness, language barriers, dementia, claustrophobia, restless legs syndrome, head tremor, musculoskeletal disorders) will influence the choice of anesthesia and the surgical plan.

The extent of the formal medical preoperative evaluation should be based on the patient's overall health and may be guided by requirements of the facility where the procedure is to take place. Screening with self-reported information gained from health questionnaires may help identify patients who are at higher risk for medical difficulties related to surgery, but this method should not be the only form of evaluation. Certainly, for all patients with risk factors related to their ability to undergo surgery, a history should be obtained and a physical examination and relevant laboratory work should be performed. However, routine medical testing before cataract surgery has not been shown to increase the safety of the procedure.

American Academy of Ophthalmology Quality of Care Secretariat, Hoskins Center for Quality Eye Care. Routine preoperative laboratory testing for patients scheduled for cataract surgery—2014. *Clinical Statement.* San Francisco: American Academy of Ophthalmology; 2014. Available at www.aao.org. Accessed October 26, 2015.

Chang DF, Braga-Mele R, Mamalis N, et al. ASCRS white paper: clinical review of intraoperative floppy-iris syndrome. *J Cataract Refract Surg.* 2008;34(12):2153–2162.

Wykoff CC, Flynn HW Jr, Han DP. Allergy to povidone-iodine and cephalosporins: the clinical dilemma in ophthalmic use. *Am J Ophthalmol.* 2011;151(1):4–6.

Pertinent Ocular History

The ocular history will help the ophthalmologist identify conditions that could affect the surgical approach and the visual prognosis. Trauma, inflammation, amblyopia, glaucoma, optic nerve abnormalities, or retinal disease might affect the visual outcome after cataract removal. In addition, an understanding of the patient's history of refractive error and spectacle or contact lens correction, as well as the patient's experience with monovision or progressive lenses, may aid refractive planning for cataract surgery.

Active uveitis should be controlled before cataract surgery so that the risk of complications from postoperative inflammation, such as macular edema and iris adhesion to the lens implant, can be minimized. Ideally, the eye is quiet without the use of topical corticosteroids for at least 3 months before surgery. Some eyes may require sustained use of topical corticosteroids even up to the time of surgery. Also, surgery may be needed before the clinician is able to get the eye completely quiet. Systemic immunomodulation may be necessary to achieve remission. The presence of zonular abnormalities, fibrin membranes, and posterior synechiae will require the surgeon to adjust his or her surgical technique, as discussed in Chapter 9.

A family history of retinal detachment or a history of retinal pathology in either of the patient's eyes is a risk factor for postoperative retinal detachment. Previous vitrectomy for the treatment of retinal disease or vitreous hemorrhage may cause intraoperative chamber fluctuations, which increase the risk of posterior capsule disruption and loss of nuclear fragments posteriorly.

In glaucoma patients, optimal control of intraocular pressure (IOP) should be achieved prior to cataract surgery. If this cannot be accomplished, the surgeon may wish to consider a combined operation (cataract surgery along with an intervention to lower IOP). New techniques combining cataract surgery with microinvasive glaucoma surgery (MIGS) may offer benefits of reducing medications while maintaining a risk profile similar to cataract surgery alone. See Chapter 9 in this volume and BCSC Section 10, *Glaucoma.*

Past records document the patient's visual acuity before the development of cataract. If the patient has had cataract surgery in the fellow eye, it is important to obtain information about the operative and postoperative course. If problems such as IFIS, elevated IOP, vitreous loss, cystoid macular edema, endophthalmitis, hemorrhage, or a refractive surprise occurred during or after the first operation, the surgical approach and postoperative follow-up could be modified for the second eye in order to reduce the risk of similar complications.

If the patient previously had refractive surgery, it is helpful to perform additional ocular measurements prior to and after the cataract surgery. See Chapter 9.

> Foster CS. Cataract surgery and uveitis. *Current Insight.* San Francisco: American Academy of Ophthalmology; 2006: Q3. Available at http://www.aao.org/current-insight/cataract-surgery-uveitis. Accessed October 26, 2015.

Social History

As discussed earlier, the decision to undertake cataract surgery is based not only on the patient's visual acuity but also on the ramifications of reduced vision on the individual's quality of life. The surgeon should be aware of the patient's occupation, hobbies, lifestyle, and any possible chemical dependencies, including nicotine and illicit (recreational) drugs, as all of these may affect postoperative recovery. Any surrogate decision makers must be identified and included in preoperative planning.

Measurements of Visual Function

Visual Acuity Testing

It is useful to measure Snellen acuity under lighted and darkened examination conditions. Although visual acuity testing in the ophthalmologist's office is commonly performed in a darkened room, diminished Snellen acuity from a symptomatic cataract is sometimes demonstrated only in a lighted room. Distance and near visual acuity must be tested and careful refraction performed so that BCVA can be determined. Visual acuity may improve after pupillary dilation, especially in patients with a PSC.

Refraction

Careful refraction must be performed on both eyes. This assessment is useful for calculating the IOL power necessary to obtain the desired postoperative refraction, as well as for determining whether a myopic shift has occurred. If the fellow eye has a clear lens and a high refractive error that requires correction, achieving emmetropia in the surgical eye might cause problems with postoperative anisometropia. The ophthalmologist should inform the patient specifically about this possibility and discuss options including refractive surgery or use of a contact lens for the noncataractous eye. Aiming for a similar myopic refractive result in the fellow eye is one option, but this will ensure long-term dependence on refractive correction. A planned monovision outcome may optimize spectacle independence, but the patient either must have experience with monovision or must be tested to find out whether adapting to unequal refractive errors will be tolerated.

Rigid contact lens overrefraction is a useful technique to assess the degree to which irregular astigmatism or other corneal irregularity is contributing to a patient's visual disability.

Glare Testing

Glare testing attempts to measure the degree of visual impairment caused by the presence of a light source located in the patient's visual field. Testing can be done with a nonprojected eye chart in ambient light conditions or with a projected eye chart and an off-axis bright light directed at the patient. Various instruments are available to standardize and facilitate this measurement. Patients with significant cataracts commonly show a decrease of 3 or more lines under these conditions, compared with results obtained when visual acuity is tested in a darkened room. Performing this assessment before the patient's pupils are dilated is recommended, as studies have shown that visual acuity decreases significantly when testing is performed after dilation. Results of any testing done after pupillary dilation must be adjusted to account for the related decrease in acuity.

Wiggins MN, Irak-Dersu I, Turner SD, Thostenson JD. Glare testing in patients with cataract after dilation. *Ophthalmology.* 2009;116(7):1332–1335.

Contrast Sensitivity Testing

Patients with cataracts may experience diminished contrast sensitivity even when Snellen acuity is preserved. Various specialized charts have been developed to test contrast sensitivity in the ophthalmologist's office. Some charts are mounted on a wall; others are handheld or incorporate the use of a monitor. Certain contrast sensitivity charts feature sine wave gratings to allow evaluation of different spatial frequencies. However, no instrument is currently considered the standard for contrast sensitivity testing. Of note, contrast sensitivity may be decreased by a wide variety of ophthalmic conditions affecting the cornea, optic nerve, and retina. It is therefore essential that the ophthalmologist identify any comorbidities before attributing an irregularity in test results solely to cataract.

Owsley C. Contrast sensitivity. *Ophthalmol Clin North Am.* 2003;16(2):171–177.

External Examination

The preoperative evaluation of a patient with cataract should include the body habitus and any abnormalities of the external eye and ocular adnexa. Such conditions as extensive supraclavicular fat, kyphosis, ankylosing spondylitis, generalized obesity, or head tremor may affect the surgical approach. The presence of enophthalmos or prominent brow may affect not only the surgical approach but also the chosen route of anesthesia.

Entropion, ectropion, or eyelid closure abnormalities, as well as abnormalities in the tear film, may have an impact on the ocular surface and thus adversely affect postoperative recovery if not addressed preoperatively. Severe blepharitis or acne rosacea may pose an increased risk of endophthalmitis and should likewise be treated before cataract surgery. Active nasolacrimal disease should also be treated, particularly if there is a history of inflammation, infection, or obstruction.

Motility

The ophthalmologist should evaluate ocular alignment and test the range of movement of the extraocular muscles. Cover testing should be performed to document any muscle deviation. Abnormal motility may suggest preexisting strabismus with amblyopia as a cause of vision loss. Patients must be made aware that they may experience diplopia after cataract surgery if they have a significant tropia resulting in disruption of fusion. Also, removal of a dense cataract may improve vision but make the patient aware of ocular misalignment.

Pupils

In addition to checking direct and consensual constriction of the pupil to light, the ophthalmologist should perform the swinging flashlight test to detect a *relative afferent pupillary defect* (*RAPD;* also known as a *Marcus Gunn pupil*), the presence of which indicates extensive retinal disease or optic nerve dysfunction. (See also BCSC Section 5, *Neuro-Ophthalmology.*) Although the vision of a patient with RAPD in the cataractous eye may improve after cataract surgery, the visual outcome may be limited by optic nerve dysfunction. The patient must be made aware of the possibility of less than complete restoration of vision.

It is important to measure the size of the pupil under different lighting conditions, because this information may affect selection of the IOL. For example, small-optic lenses may be inappropriate for a patient who has a large pupil in moderate or dim illumination. The edge of the optic can fall inside the pupil border, allowing light to pass around the optic edge, with resultant glare or dysphotopsias. Also, the function of a multifocal IOL may be affected by a pupil that is small, atonic, or eccentric. It is helpful to assess pupil size before and after dilation, because the risk of surgical complications is higher in small pupils that do not dilate adequately (eg, in patients with diabetes mellitus, posterior synechiae, pseudoexfoliation syndrome, or a history of systemic α_1-adrenergic antagonist or long-term topical miotic use); in such cases, the surgeon may need to use expansion techniques. These techniques are discussed in Chapters 7 and 9.

Slit-Lamp Examination

Conjunctiva

Vascularization or scarring of the conjunctiva due to previous inflammation, injury, or ocular surgery may indicate compromised healing and limit surgical exposure. Symblepharon or shortening of the fornices may be associated with underlying systemic or ocular surface diseases. Infectious processes should receive appropriate treatment before cataract surgery in order to ensure optimal postoperative healing.

Cornea

The clinician should assess corneal thickness and look for the presence of corneal dystrophy, as abnormalities could increase the risk of poor healing and decompensation postoperatively. Preoperative corneal thickness greater than 640 μm is associated with a higher risk of postoperative corneal decompensation. Specular reflection with the slit lamp may provide an estimate of the endothelial cell count and information regarding cell morphology. Descemet membrane irregularity associated with cornea guttae, as well as any central opacity, may affect the surgeon's view of the lens during surgery and limit visual acuity after surgery. In patients with pannus due to long-term contact lens use or other conditions, the surgeon should plan to avoid making corneal incisions in areas of vascularization, if possible. Also, weakened or thinned areas in the cornea should be identified so that they can be avoided intraoperatively.

The ocular surface is the first and principal refracting interface of the eye. Tear film quantity and quality are thus critical to visual results. Diagnosis and management of keratitis sicca, blepharitis, and epithelial basement membrane dystrophy are of critical importance in cataract patients.

Areas of scarring possibly consistent with a history of herpetic eye disease should prompt further questioning of the patient, as prophylactic antiviral medication and careful monitoring of steroid therapy in the perioperative period may be advisable to prevent reactivation.

If the patient has undergone previous corneal refractive surgery, the surgeon should document the placement of radial or astigmatic incisions, as well as any apparent problems with healing. If the patient has undergone previous radial keratotomy (RK), the surgeon must take care to develop a surgical plan that avoids corneal splitting at the site of the RK incisions. See also Chapter 9 in this volume and BCSC Section 13, *Refractive Surgery.*

Anterior Chamber and Iris

Knowing the depth of the anterior chamber and the axial thickness of the lens aids in surgical planning. A shallow anterior chamber may indicate anatomically narrow angles, nanophthalmos, short axial length, an intumescent lens, or a weak lens zonule.

The clinician should consider performing gonioscopy preoperatively to rule out angle abnormalities, including peripheral anterior synechiae, neovascularization, or a prominent major arterial circle. Use of a 3-mirror lens helps in the evaluation of the lens zonule for traumatic or congenital dehiscence. Gonioscopy is essential if anterior chamber IOL implantation is anticipated.

The presence of iridodonesis or exfoliation at the margin of the undilated pupil indicates weakened or absent zonular attachments and may affect the surgical plan. In addition, careful examination of the iris is important, as iris coloboma is often accompanied by lens coloboma and localized absence of zonular attachments.

Crystalline Lens

The clinician should carefully note the appearance of the lens both before and after dilation of the pupil. The impact of "oil droplet" nuclear cataracts and small PSCs is most closely correlated with visual symptoms before pupil dilation. After dilation, nuclear density can be evaluated, pseudoexfoliation syndrome can be detected, and opacities and distortion of the retinoscopic reflex can be visualized more easily.

To assess the lenticular contribution to the visual deficit, the clinician should evaluate the clarity of the media in the visual axis with the slit lamp. Dense, brunescent nuclear sclerotic cataracts may permit remarkably good vision, especially at near, whereas vacuolar cataracts, which may be detected by red reflex examination, can cause surprisingly severe vision loss. When dense cortical opacification is present, the intraoperative use of capsular dye to enhance visualization of the capsulorrhexis should be considered. The presence of a congenital posterior polar opacity is associated with a significant risk of capsule rupture and should be identified before surgery.

The position of the lens and the integrity of the zonular fibers should also be evaluated. Lens coloboma, lens decentration, phacodonesis, or excessive distance between the lens and the pupillary margin indicates zonular disruption due to conditions such as lens subluxation as a result of previous trauma, metabolic disorders, or hypermature cataract. An indentation or flattening of the lens periphery may indicate focal loss of zonular support. For patients with these types of zonular disruption, the surgeon should be prepared to alter surgical technique, including by using capsular tension rings or other capsular or iris support devices intraoperatively (see Chapter 9).

Ozturk F, Osher RH. Capsular staining: recent developments. *Curr Opin Ophthalmol.* 2006; 17(1):42–44.

Limitations of Slit-Lamp Examination

Some visually significant cataracts may appear minimal on slit-lamp biomicroscopy. However, examination of the lens with the retinoscope may clarify the lenticular contribution to the patient's vision changes. By examining the retinoscopic reflex, the clinician may detect posterior subcapsular opacities, refractile nuclear changes, or even diffuse cataracts. Similarly, examination using the direct ophthalmoscope through a +10.00 D lens at a distance of 2 ft will enhance the portions of the cataractous lens that are producing optical aberrations. This technique is particularly useful for identifying oil droplet cataracts.

Fundus Evaluation

Ophthalmoscopy

The ophthalmologist must perform a full fundus examination to evaluate the macula, optic nerve, vitreous, retinal vessels, and retinal periphery. Particular attention should be paid to early macular degeneration or other maculopathy that may limit visual outcome after an otherwise uneventful cataract extraction. The indirect ophthalmoscope is not useful for judging the visual significance of cataract. Although the direct ophthalmoscope, retinal contact lens, and noncontact fundus lens are more useful in judging media clarity, the ophthalmologist must keep in mind that they, too, provide light that is more intense than that available to the patient under ambient lighting conditions.

Patients with diabetes mellitus should be examined carefully for the presence of macular edema, retinal ischemia, and background and proliferative retinopathy. Even in uncomplicated cataract surgery and in patients with minimal or no retinopathy, diabetic eye disease can progress postoperatively. Retinal ischemia may potentiate posterior or anterior neovascularization postoperatively, especially if the surgeon uses an intracapsular technique or ruptures the posterior capsule during extracapsular cataract extraction. Careful examination of the retinal periphery may reveal the presence of vitreoretinal traction or preexisting retinal holes and lattice degeneration that may warrant preoperative treatment.

Hong T, Mitchell P, de Loryn T, Rochtchina E, Cugati S, Wang JJ. Development and progression of diabetic retinopathy 12 months after phacoemulsification cataract surgery. *Ophthalmology.* 2009;116(8):1510–1514.

Safran SG. SD-OCT: a quantum leap for anterior segment surgeons. *Current Insight.* San Francisco: American Academy of Ophthalmology; 2009: Q4. Available at www.aao.org /current-insight/sdoct-quantum-leap-anterior-segment-surgeons. Accessed October 26, 2015.

Optic Nerve

The ophthalmologist should examine the optic nerve for cupping and pallor, as well as other abnormalities. Visual acuity, measurement of IOP, and the results of confrontation testing and the pupillary examination will help determine whether other adjunctive testing is warranted.

Fundus Evaluation With Opaque Media

B-scan ultrasonography of the posterior segment of the eye is useful whenever a dense cataract makes visualization of the retina impossible. Ultrasonography can elucidate whether a retinal detachment, vitreous opacity, posterior pole tumor, or staphyloma is present. (See also BCSC Section 3, *Clinical Optics.*) Tests such as light projection, 2-point discrimination, gross color vision, photostress recovery, blue-light entoptoscopy, or the Maddox rod test may also be useful in detecting retinal pathology. Electroretinography and visually evoked response testing are warranted when other modalities are inconclusive and the surgeon must decide whether cataract removal would provide any benefit.

See BCSC Section 12, *Retina and Vitreous,* for discussion of these tests.

Special Tests

Potential Acuity Estimation

Potential acuity estimation can be helpful in assessing the lenticular contribution to vision loss. The potential acuity pinhole test is a simple but accurate method of evaluation for patients who do not have other ocular pathology and whose visual acuity is better than 20/200. For this test, the patient is asked to read a brightly illuminated near card through a pinhole aperture. The Retinal Acuity Meter, or RAM (AMA Optics, Miami Beach, FL), functions in a similar manner.

The Potential Acuity Meter, or PAM (Mentor Graphics/Marco, Jacksonville, FL), is one of several instruments that project a numerical or Snellen vision chart through a small entrance pupil. The image can be projected onto the retina, around lenticular opacities, allowing for an estimate of what the BCVA would be if the media abnormality were absent.

It is important to note that these tests can be misleading in the presence of several disorders, including age-related macular degeneration, amblyopia, macular edema, glaucoma, small macular scars, and serous retinal detachment. An accurate clinical examination of the eye is often the best predictor of visual outcome.

Melki SA, Safar A, Martin J, Ivanova A, Adi M. Potential acuity pinhole: a simple method to measure potential visual acuity in patients with cataracts, comparison to potential acuity meter. *Ophthalmology.* 1999;106(7):1262–1267.

Visual Field Testing

Confrontation field testing should be performed in all cataract patients; however, formal visual field testing is not indicated for every patient with lens opacity. Visual field testing may help the ophthalmologist identify vision loss resulting from disease processes other than cataract. Patients with a history of glaucoma, optic nerve disease, or retinal abnormality may benefit from visual field evaluation to document the degree of visual field loss. Preoperative visual field loss does not preclude improvement in visual function following cataract surgery. Progressive cataracts may induce diffuse visual field depression that disappears after cataract removal.

Objective Tests of Macular Function

Optical coherence tomography is increasingly performed as part of the preoperative testing regimen for cataract surgery in the United States. It may be useful in the assessment or detection of macular pathology, including neovascularization, edema, holes, and traction. Screening macular OCT to detect occult macular pathology may be of particular benefit for patients undergoing surgery with premium IOLs or when the vision is poorer than the degree of cataract would suggest.

Fluorescein angiography can be used to assess vascular and exudative abnormalities.

Preoperative Measurements

Accurate preoperative measurements of the eye are essential to achieving the desired postoperative refractive result.

Biometry

Ocular axial length (AL) is a key component of IOL power calculations, discussed later in this chapter. Several techniques are available to measure AL. No matter which is used, it is helpful to obtain data for both eyes, even if surgery is planned for only 1 eye. The difference in AL between the 2 eyes should be no greater than 0.3 mm, unless there is a refractive difference or there are other relevant ocular findings. The clinician should document any significant disparity in AL.

Optical biometers are noncontact instruments that use optical coherence reflectometry instead of ultrasound to measure multiple parameters, such as AL, corneal curvature, anterior chamber depth, and horizontal white-to-white distance (corneal diameter). Because the level of patient cooperation varies, the technician or physician performing biometry should be adept at working with patients to obtain the most accurate measurements. Biometers are optical devices; therefore, measurements may be confounded by corneal scarring, mature or posterior subcapsular cataracts, or vitreous hemorrhage. *A-scan*

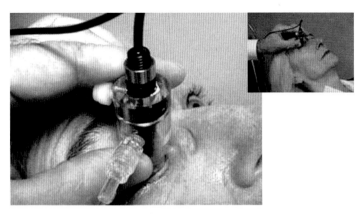

Figure 6-1 Immersion shell (Prager design/infusion shell). Although there are other immersion shells, they are now rarely used in the United States, as visual axis alignment is more easily achieved with infusion shells than with cup shells. Infusion shells are also easier to use. *(Courtesy of ESI, Inc.)*

ultrasonography measures AL by using either an immersion technique (Fig 6-1) or a contact applanation method. With the immersion technique, a shell is placed on the eye between the eyelids to provide a watertight seal over the cornea. An ultrasound transducer is mounted in the shell. With the contact applanation method, the examiner must be careful not to compress the cornea, because corneal compression results in an artificially shortened AL measurement. Though generally not clinically significant in the patient with an "average" refraction, such errors become more important in patients with high hyperopia (AL of 20 mm or less); in the short eyes of these patients, each millimeter of error results in up to 3.75 D of inaccuracy in IOL power. The immersion technique avoids this problem.

Note that ultrasonographic measurement of AL is actually determined by calculation. The ultrasonic biometer measures the transit time of the ultrasound pulse. Using an estimated average velocity through the various ocular media (cornea, aqueous, lens, and vitreous), the biometric software calculates the AL. This value should be altered when velocities differ from the norm. For example, in performing AL measurements in a patient with silicone oil in the posterior chamber, the clinician must take into account the different velocity of sound waves in vitreous (1532 m/s) and in silicone oil (980 m/s), as well as the change in transit time, which is extended when silicone oil is present. Also, the index of refraction of silicone oil is much lower than that of vitreous; thus, the refractive index of the oil (and the design of the IOL) must be figured into IOL calculations for these eyes.

Bjeloš Rončević M, Bušić M, Cima I, Kuzmanović Elabjer B, Bosnar D, Miletić D. Intraobserver and interobserver repeatability of ocular components measurement in cataract eyes using a new optical low coherence reflectometer. *Graefes Arch Clin Exp Ophthalmol.* 2011;249(1):83–87.

Ianchulev T, Hoffer KJ, Yoo SH, et al. Intraoperative refractive biometry for predicting intraocular lens power calculation after prior myopic refractive surgery. *Ophthalmology.* 2014;121(1):56–60.

Roessler GF, Huth JK, Dietlein TS, et al. Accuracy and reproducibility of axial length measurement in eyes with silicone oil endotamponade. *Br J Ophthalmol.* 2009;93(11):1492–1494.

Sahin A, Hamrah P. Clinically relevant biometry. *Curr Opin Ophthalmol.* 2012;23(1):47–53.

Corneal Topography

Topography provides a map of the corneal contour. Various methods, including Placido disk–based topography, Scheimpflug imaging, or light-emitting diode (LED) reflection, provide additional information about the corneal surface and power. Corneal topography is particularly helpful if the patient has irregular astigmatism or early keratoconus, has previously undergone keratorefractive surgery, desires a toric or presbyopic IOL, or might benefit from astigmatism-correcting corneal incisions. Posterior corneal astigmatism, which is difficult to measure, is increasingly recognized as an important factor in refractive surprises following IOL surgery.

Corneal power calculations are problematic in eyes that have undergone refractive surgery, since traditional measures assume a particular relationship between anterior and posterior curvature. Laser refractive surgery modifies this relationship by altering the anterior curvature.

Koch DD, Jenkins RB, Weikert MP, Yeu E, Wang L. Correcting astigmatism with toric intraocular lenses: effect of posterior corneal astigmatism. *J Cataract Refract Surg*. 2013; 39(12):1803–1809.

Additional Evaluation of the Cornea

In patients with a history of endothelial dystrophy, previous ocular surgery, or trauma, additional corneal measurements may be useful. These data may aid the surgeon in counseling the patient regarding the possibility of postoperative corneal decompensation. In some cases, consideration of a combined surgery incorporating removal of the cataract and transplantation of corneal tissue may be in order.

Corneal pachymetry, a method employed to measure corneal thickness, is useful for indirectly assessing the function of the endothelium. Significantly increased central corneal thickness (>640 μm) in patients with endothelial dysfunction is associated with a greater risk of postoperative corneal decompensation.

Specular microscopy is used to determine the number of corneal endothelial cells per square millimeter and evaluate their regularity. Because cataract surgery results in some loss of endothelial cells, the risk of postoperative corneal decompensation is increased if the preoperative endothelial cell count is low. Abnormal endothelial cell morphology, including enlargement (polymegathism) and irregularity (pleomorphism), may limit the cornea's ability to withstand stress. (See also BCSC Section 8, *External Disease and Cornea.*)

IOL Power Determination

Formulas used for calculating the appropriate IOL power are based on the refracting power of the cornea, the anticipated postoperative distance between the anterior surface of the cornea and the anterior surface of the IOL (anterior chamber depth), and the AL of the eye. The refracting power of the cornea is determined by keratometry (manual or automatic) or by optical coherence biometry.

Anterior chamber depth is estimated from measurements made on eyes with implants similar to the style of IOL to be used, or it is measured using biometry. The AL is the distance between the anterior surface of the cornea and the fovea as measured by A-scan ultrasonography or optical coherence reflectometry. For every IOL, an "A constant," a theoretical value relating the lens power to AL and keratometry, is specified by the manufacturer. This constant is not expressed in units, and it is specific to the design of the IOL and its intended location and orientation within the eye.

Intraoperative aberrometry may be used to directly determine the IOL power without using measurements of corneal power and AL. Therefore, it has benefits in measuring eyes that have undergone corneal refractive surgery.

Prager TC, Hardten DR, Fogal BJ. Enhancing intraocular lens outcome precision: an evaluation of axial length determinations, keratometry, and IOL formulas. *Ophthalmol Clin North Am.* 2006;19(4):435–448.

IOL Calculation

Prior to surgery, the ophthalmologist needs to determine the power of the IOL that should be implanted to achieve the desired refractive result. The earliest formulas (eg, Binkhorst, Colenbrander, Fyodorov) were theoretical. Newer formulas incorporate regression analyses based on large numbers of postoperative results. Popular third-generation formulas include Hoffer Q, Holladay 1, Haigis L, and SRK/T. The dependability of the calculations often varies among subgroups of patients. For example, the Hoffer Q formula has been shown to be more reliable for eyes with a short AL, while the SRK/T formula has shown more reliability in long eyes. Fourth-generation formulas (Holladay 2, Preussner, Barrett, and Olsen) utilize additional measurements to refine refractive results. IOL formulas in this latest generation are also more complex. For example, they incorporate the concept that the postoperative anterior chamber depth is not identical to preoperative measurements but varies with factors such as corneal curvature and IOL position. In addition, some formulas allow the ophthalmologist to adjust IOL calculations based on personal experience with a particular lens.

Despite ophthalmologists' intense dedication to determining the best IOL calculation formulas, several large series have shown that approximately 25% of postoperative results miss the refractive target by more than 0.50 D. And as previously discussed, IOL calculation in eyes that have undergone refractive surgery is especially problematic, as the alteration in anterior corneal curvature yields incorrect results if traditional determination of corneal power is used. Acknowledging that no single formula is perfect, many surgeons use multiple IOL calculations to hone in on the best choice. The American Society of Cataract and Refractive Surgery (ASCRS) hosts a website (http://iolcalc.org/) that allows surgeons to run several calculations simultaneously.

Narváez J, Zimmerman G, Stulting RD, Chang DH. Accuracy of intraocular lens power prediction using the Hoffer Q, Holladay 1, Holladay 2, and SRK/T formulas. *J Cataract Refract Surg.* 2006;32(12):2050–2053.

IOL calculation following refractive surgery

Calculating the IOL power for eyes that have undergone refractive surgery presents problems for both patients and surgeons. These patients were initially motivated to have refractive surgery because they did not want to be dependent on glasses. They may have higher expectations regarding postoperative refractive results. However, determining the central keratometric power, a key element in lens power calculation, is complicated because of the corneal change that occurred as a result of the original refractive procedure. For example, the refractive outcomes of cataract surgery patients who have previously undergone RK have historically been fraught with undercorrections.

Manual keratometers and corneal topography units (videokeratography) do not measure corneal power directly but rather calculate the curvature of the anterior cornea. Following corneal refractive surgery, the cornea becomes aspheric. This asphericity invalidates the anterior corneal curvature measurements obtained by either type of instrument.

In addition, although RK did not alter the relative positions of the anterior and posterior corneal surfaces, photorefractive keratectomy (PRK) and laser in situ keratomileusis (LASIK) do. For these reasons, different techniques must be employed to accurately estimate the anterior corneal surface curvature following these types of refractive surgery. Newer corneal topography systems that measure both anterior and posterior corneal curvatures can improve the accuracy of IOL power calculation. Because intraoperative aberrometry relies not on keratometric power but rather on the total refractive error of the eye, it is a good option for determining IOL power in post-LASIK eyes.

Patients who have undergone previous corneal refractive surgery should be informed of potential problems with IOL selection. The surgeon should mention that refractive surprise due to overcorrection or undercorrection is a possibility and may require refractive correction with glasses, contact lenses, refractive surgery, or IOL exchange. Documenting this discussion is extremely important.

A variety of methods have been developed to better estimate the central corneal power after refractive surgery. As each method has advantages and disadvantages, the ophthalmic surgeon should use more than one method to calculate the corneal power. Selecting the highest IOL power of a tightly clustered group may avoid undercorrection. The ASCRS website offers a calculator for selecting IOL power for eyes that have previously undergone refractive surgery (http://iolcalc.ascrs.org). See also BCSC Section 13, *Refractive Surgery*.

Seitz B, Langenbucher A, Nguyen NX, Kus MM, Küchle M. Underestimation of intraocular lens power for cataract surgery after myopic photorefractive keratectomy. *Ophthalmology.* 1999;106(4):693–702.

Wang L, Booth MA, Koch DD. Comparison of intraocular lens power calculation methods in eyes that have undergone LASIK. *Ophthalmology.* 2004;111(10):1825–1831.

Historical methods If the patient's pre–refractive surgery data are available, the surgeon can use the clinical history method to calculate the IOL power.

One such method (after Hoffer) involves calculating the corneal power from the refractive and keratometry measurements made before and after the patient's refractive surgery.

Another historical method (after Feiz and Mannis) calculates the IOL power from the pre–refractive surgery data and then increases this power by a factor related to the amount of refractive change in the spectacle plane produced by the refractive surgery:

IOL pre–refractive surgery – (change in refraction/0.7) = IOL desired for patient

A potential problem with using certain regression formulas in post–refractive surgery cases is that reduced central corneal power may be linked in the formula to an anterior chamber depth that is assumed to be less than it actually is, resulting in the calculation of a lower IOL power than is really required. The Holladay 2 formula includes pre–refractive surgery corneal data that may correct for this error. Otherwise, the keratometric value may be modified so that undercorrections are reduced.

> Shammas HJ. IOL power calculation in patients with prior corneal refractive surgery. *Focal Points: Clinical Modules for Ophthalmologists.* San Francisco: American Academy of Ophthalmology; 2013, module 6.

Preventing Errors in IOL Calculation, Selection, and Insertion

The A-scan transducer should be calibrated before use each day. Several scans should be done on each patient, and the measurements should cluster around a value, with a variance no greater than 0.2 mm. Both eyes should be checked, especially if the first eye measures longer or shorter than anticipated. The difference between the eyes should be no greater than 0.3 mm, unless there is a refractive or other anatomical explanation. The surgeon should make sure that the patient name and K-readings, as well as AL and white-to-white measurements, are appropriately documented. The lens power and the manufacturer's model number should also be specified. In addition, lenses and powers for placement in the capsular bag, sulcus, or anterior chamber angle should be selected and carefully identified.

All this information should be accessible to the surgeon in the operating room, and the lenses should be located and set aside preoperatively. The surgeon should check the IOL calculations to verify that the lenses are the correct ones. In the operating room, a "time-out" should be performed with the entire surgical team before the procedure begins to confirm the patient's identity, the operative eye, the procedure, and the IOL to be implanted.

Improving Outcomes

The cataract surgeon should track his or her refractive outcomes, asking questions such as the following: Are there overcorrections or undercorrections, and do they occur more often with longer eyes or shorter eyes or roughly as frequently in both? Does the incision routinely induce cylinder? Are toric lenses correcting as calculated? If limbal relaxing incisions have been used intraoperatively for the correction of astigmatism, have they been effective? Commercially available programs may be useful for tracking outcomes.

After the surgeon has analyzed these factors, he or she may make adjustments to improve refractive outcomes, such as including a "surgeon factor" (a modification of the parameters used that reflects the surgeon's experience) in lens power calculation, changing the calculation software, or using immersion or optical biometry. Improving outcomes is important for increasing not only patient satisfaction but also surgeon confidence.

Patient Preparation and Informed Consent

When planning cataract surgery, the surgeon must evaluate the patient's ability to adhere to the postoperative care regimen. The surgeon should inform the patient (and caregivers, if appropriate) of the importance of using prescribed medication, maintaining proper ocular hygiene, and keeping required appointments. It is helpful to provide written instructions, along with appropriate illustrations or video presentations, and include a family member or friend in preoperative discussions in order to reinforce the patient's memory. The patient should understand that there are activity restrictions during the immediate postoperative period, although the advent of small-incision surgery has significantly minimized these limitations. The surgeon should also assess the patient's ability to function with only the fellow eye in the event that vision rehabilitation of the surgical eye is prolonged.

The surgeon must obtain informed consent preoperatively. Before deciding to proceed with cataract surgery, the patient should have a clear understanding of the indications for surgery, the risks and benefits, the alternatives to surgery, the surgical technique, and IOL options. The surgeon should identify any risk factors for decreased visual outcome. In addition, the surgeon and patient should discuss the anticipated postoperative refractive status, the limitations of pseudophakic correction, and the proposed date for providing the final optical correction.

Any costs associated with the surgery (eg, those related to medications or the use of premium IOL implants) should also be clearly outlined preoperatively. In addition, if co-management with an optometrist or another ophthalmologist is planned, the patient must be explicitly notified and must give consent in writing.

American Academy of Ophthalmology Cataract and Anterior Segment Panel. Preferred Practice Pattern Guidelines. *Cataract in the Adult Eye.* San Francisco: American Academy of Ophthalmology; 2011. Available at www.aao.org/ppp.

Comprehensive guidelines for the co-management of ophthalmic postoperative care. American Academy of Ophthalmology website. http://www.aao.org/ethics-detail/guidelines -comanagement-postoperative-care. Published 2016. Accessed September 19, 2016.

Moseley TH, Wiggins MN, O'Sullivan P. Effects of presentation method on the understanding of informed consent. *Br J Ophthalmol.* 2006;90(8):990–993.

CHAPTER **7**

Surgery for Cataract

▶ *This chapter includes related videos, which can be accessed by scanning the QR codes provided in the text or going to www.aao.org/bcscvideo_section11.*

Historical Overview of Cataract Surgery

Ancient and medieval treatment of cataract included *couching,* a technique with a colorful history dating to approximately the fifth century BC. This procedure, which was used throughout the Roman Empire, Europe, India, and sub-Saharan Africa, was performed on mature cataracts. With the patient in a seated position, the surgeon inserted a needle or knife posterior to the corneoscleral junction and then pushed the lens inferiorly (Fig 7-1).

By the 17th century, a better understanding of anatomy led to a fundamental improvement in technique. Jacques Daviel (1696–1762) is credited with propelling cataract surgery toward the modern era by introducing a method to extract the cataract rather than simply displace it. His method involved creating an incision through the inferior

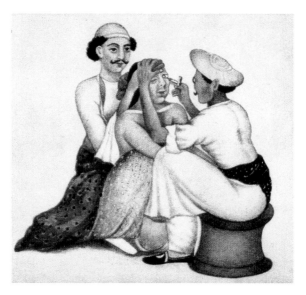

Figure 7-1 Couching. *(Reproduced from Duke-Elder S. Diseases of the Lens and Vitreous; Glaucoma and Hypotony. St Louis: Mosby; 1969. System of Ophthalmology; vol II.)*

cornea, enlarging the wound with scissors, incising the lens capsule, expressing the nucleus, and removing the cortex by curettage (Fig 7-2). This *extracapsular cataract extraction,* or *ECCE,* became the new standard of care. Subsequently, Albrecht von Graefe (1828–1870) advanced this technique by developing a corneal knife that created a cleaner incision and led to improved wound healing. The development of fine suture material, the invention of the binocular operating microscope, and the introduction of modern sterilization techniques reduced the incidence of surgical complications, and variations on manual ECCE continue to be employed to this day. See the appendix for a more detailed discussion of ECCE.

Removal of a cataractous lens via *intracapsular cataract extraction,* or *ICCE,* was first performed in 1753 by Samuel Sharp. This procedure involved removing the lens with the capsule intact through a limbal incision by using various means to break or dissolve the zonular fibers, which attach the lens to the ciliary body. See the appendix for further discussion of the modern ICCE procedure, including a figure showing ICCE performed with a cryoprobe to remove the encapsulated lens.

The invention of phacoemulsification by Charles Kelman in 1967 marked the beginning of the modern era of cataract surgery. Though initially met with strong resistance, phacoemulsification gained popularity by the 1990s. In this procedure, an ultrasonically driven tip is used to emulsify the lens nucleus and remove the fragments with an automated aspiration system. This paradigm shift allowed cataract surgery to be performed

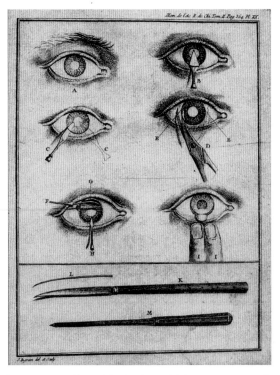

Figure 7-2 Daviel J. Sur une nouvelle méthode de guérir la cataracte par l'extraction du cristalin. *(Reproduced from Louis M, et al.* Memoires de l'Académie Royale de Chirurgie. *Paris: Théophile Barrois Lejeune; 1787.)*

via relatively small corneal incisions, resulting in a lower incidence of wound-related and vitreous-related complications and more rapid rehabilitation of vision. This advance also coincided with the invention of ophthalmic viscosurgical devices, the evolution of intraocular lens design, and a change to performance of cataract surgery on an outpatient basis.

> Kelman CD. *Through My Eyes: The Story of a Surgeon Who Dared to Take On the Medical World.* New York: Crown Publishing; 1985.

Anesthesia for Cataract Surgery

Consideration of the options for anesthesia is an important part of preoperative planning. A general review of the advantages and risks of the different types of anesthesia should accompany the informed consent process. A discussion of what the patient will experience in the operating room increases the likelihood of comfort and cooperation on the day of surgery. (See also BCSC Section 1, *Update on General Medicine,* for a discussion of perioperative management in ocular surgery.)

Retrobulbar anesthesia for cataract surgery provides excellent ocular akinesia and anesthesia. The modern technique of retrobulbar injection (Fig 7-3), first described in 1945 by Walter Atkinson, involves administration of lidocaine into the muscle cone via a 25-gauge, 1.5-inch (38-mm) blunt retrobulbar needle. Complications of retrobulbar anesthesia are uncommon but include retrobulbar hemorrhage; globe penetration; optic nerve trauma; extraocular muscle toxicity; inadvertent intravenous injection associated with cardiac arrhythmia; and inadvertent intradural injection with associated seizures, respiratory arrest, and brainstem anesthesia.

Peribulbar anesthesia theoretically eliminates the risk of complications such as optic nerve injury and intradural injection. However, it is slightly less effective than the retrobulbar method for providing akinesia and anesthesia. In this technique, a shorter (1-inch) 25- or 27-gauge needle is used to introduce anesthetic solution external to the muscle cone, underneath the Tenon capsule.

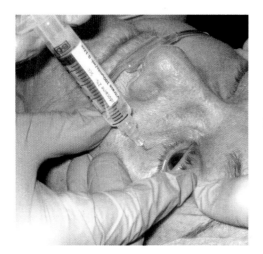

Figure 7-3 Retrobulbar injection. *(Courtesy of Michael N. Wiggins, MD.)*

Sub-Tenon infusion of lidocaine may be used for supplemental anesthesia during surgery. A small, posterior incision is made through anesthetized conjunctiva and the Tenon capsule, and a small cannula is used to administer the anesthetic (Fig 7-4).

Topical anesthesia has been increasingly utilized as surgical techniques have advanced. The use of topical anesthesia eliminates the risk of ocular perforation, extraocular muscle injury, and central nervous system depression. Visual recovery is accelerated, and patients are often able to leave the operating room without being patched. Topical anesthesia is administered via proparacaine or tetracaine drops, cellulose pledgets soaked in anesthetic, or lidocaine jelly. These agents may be supplemented with intravenous sedation and/or intracameral preservative-free lidocaine. Only nonpreserved 1% or 2% lidocaine should be used for anterior chamber instillation, because of the toxic effect of some preservative agents on intraocular structures. Disadvantages of topical anesthesia include blepharospasm, lack of akinesia, and potential patient discomfort, which can interfere with the surgeon's ability to perform delicate maneuvers. Topical anesthesia should be reserved for the cooperative cataract patient who, with a dilated pupil, can tolerate the microscope light.

A *facial nerve block,* common in the era of large-incision ICCE and ECCE, is not generally necessary with small-incision surgery. However, patients with essential or reactive blepharospasm may benefit from a facial nerve block to control squeezing during surgery. Types of facial nerve blocks include the O'Brien block, directed proximally and peripherally at the nerve trunk; the van Lint block, directed proximally and peripherally at the terminal branches; and the Atkinson block, directed between these two regions (Fig 7-5).

General anesthesia, with clearance from the patient's primary care physician or an anesthesiologist, is appropriate to consider for pediatric patients and for patients who have any condition that would prevent their cooperation and ability to lie flat during surgery, including dementia, head tremor, deafness, language barrier, musculoskeletal disorder, restless legs syndrome, or claustrophobia.

Schimek F, Fahle M. Techniques of facial nerve block. *Br J Ophthalmol.* 1995;79(2):166–173.

Zhao LQ, Zhu H, Zhao PQ, Wu QR, Hu YQ. Topical anesthesia versus regional anesthesia for cataract surgery: a meta-analysis of randomized controlled trials. *Ophthalmology.* 2012; 119(4):659–667.

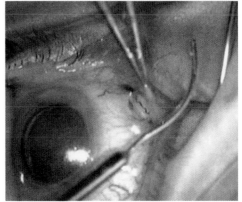

Figure 7-4 Sub-Tenon injection. *(Courtesy of University of Iowa, Dept of Ophthalmology.)*

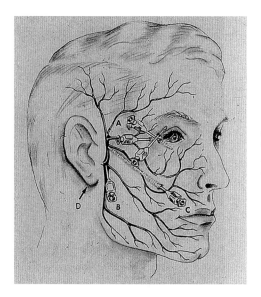

Figure 7-5 Akinesia of orbicularis oculi. **A,** Van Lint akinesia. **B,** O'Brien akinesia. **C,** Atkinson akinesia. **D,** Nadbath-Ellis akinesia. *(Modified with permission from Jaffe NS, Jaffe MS, Jaffe GF. Cataract Surgery and Its Complications. 5th ed. St Louis: Mosby; 1990.)*

Antimicrobial Prophylaxis

Endophthalmitis remains one of the most serious complications of cataract surgery (see Chapter 8). Therefore, a major objective of preoperative preparation and intraoperative management of the patient is to reduce the introduction of pathogenic organisms into the anterior chamber.

Before Surgery

Before the day of surgery, the surgeon should identify and reduce infectious risk factors as much as possible through preoperative treatment of coexisting eyelid disorders such as conjunctivitis, blepharitis, hordeolum, and chalazion. Systemic infections should also be identified and treated.

Cataract surgery is not considered to be an invasive procedure that induces transient bacteremia; thus, systemic antibiotic prophylaxis is not required. If questions arise about whether antibiotic prophylaxis is advisable in the perioperative period, the surgeon should consult with the physicians involved in the patient's systemic care.

Although no studies have convincingly demonstrated the efficacy of topical antibiotics in reducing the risk of endophthalmitis in routine cataract surgery, there is some evidence supporting an association between the use of preoperative topical antibiotics and a reduction in ocular surface bacterial counts, as well as a lower incidence of positive aqueous cultures after surgery. Many cataract surgeons prescribe preoperative topical antibiotics.

For patients with a history of herpetic eye disease, the surgeon should consider prescribing prophylactic antiviral medications. This topic is further discussed in Chapter 9.

Sykakis E, Karim R, Parmar DN. Management of patients with herpes simplex virus eye disease having cataract surgery in the United Kingdom. *J Cataract Refract Surg.* 2013; 39(8):1254–1259.

Yoshida J, Kim A, Pratzer KA, Stark WJ. Aqueous penetration of moxifloxacin 0.5% ophthalmic solution and besifloxacin 0.6% ophthalmic suspension in cataract surgery patients. *J Cataract Refract Surg.* 2010;36(9):1499–1502.

In Surgery

In the operating room, sterilization of the fornix is important. A 5% povidone-iodine solution (not scrub or soap) placed in the conjunctival fornix prior to surgery has been associated with a reduction in bacterial colony counts in cultures from the ocular surface at the time of surgery and a decreased risk of culture-proven endophthalmitis. In addition, preparation of the skin around the eye with a 10% povidone-iodine solution can reduce bacterial counts on the eyelid margins. Because eyelid margins may harbor pathogens, care should be taken to drape the eyelashes out of the operative field (Fig 7-6).

It is important not only to limit the number of times that instruments are introduced into the eye but also to check for signs of lint, cilia, and other debris on the tips of all instruments inserted. Intraoperative manipulation should be reduced as well. Meticulous wound closure is imperative. Despite surgeons' best efforts, however, 7%–35% of cataract surgeries result in bacterial inoculation of the anterior chamber. The low incidence of endophthalmitis is a testament to the ability of the anterior chamber to clear itself of a potentially pathologic inoculum. The surgeon should also be aware that the risk of endophthalmitis increases with a torn posterior lens capsule, vitreous loss, and prolonged surgery.

Some surgeons add antibiotics to the irrigating solution or inject them into the anterior chamber at the conclusion of the operation. The Endophthalmitis Study Group reported a significant reduction in endophthalmitis with the use of intracameral cefuroxime. The use of intracameral cefuroxime has not been universally adopted, however, because of the lack of commercial antibiotic preparations for intracameral use.

Whether the risk of endophthalmitis is increased after cataract surgery performed using a sutureless clear corneal wound is controversial. By tracking the flow of fluorescein into the anterior chamber, some have suggested that inflow of bacteria from the ocular surface may be possible via a sutureless incision. For this reason, hydrating the corneal stroma to reapproximate the anterior and posterior aspects of the wound may reduce the risk of wound separation. Any possibility of leakage should be addressed with wound closure by suture or tissue adhesive.

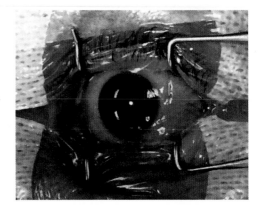

Figure 7-6 Sterile draping of the eye for surgery. *(Courtesy of Lisa Park, MD.)*

Chang DF, Braga-Mele R, Henderson BA, Mamalis N, Vasavada A; ASCRS Cataract Clinical
  Committee. Antibiotic prophylaxis of postoperative endophthalmitis after cataract
  surgery: results of the 2014 ASCRS member survey. *J Cataract Refract Surg.* 2015;41(6):
  1300–1305.
Endophthalmitis Study Group, European Society of Cataract & Refractive Surgeons (ESCRS).
  Prophylaxis of postoperative endophthalmitis following cataract surgery: results of the
  ESCRS multicenter study and identification of risk factors. *J Cataract Refract Surg.* 2007;
  33(6):978–988.
Gower EW, Keay LJ, Stare DE, et al. Characteristics of endophthalmitis after cataract surgery
  in the United States Medicare population. *Ophthalmology.* 2015;122(8):1625–1632.
Nentwich MM, Ta CN, Kreutzer TC, et al. Incidence of postoperative endophthalmitis from
  1990 to 2009 using povidone-iodine but no intracameral antibiotics at a single academic
  institution. *J Cataract Refract Surg.* 2015;41(1):58–66.

After Surgery

After routine cataract surgery, use of antibiotic eyedrops is commonly continued or instituted. Although reduced bacterial counts have been documented with the administration
of topical antibiotics, there is no definitive evidence that their use reduces the incidence of
endophthalmitis. The studies cited in this section indicate the complexity of the issues
involved in preventing postoperative infection.

Behndig A, Cochener B, Güell JL, et al. Endophthalmitis prophylaxis in cataract surgery:
  overview of current practice patterns in 9 European countries. *J Cataract Refract Surg.*
  2013;39(9):1421–1431.

Ophthalmic Viscosurgical Devices

Ophthalmic viscosurgical devices (OVDs), also referred to as *viscoelastic agents,* have
been employed in anterior segment surgery since 1979. They play an important role in
maintaining the anterior chamber and protecting the corneal endothelium during surgery, and their use has had a profound influence on the evolution of extracapsular and
phacoemulsification surgery.

OVDs contain one or more of the following substances in varying concentrations:
sodium hyaluronate, chondroitin sulfate, and hydroxypropyl methylcellulose. *Sodium
hyaluronate* is a biopolymer that occurs in many connective tissues throughout the body,
such as synovial (joint) fluid and vitreous. It was originally isolated from human umbilical
cord and rooster combs. Sodium hyaluronate has a half-life of approximately 1 day in aqueous and 3 days in vitreous. *Chondroitin sulfate* is a sulfated glycosaminoglycan, which is an
important component of cartilage. *Hydroxypropyl methylcellulose (HPMC)* does not occur
naturally in animal tissues, but cellulose is widely distributed in plant fibers such as cotton and wood. The commercial product is a cellulose polymer modified by the addition
of hydroxypropyl and methyl groups to increase the hydrophilic property of the material.
Methylcellulose is a nonphysiologic compound that does not appear to be metabolized
intraocularly. It is eventually eliminated in the aqueous but can easily be irrigated from
the eye.

Physical Properties

The physical properties of OVDs are not necessarily due to the specific biopolymer composition; rather, they are the result of chain length and molecular interactions both within chains and between chains and ocular tissue. There are 4 general physical properties:

1. *Viscosity* describes resistance to flow and can be thought of as the "thickness" or "thinness" of a fluid. It is determined primarily by molecular weight and concentration, so that substances with high molecular weight and high concentration have the highest viscosity. The higher the viscosity, the better the OVD is at displacing tissue and staying in place.
2. *Elasticity* refers to the ability of a material to return to its original shape after being stressed. It describes the OVD's ability to re-form after an external force is applied to the anterior chamber and then removed. A highly elastic substance is excellent for maintaining space.
3. *Pseudoplasticity* refers to the ease with which a material can change from being highly viscous at rest to being watery at increasing rates of shear stress. This property is found in certain everyday substances such as toothpaste; when squeezed out of a tube, toothpaste flows easily, but it retains its shape when it is at rest on the toothbrush. In clinical terms, at zero shear force an OVD is a lubricant and coats tissues well, but when forced through a small-gauge cannula it functions like a liquid.
4. *Surface tension* describes how the surface of a fluid tends to stick to another surface. This property is also referred to as coatability, which is inversely proportional to surface tension. Thus, an OVD with low surface tension is better at coating tissue but is harder to remove from the eye.

Given the different combinations of all of these properties, OVDs can be classified into 2 general categories:

1. *Cohesive OVDs* are long-chain, high-molecular-weight, high-viscosity substances. These agents maintain space well at no or low shear rates, whereas at high shear rates they are easily displaced. Cohesive OVDs are easier to remove from the eye because they stick together and are aspirated as long pieces (similar to spaghetti). However, they have minimal coating ability and therefore afford less tissue protection during surgery.
2. *Dispersive OVDs* are short-chain, low-molecular-weight, low-viscosity substances with low surface tension. These agents provide excellent coating and protection at high shear rates; however, they are more difficult to remove from the eye because they do not stick together and are aspirated in short fragments (similar to macaroni). They are more likely to be retained in the eye after cataract surgery, increasing the likelihood of angle obstruction with reduced outflow and subsequent IOP elevation.

Cohesive agents include Healon, Healon GV (Abbott Medical Optics, Santa Ana, CA); Amvisc, Amvisc Plus (Bausch + Lomb, Rochester, NY); and Provisc (Alcon, Ft Worth, TX). Dispersive agents include OcuCoat (Bausch + Lomb), Viscoat (Alcon), and Healon

Endocoat (Abbott Medical Optics). Discovisc (Alcon) combines qualities of dispersive and cohesive agents.

Some additional OVDs, such as the viscoadaptive agent Healon5 (Abbott Medical Optics), may need separate classification. Healon5 is a long, fragile chain with high molecular weight that changes its behavior at different flow rates. The lower the flow rate, the more viscous and cohesive the OVD is, and the higher the flow rate, the more the chains fracture. As a result, this OVD acts as a pseudodispersive agent. However, it must be carefully removed at the end of surgery because it can cause extremely elevated IOP if left in the eye.

Oshika T, Eguchi S, Oki K, et al. Clinical comparison of Healon5 and Healon in phacoemulsification and intraocular lens implantation: randomized multicenter study. *J Cataract Refract Surg.* 2004;30(2):357–362.

Pape LG, Balazs EA. The use of sodium hyaluronate (Healon) in human anterior segment surgery. *Ophthalmology.* 1980;87(7):699–705.

Uses of Ophthalmic Viscosurgical Devices

The *space maintenance ability* of OVDs keeps the anterior chamber formed despite the presence of one or more corneal incisions. With expansion of the chamber, manipulations can be made away from the corneal endothelium and posterior lens capsule. A cohesive OVD can be used to enlarge a marginally dilated pupil (viscomydriasis). It can also be used to keep the plane of the anterior capsule flat to assist a controlled continuous curvilinear capsulorrhexis. Lens implantation is less traumatic to the zonular fibers and the posterior capsule when the capsular bag is inflated with an OVD.

The *coatability* of OVDs can be used to protect the corneal endothelium from phaco energy, particularly in dense cataracts or during long operations. The surgeon must take care to remove dispersive OVDs completely to reduce the risk of an ocular hypertensive period caused by angle outflow obstruction. In the presence of an open posterior lens capsule, a dispersive OVD can be injected over the tear to provide a vitreous tamponade and prevent prolapse of vitreous anteriorly.

The *optical clarity* of OVDs has prompted some surgeons to use a layer of OVD on the surface of the cornea. When slightly moistened with balanced salt solution, the agent coats the epithelium. This maneuver prevents drying and eliminates the need to irrigate the corneal surface. It also provides a slightly magnified view of anterior segment structures.

The choice of OVD varies depending on the clinical scenario. A survey showed that 97% of surgeons vary their choice of OVD in complicated cases. For example, in pediatric cataracts or cases with a low endothelial cell count, shallow anterior chamber, or intraoperative floppy iris syndrome, the choice of OVD can play a critical role in management.

Buratto L, Giardini P, Bellucci R. *Viscoelastics in Ophthalmic Surgery.* Thorofare, NJ: Slack; 2005:5.

Lane SS, Lindstrom RL. Viscoelastic agents: formulation, clinical applications, and complications. In: Steinert RF, ed. *Cataract Surgery: Technique, Complications, and Management.* Philadelphia: Saunders; 1995:37–45.

Riedel PJ. Ophthalmic viscosurgical devices. *Focal Points: Clinical Modules for Ophthalmologists.* San Francisco: American Academy of Ophthalmology; 2012, module 7.

Phacoemulsification: Instrumentation, Terminology, and Key Concepts

Instrumentation

There are several types of phaco machines, but their major components are essentially the same. These include the handpiece, foot pedal, irrigation system, and vacuum pump.

Phacoemulsification makes use of ultrasound technology, as well as vacuum (defined in the section Fluidics and Phacodynamics). The phaco handpiece (Fig 7-7) has been likened to a combination of a jackhammer, vacuum, and garden hose. The surgeon uses the handpiece to simultaneously emulsify and aspirate the crystalline lens while keeping the tip cool and maintaining anterior chamber depth. The mechanical energy

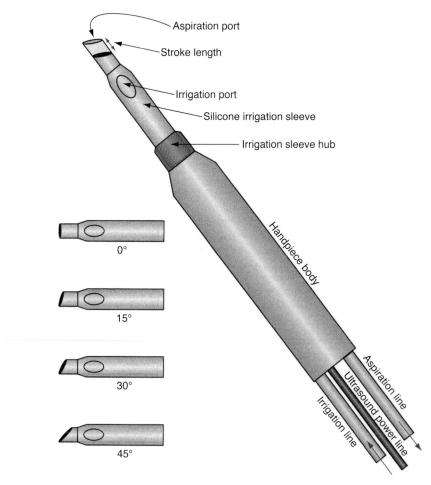

Figure 7-7 Parts of a phaco handpiece. The smaller drawings depict the different tip bevels available. *(Reprinted with permission from Seibel BS. Phacodynamics: Mastering the Tools and Techniques of Phacoemulsification Surgery. 3rd ed. Thorofare, NJ: Slack; 1999.)*

of phacoemulsification is produced by a to-and-fro oscillation generated by *piezoelectric crystals* in the phaco handpiece. The amplitude of the movement, or *stroke length,* is variable and increases when the power is raised. As the phaco tip moves forward, compression of gas atoms in solution occurs; as the tip moves backward, expansion of gas atoms occurs, and bubbles of gas form (cavitation; see the section Ultrasonic Technology Terminology). The bubbles are subject to the same compression and expansion. When the bubbles implode, they release heat and shock waves, which contribute to activity that disassembles the nucleus at the phaco tip. Nonaxial vibrations generated by a torsional or elliptical motion of the tip can augment the primary oscillation and cause the mechanical breakdown of nuclear material. These mechanisms are specific to the type of phaco machine used.

The phaco foot pedal is an important component for mastering the phacoemulsification technique. All current phaco machines have foot-pedal controls with at least 3 positions. Position 1 produces irrigation, whereas position 2 engages the aspiration mode at a constant or variable rate. Position 3 adds phaco power at a variable or fixed level. When fixed, the power level may be set from 0% to 100%, and the chosen power level is delivered immediately when the foot pedal is depressed to position 3. With linear ultrasound, the surgeon controls the amount of phaco power delivered by varying the depth of depression of the foot pedal while it is in position 3.

Ultrasonic Technology Terminology

The following terms are commonly used in reference to ultrasonic technology.

Cavitation The formation of gas bubbles arising from the aqueous in response to pressure changes at the tip of the phaco needle; these bubbles expand and contract. Implosion of the bubbles causes localized intense heat and pressure liberation at the tip, resulting in emulsification of lens material. Continuous cavitation, produced by continuous ultrasound delivery, is less efficient than the transient cavitation of intermittent ultrasound delivery.

Chatter Occurs when the ultrasonic stroke overcomes the vacuum, or "holding power." This process causes the nuclear fragments to be repelled by the ultrasonic tip until the vacuum reaches levels sufficient to neutralize the ultrasonic tip's repulsive energy and once again attract the material. This back-and-forth movement of lens material from the tip inhibits followability (see the section Fluidics and Phacodynamics Terminology, later in this chapter). A reduction in phaco power can diminish chatter by decreasing the stroke length of the tip excursion, thereby reducing forces that push the fragment away from the tip.

Energy Power multiplied by time. Surgeons may reduce the amount of energy released inside the eye by decreasing either the phaco power or the length of time that the phaco power is on. Thus, energy and power are not the same.

Frequency The speed at which the phaco needle moves back and forth. The term *ultrasonic* is used for frequencies above the range of human audibility, or greater than 20,000 Hz. The frequency of phaco handpieces is between 27,000 Hz and 60,000 Hz.

Piezoelectric crystal A type of transducer used in ultrasonic handpieces that transforms electrical energy into mechanical energy. Linear motion is generated when a tuned, highly refined crystal is deformed by the electrical energy supplied by the console.

Power The ability of the phaco needle to vibrate and cavitate the adjacent lens material. Power is noted as a linear percentage of the maximum stroke length of the phaco needle. Phaco power is produced when the foot pedal is depressed to position 3.

Stroke The linear distance that the tip traverses to produce an impact on lens material. In phacoemulsification, the stroke length varies among devices, from 0.05 to 0.10 mm (or 0.002 to 0.004 inches).

Key Concepts and Advances in Phaco Power Delivery

The delivery of phaco power can have both favorable and unfavorable consequences. Certainly, cavitation, shock waves, shear forces, and heat buildup at the tip may all facilitate disassembly of the lens nucleus. However, more power is not necessarily better; the longitudinal stroke of the phaco tip tends to push nuclear fragments away even as the aspiration attracts them, resulting in *chatter*. In addition, heat buildup from the delivery of phaco power may cause wound burns and damage to the corneal endothelium. The goal is to achieve the correct balance of safety and phaco power. Many parameters can be adjusted to deliver phaco power more efficiently and safely. The size and angle of the phaco tip can be altered to increase cutting efficiency. Modes of intermittent rather than continuous phacoemulsification, such as pulse and burst, can also be used. Various mechanical strategies, including torsional and elliptical movement of the phaco tip, may also minimize heat generation.

Phaco tip

Phaco tips vary according to the angle of the tip and the size of the lumen. Phaco tips are available with bevels of 0°, 15°, 30°, 45°, and 60° (see Fig 7-7). End configurations can be round, ellipsoid, bent, or flared. In general, the surgeon chooses the bevel angle of the phaco tip according to personal preference. A tip with a steeper bevel has an oval port with a larger surface area, which can generate more holding force (Fig 7-8) and greater cutting efficiency. The disadvantage of steeper bevels is that the larger opening may be more difficult to occlude to achieve full vacuum.

Pulse and burst

To reduce the total energy delivered to the corneal endothelium, the surgeon may use modes of intermittent rather than continuous phacoemulsification.

Pulsed phacoemulsification involves setting the number of pulses per second while in position 3. The term *pulse* describes an interval of phaco power turned on alternating with an interval during which phaco power is off. The amount of power delivered depends on the foot-pedal excursion in position 3. The delivery of phaco power for only a portion of the cycle reduces repulsion of material by the vibrating tip and improves followability. Duty cycle refers to the ratio of on:off pulses. If the time of "power on" equals the time of "power off," the duty cycle is 50%.

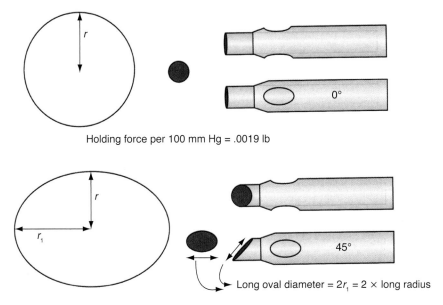

Holding force per 100 mm Hg = .0019 lb

0°

Long oval diameter = $2r_1$ = 2 × long radius

45°

Holding force per 100 mm Hg = .0027 lb

Figure 7-8 Drawing depicting the relationship between the phaco tip bevel and holding force. r = radius of the tip. *(Reprinted with permission from Seibel BS.* Phacodynamics: Mastering the Tools and Techniques of Phacoemulsification Surgery. *3rd ed. Thorofare, NJ: Slack; 1999.)*

Burst-mode phacoemulsification involves delivery of preset power (0%–100%) in single bursts that are separated by decreasing intervals as the foot pedal is depressed through position 3. At the end of the position 3 excursion, the power is no longer delivered in bursts but is continuous. Burst mode allows the tip of the phaco needle to be buried into the lens, an essential step for chopping techniques.

Torsional and elliptical phacoemulsification

Advances in phacoemulsification technology have resulted in reductions in the total amount of phaco energy delivered to achieve emulsification. For example, in torsional phacoemulsification (Ozil Torsional, Alcon, Ft Worth, TX), the piezoelectric crystals of the phaco handpiece produce an oscillatory (torsional) movement, which is amplified by use of a bent Kelman phaco tip. The greater side-to-side movement at the tip allows for greater shearing forces to assist in nucleus disassembly. Another system utilizes a combination of transverse and longitudinal modalities (Ellips FX Technology, Abbott Medical Optics, Abbott Park, IL); the resulting elliptical cutting pattern enhances nucleus emulsification.

Irrigation

The fluid dynamics of phacoemulsification require constant irrigation through the sleeve around the ultrasound tip with some egress of fluid through the incisions. Coaxial irrigation with balanced salt solution cools the phaco tip, preventing heat buildup and consequent damage to adjacent tissue.

Another important purpose of irrigation is maintenance of the anterior chamber during surgery. The surgeon generally adjusts intraocular pressure and anterior chamber depth by changing the height of the irrigation bottle, with gravity providing the force necessary to increase the level of irrigation. In newer phaco machines, a collapsible saline bag is compressed by pressure plates. Sensors on the plates provide continuous feedback, allowing for active control of fluidics and resulting in a more stable anterior chamber.

Some surgeons put additives in the irrigation bottle to maintain pupillary dilation. Others add antibiotics to the bottle as prophylaxis against endophthalmitis (see the section Antimicrobial Prophylaxis, earlier in this chapter).

Lindstrom RL, Loden JC, Walters TR, et al. Intracameral phenylephrine and ketorolac injection (OMS302) for maintenance of intraoperative pupil diameter and reduction of postoperative pain in intraocular lens replacement with phacoemulsification. *Clin Ophthalmol.* 2014;8: 1735–1744.

Fluidics and Phacodynamics Terminology

The following terms are commonly used in the discussion of fluidics and phacodynamics.

Aspiration The withdrawal of fluid and lens material from the eye; produced by depressing the foot pedal to position 2 and continuing in position 3.

Flow rate The flow of fluid through the tubing, measured in milliliters per minute (mL/min). Fluid flow occurs when the phaco tip is not occluded, and the rate helps determine how quickly fragments flow to the phaco tip.

Followability The ability of a fluidic system to attract and hold nuclear or cortical material onto the tip of an ultrasonic or irrigation/aspiration (I/A) handpiece until vacuum forces achieve evacuation.

Occlusion An obstruction of the aspiration port or aspiration tubing. When lens material occludes the tip of the phaco needle, vacuum builds until it reaches the machine's preset value or until the material is evacuated.

Rise time The rate at which vacuum builds once the aspiration port has been occluded. Rise time is related to the aspiration flow rate, which is related to the speed of the aspiration pump (see the section Aspiration Pumps). The faster the aspiration flow rate (or pump speed), the faster is the rise time.

Surge A phenomenon that occurs when a vacuum has built up because of an occlusion and the occlusion is suddenly broken, causing the fluid in the higher-pressure (positive) anterior chamber to rush into the lower-pressure (negative) phaco tip. If the negative surge exceeds the inflow capability of the irrigation line, fluctuations in anterior chamber depth may occur, and the iris or posterior capsule may be drawn into the tip. Changes made in phaco equipment in order to limit surge include higher irrigation, lower vacuum, low-compliance tubing of smaller diameter, a smaller tip, coiled aspiration tubing, and occlusion-mode software. In addition, improvements in software allow automatic modification of aspiration and flow.

Vacuum A parameter measured in millimeters of mercury (mm Hg) or inches of water and defined as the magnitude of negative pressure created in the tubing. Vacuum is generated when the phaco tip is occluded and measures how well particulate material will be held onto it.

Aspiration Pumps

The aspiration system of the phaco machine is a critical element in the performance of various phaco maneuvers. An understanding of this system, therefore, can greatly affect the efficiency of the surgeon's phaco technique. Adjusting the flow rate can help attract nuclear or cortical material onto the distal end of the handpiece. Adjusting vacuum determines how tightly particulate material that has occluded the phaco tip will be grasped. The objectives are to utilize fluidics to maximize phaco efficiency and to grasp nuclear fragments without inadvertently damaging the iris, capsule, or other intraocular tissues.

There are 3 main types of aspiration pumps that are used in phaco machines: peristaltic pumps, diaphragm pumps, and Venturi pumps. A *peristaltic pump* consists of a set of rollers that move along flexible tubing, forcing fluid through the tubing and creating a relative vacuum at the aspiration port of the phaco tip (Fig 7-9). The vacuum response time with this type of pump is relatively rapid; linear control is achieved as the speed of the rollers is increased. Vacuum is flow based and does not build up until the tip is occluded.

A *diaphragm pump* consists of a flexible diaphragm overlying a fluid chamber with 1-way valves at the inlet and outlet. The diaphragm moves out, creating a relative vacuum in the chamber that closes the exit valve, causing the fluid to flow into the chamber. The diaphragm then moves in, increasing the pressure in the chamber and closing the intake valve while opening the exit valve (Fig 7-10). This type of pump system produces a slower rise in vacuum. With continued occlusion of the aspiration port, however, the vacuum will continue to increase in an exponential manner.

A *Venturi pump* (Fig 7-11) creates a vacuum based on the Venturi principle: a flow of gas or fluid across a port creates a vacuum proportional to the rate of flow of the gas. This system produces a rapid, linear rise in vacuum and enables instantaneous venting to the atmosphere, immediately stopping the flow through the port. The vacuum is not flow based and builds according to the machine setting.

In general, all of these pumps are effective. The vacuum rise time (the amount of time required to reach a given level of vacuum) varies among the different pump designs. The latest generation of machines employs continuous feedback sensors that measure flow and make immediate adjustments.

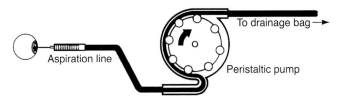

To drainage bag
Aspiration line
Peristaltic pump

Figure 7-9 The peristaltic pump. *(Redrawn with permission from* Practical Phacoemulsification: Proceedings of the Third Annual Workshop. *Montreal, Quebec: Medicopea International; 1991:43–48.)*

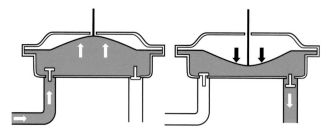

Figure 7-10 The diaphragm pump. A flexible diaphragm overlies a fluid chamber with 1-way valves. The *white arrows* show the influx of fluid as the diaphragm pulls up and the outflow of fluid as the diaphragm pushes down on the chamber. *(Redrawn with permission from* Practical Phacoemulsification: Proceedings of the Third Annual Workshop. *Montreal, Quebec: Medicopea International; 1991:43–48.)*

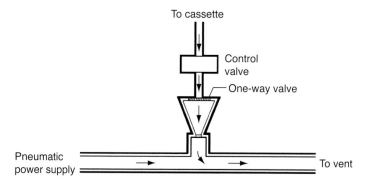

Figure 7-11 The Venturi pump. *(Redrawn with permission from* Practical Phacoemulsification: Proceedings of the Third Annual Workshop. *Montreal, Quebec: Medicopea International; 1991:43–48.)*

Devgan U. Basic principles of phacoemulsification and fluid dynamics. *Focal Points: Clinical Modules for Ophthalmologists.* San Francisco: American Academy of Ophthalmology; 2010, module 8.

Seibel BS. *Phacodynamics: Mastering the Tools and Techniques of Phacoemulsification Surgery.* 4th ed. Thorofare, NJ: Slack; 2005.

Outline of the Phacoemulsification Procedure

Eye Marking and Time-Out

Prior to surgery, a designated member of the surgical team, typically the surgeon, marks the operative eye to prevent errors in surgical site (eg, wrong eye). Standard practice includes using marking pens or stickers to identify the operative eye. Depending on the surgical drape being used, it may be beneficial to place the mark on the cheek or under the eyebrow, rather than on the forehead. In this way, the surgeon can see the identifying mark immediately before placing the surgical drape.

The "time-out" is an opportunity for the surgeon and the rest of the operating room team, including the anesthesiologist and nursing staff, to ensure that everyone is prepared for the correct surgical procedure on the correct eye, with the correct implant. Informa-tion typically reviewed during the time-out includes patient name, patient date of birth, procedure, operative eye, and the type and power of intraocular lens (IOL). Using 2 pa-tient identifiers (eg, name and date of birth) will help prevent errors in cases where 2 patients share the same name. Also, verifying the IOL at this time reduces the risk of implanting an incorrect lens.

Exposure of the Globe

After the anesthesia has been administered and the eye is prepared and draped in sterile fashion (see the section Antimicrobial Prophylaxis, earlier in this chapter, and Fig 7-6), the eyelids are held apart with an eyelid speculum. When selecting the speculum, the surgeon should make sure that it will accommodate the phaco handpiece and other in-struments (Fig 7-12).

The surgeon may choose to be seated superiorly or temporally. This preference may be dictated by the prominence of the patient's brow, the presence of a large pterygium or filtering bleb, or a history of previous ocular surgery. Another factor to consider is the axis of astigmatism, with mild flattening induced at the site of a clear corneal wound.

Paracentesis

The paracentesis incision is used for multiple purposes, including insertion of a second instrument, introduction of intracameral additives, and placement of iris hooks. A small sharp blade, such as a 15° superblade or microvitreoretinal (MVR) blade, is used to cre-ate 1 or 2 small paracentesis incisions placed approximately 2 or 3 clock-hours away from the site where an incision will be made for the phaco handpiece. A straight entry plane is made parallel to the iris or at a slight downward angle. Alternatively, these incisions may be made by femtosecond laser. Once the paracentesis is complete, an OVD is instilled to protect intraocular structures and to give the surgeon more control during creation of the phaco incision.

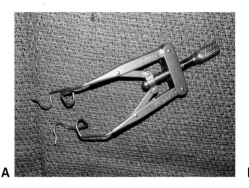
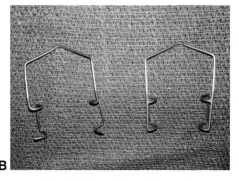

A   **B**

Figure 7-12 **A,** Lieberman speculum. **B,** Open-loop speculum *(left)* and closed-loop wire spec-ulum *(right)*. *(Courtesy of Lisa Park, MD.)*

Clear Corneal Incision

Most phaco surgeons use a clear corneal approach for the main incision (Fig 7-13). These small incisions are typically 2.4–3.2-mm wide, just large enough to accommodate the phaco handpiece and allow for insertion of the IOL. Globe stabilization is important in clear corneal incisions, especially if the procedure is performed with topical anesthesia. Fixation rings, 0.12-mm toothed forceps, or instruments supplying counterpressure can be used to stabilize the globe as the incisions are made.

Various types of corneal phaco incisions, including biplanar and multiplanar incisions, have been described. Regardless of which type of clear corneal incision is used, an important objective is to create a stable, watertight incision in order to minimize the risk of wound leak and endophthalmitis. In the multiplanar technique introduced by David Langerman, a diamond or metal knife is used to create a 0.3-mm-deep groove perpendicular to the corneal surface. Another blade is inserted into the groove, and its tip is then directed tangentially to the corneal surface, creating a tunnel through clear cornea into the anterior chamber. This multiplanar incision architecture usually results in a wound that is watertight.

Another approach is the beveled, biplanar self-sealing incision, as advocated by Shimuzu and Fine. A beveled blade is flattened against the eye, and the tip is used to enter the cornea just anterior to the vascular arcade. The blade is advanced tangentially to the corneal surface until the shoulders of the blade are fully buried in the stroma. The point of the blade is then redirected posteriorly so that the point and the rest of the blade enter

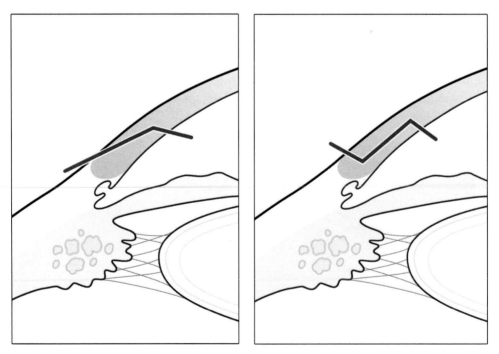

Figure 7-13 Architecture of clear corneal incisions: biplanar *(left)* and triplanar *(right)*. *(Illustration developed by Lisa Park, MD, and rendered by Christine Gralapp.)*

the anterior chamber parallel to the iris. This technique ideally creates a tunneled corneal incision that is watertight.

Beveled, trapezoidal diamond blades have been developed for creating self-sealing clear corneal incisions. Such blades can be advanced in one motion and in one plane, from clear cornea into the anterior chamber. The blade is oriented parallel to the iris, and the tip is placed at the start of the clear cornea, just anterior to the vascular arcade. The blade is tilted up and the heel down so that the blade is angled 10° from the iris plane; it is then advanced into the anterior chamber in one smooth, continuous motion.

Another type of incision is the "near clear" approach, in which the incision begins within the vascular arcade. Proponents of this approach cite better wound closure and a reduced incidence of induced astigmatism. However, slight bleeding may take place during surgery; conjunctival ballooning may occur; and a subconjunctival hemorrhage may be present postoperatively.

Regardless of which type of clear corneal incision is used, the length of the wound should permit optimal visualization and instrument manipulation during phacoemulsification. If the corneal incision is too long, the surgeon may have problems manipulating the phaco tip within the anterior chamber and corneal striae may reduce visibility as the surgeon manipulates the handpiece. If the tunnel is too short, the incision may not seal postoperatively. The phaco tip may also abrade the iris, causing atrophy and possible pupil distortion.

Scleral Tunnel Incision

An alternative to the clear corneal incision is a scleral tunnel incision (Fig 7-14). One advantage of this type of incision is that it creates an internal corneal lip, which may reduce

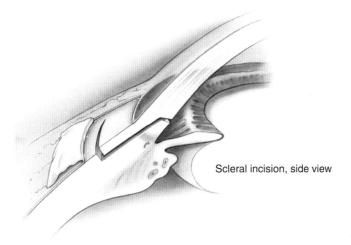

Scleral incision, side view

Figure 7-14 Illustration showing scleral tunnel incision, side view: The initial groove is one-third to one-half of the scleral depth. The incision is traditionally 2–3 mm posterior to the limbus. The tunnel is traditionally dissected past the vascular arcade. A short third plane is made by changing the angle of the blade before entering the anterior chamber. *(Reproduced with permission from Johnson SH. Phacoemulsification. Focal Points: Clinical Modules for Ophthalmologists. San Francisco: American Academy of Ophthalmology; 1994, module 6. Illustration by Christine Gralapp.)*

the incidence of both early and late surgically induced astigmatism. Another advantage may be more-controlled conversion to ECCE, if this becomes necessary.

A limited conjunctival peritomy is created over the intended incision site. The surgeon then clears the overlying Tenon capsule from the sclera and applies light bipolar cautery to achieve hemostasis. Excessive cautery should be avoided because it may cause scleral shrinkage and postoperative astigmatism.

The scleral incision is usually linear, but it may be either curvilinear (smile-shaped, following the limbus, or frown-shaped, following the curve opposite the limbus) or chevron-shaped. After making the incision, the surgeon uses a blade to enter the scleral groove at a depth of half the scleral thickness, dissecting anteriorly into clear cornea just anterior to the vascular arcade, creating a partial-thickness scleral tunnel. If the scleral groove is entered too deeply, the scleral flap will be very thick, and the blade may penetrate the anterior chamber earlier than anticipated, closer to the vascular iris root. If the scleral groove is entered too superficially, the scleral flap will be very thin and prone to tears or buttonholes.

To enter the anterior chamber from beneath the scleral flap, the surgeon uses a keratome sized to match the width of the phaco tip. The keratome is inserted into the corneal stroma until the tip reaches the clear cornea beyond the vascular arcade. The heel of the keratome is elevated, and the tip of the keratome is pointed posteriorly, aiming toward the center of the lens and creating a dimple in the peripheral cornea. The keratome is then slowly advanced in this posterior direction, creating an internal corneal lip as it enters the anterior chamber.

Ernest PH, Neuhann T. Posterior limbal incision. *J Cataract Refract Surg.* 1996;22(1):78–84.

Fine IH. Corneal tunnel incision with a temporal approach. In: Fine IH, Fichman RA, Grabow HB, eds. *Clear-Corneal Cataract Surgery & Topical Anesthesia.* Thorofare, NJ: Slack; 1993:50–51.

Langerman DW. Architectural design of a self-sealing corneal tunnel, single-hinge incision. *J Cataract Refract Surg.* 1994;20(1):84–88.

Continuous Curvilinear Capsulorrhexis

After the incision has been made, the next step is to open the lens capsule. Opening the capsule with a continuous curvilinear capsulorrhexis (CCC) gives the surgeon a wide range of phacoemulsification techniques from which to choose (Fig 7-15).

A CCC resists radial tears that could extend around and open the posterior capsule, setting the stage for complications. In addition, a CCC stabilizes the lens nucleus, allowing maneuvers to disassemble it within the capsular bag and thereby reducing trauma to the corneal endothelium. A CCC also transfers haptic forces circumferentially and helps stabilize and center the lens implant. A CCC sized just smaller than the IOL optic may allow for tighter contact between the posterior surface of the posterior chamber IOL (PCIOL) and the posterior capsule, possibly reducing the incidence of posterior capsule opacification.

The surgeon begins a CCC with a central, radial cut in the anterior capsule by using a cystotome needle or capsulorrhexis forceps with special tips for grasping and tearing.

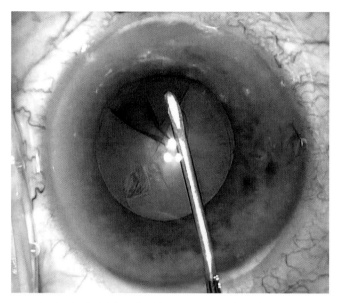

Figure 7-15 A capsulorrhexis is initiated with a puncture into the anterior capsule, which is then extended radially, and a flap turned over. A cystotome or forceps is then used to grasp this flap and tear circumferentially. *(Courtesy of Lisa Park, MD.)*

At the end of the radial cut, the needle is either pushed or pulled in the direction of the desired tear, allowing the anterior capsule to fold over on itself. The surgeon then engages the free edge with either forceps or the cystotome needle, and the flap is carried around in a circular manner (Video 7-1). For maximum control of the size of the capsulotomy, frequent regrasping of the flap near the tear is helpful. An OVD may be added to keep the lens surface flat in order to reduce the likelihood of peripheral extension.

 VIDEO 7-1 Continuous curvilinear capsulorrhexis.
Courtesy of Lisa Park, MD.
Access all Section 11 videos at www.aao.org/bcscvideo_section11.

The tear should not be allowed to turn either inward (which results in a central opening that is too small) or outward (which leads either to an opening that is too large or to extension of the tear to the posterior capsule). An opening that is too small complicates most nucleus disassembly techniques and may contract postoperatively (capsular phimosis). The overlapping anterior capsule is prone to opacification, especially in patients with diabetes mellitus. A capsulorrhexis that is too large may allow the IOL optic or haptic to dislocate anteriorly. For these reasons, many surgeons advocate a size that allows the capsular rim to cover the optic edge. This technique may become increasingly important with the use of premium IOLs, which require a stable position within the eye for optimal refractive results.

If a CCC cannot be completed, conversion to a can-opener capsulotomy is an acceptable strategy (see the appendix, Fig A-1). However, this type of anterior capsulotomy makes hydrodissection, hydrodelineation, and endocapsular phacoemulsification more challenging because of a higher likelihood of posterior capsule extension. A can-opener capsulotomy is performed by using a cystotome or bent 27-gauge needle to create multiple small tears or punctures in the anterior capsule. These are circumferential to the equator and pulled centrally in a clockwise or counterclockwise direction in order to create a complete opening.

Mackool RJ. Capsule stabilization for phacoemulsification. *J Cataract Refract Surg.* 2000; 26(5):629.

Hydrodissection

Hydrodissection is performed to separate the peripheral and posterior cortex from the underlying posterior lens capsule. In addition to loosening the lens-cortex complex, this procedure facilitates nucleus rotation during phacoemulsification and hydrates the peripheral cortex, making it easier to aspirate after nucleus removal.

The surgeon places a bent, blunt-tipped 25- to 30-gauge cannula or flattened hydrodissection cannula attached to a 3–5-mL syringe under the anterior capsule flap. While carefully lifting the capsular flap, the surgeon injects balanced salt solution in a radial direction. Exerting gentle posterior pressure on the nucleus will express posterior fluid and prevent fluid pressure from rupturing the posterior capsule. Gentle irrigation should continue until the surgeon sees a wave of fluid moving under the nucleus and across the red reflex (Video 7-2). In mature cataracts or in cases without a red reflex, careful hydrodissection should continue until nucleus rotation can be performed. Irrigation in the subincisional area may require a right-angled or J-shaped hydrodissection cannula.

 VIDEO 7-2 Hydrodissection.
Courtesy of Linda Tsai, MD.

If the nucleus is displaced into the anterior chamber, it can be reposited into the posterior chamber with injection of OVD and application of slight posterior pressure. Alternatively, a supracapsular phacoemulsification technique may be selected in this situation. Hydrodissection is riskier after a can-opener capsulotomy has been performed, with zonular fibers that are weakened, or in a patient who has a posterior polar cataract.

Hydrodelineation

Some surgeons also inject balanced salt solution into the substance of the nucleus to *hydrodelineate,* or separate, the various layers of the nucleus after hydrodissection. This separates the harder nucleus from the softer epinucleus, which can be left to act as a cushion to protect the underlying posterior capsule. In less brunescent cataracts, a fluid wave can be seen to separate the endonucleus from the epinucleus and produce the "golden ring" sign. In cataracts with a white or densely brunescent nucleus, the epinucleus layer may not be present, making hydrodelineation ineffective.

Nucleus Rotation

If hydrodissection has succeeded in breaking the attachments between peripheral and posterior cortex and the posterior capsule, the surgeon should be able to rotate the nucleus within the capsular bag. Because phacoemulsification techniques are easier to perform when the lens rotates freely, the surgeon should confirm nucleus rotation before proceeding with the procedure. Difficulty in rotation may suggest inadequate hydrodissection.

These maneuvers must be approached with caution in patients with loose zonular fibers. Attempting to rotate the nucleus in such cases will weaken the stability of the capsular bag. Hydrodissection and nucleus rotation may also be avoided in patients with posterior polar cataracts, as adhesions of the lens to the posterior capsule increase the risk of capsular tears or rupture. (See also Chapter 9.)

Nucleus Disassembly and Removal

Most methods of nucleus disassembly and removal consist of several distinct steps; these include sculpting, cracking, chopping, grasping, and emulsifying. With modern phaco machines, all parameters (power levels and intervals of delivery, aspiration flow rate, and vacuum) can be adjusted for each step of the procedure as well as for the density of the cataract, giving the surgeon maximum control of the process.

There are 2 main modes or settings that are used during phacoemulsification: sculpt and segment removal. With the *sculpt* setting, the central nucleus is debulked. This process involves a shaving maneuver in which the tip of the phaco needle is never fully occluded in order to generate minimal vacuum. Thus, the portion of the phaco needle that is in contact with the lens passes through without grabbing, and the lens material can be emulsified and aspirated in a controlled fashion. Sculpting is usually performed with modest vacuum, low aspiration flow, and high phaco power.

The *segment removal* setting is employed once the nucleus has been divided (using one of the techniques described later in this chapter); the resulting fragments are grasped using high vacuum and pulled centrally for emulsification. Full occlusion of the phaco tip is necessary to allow the vacuum to build to the desired level. Once this level has been reached, ultrasound power may be applied. After the nucleus is emulsified, the epinuclear material may be removed with lower flow and aspiration settings with either the phaco handpiece or the I/A instrument (discussed in Irrigation and Aspiration, later in this chapter).

Location of Emulsification

The nucleus may be emulsified at various locations within the eye, including the posterior chamber, iris plane, and anterior chamber. The location determines which techniques are used to emulsify the nucleus.

Posterior chamber

The posterior chamber is a common location for nucleus disassembly and emulsification. Removal of the nucleus at this location is facilitated by hydrodissection and nucleus rotation. The advantages of posterior chamber phacoemulsification include the reduced risk of corneal endothelial trauma and the ability to minimize the size of the capsulorrhexis opening, which is helpful with suboptimal pupil dilation. Disadvantages include an increased risk of complications due to the fact that emulsification takes place closer to the posterior capsule, greater stress placed on the capsule and zonular fibers when the nucleus is being manipulated, and the need for sophisticated methods of nucleus splitting.

Iris plane

When phacoemulsification is performed at the iris plane, one pole of the nucleus is prolapsed anteriorly. Once prolapsed, the nucleus can be manipulated with less stress on the posterior capsule and zonular fibers. Emulsification occurs between the corneal endothelium and the posterior capsule, thereby reducing the risk of damage to either structure.

This location is often suitable for the beginning phaco surgeon and advantageous in patients who have compromised capsular or zonular integrity. In patients with small pupils, this technique permits good visualization and enables safe emulsification. The disadvantages of working at the iris plane include difficulty prolapsing the nucleus and the risk of potential damage to the corneal endothelium if the surgeon emulsifies the nucleus too close to the cornea.

Anterior chamber

This technique involves prolapsing the nucleus through the capsulorrhexis during hydrodissection, which requires a medium to large capsulorrhexis and a relatively soft nucleus. This approach theoretically reduces the stress on the zonular fibers during manipulation of the nucleus. The risks of this technique include a greater chance of aspirating the iris in the phaco tip, as well as damaging the corneal endothelium. However, phacoemulsification in a supracapsular location is a useful technique in certain settings, such as the presence of posterior chamber rupture. Using an OVD to protect the endothelium and minimizing phaco energy are recommended.

Techniques of Nucleus Disassembly

Phaco fracture technique

The most widely used 2-handed technique, developed by Howard Gimbel and John Shepherd and referred to as "divide and conquer nucleofractis," can be effectively applied to all but very soft cataracts.

After adequate hydrodissection and hydrodelineation, continuous ultrasound is used to sculpt a deep central linear groove or trough in the nucleus. Signs that the groove depth is adequate include smoothing of the striations in the groove, brightening of the red reflex in the groove, and sculpting to a depth of 2–3 phaco tip diameters (Fig 7-16).

At this point, the surgeon can either separate the nucleus into 2 pieces (nucleus cracking) or rotate the nucleus 90° and sculpt a perpendicular groove (Video 7-3). The phaco tip and second instrument are then inserted into each groove and spread apart with a cross action or parallel action, thereby achieving complete separation of the pieces (Fig 7-17).

VIDEO 7-3 Nucleus cracking.
Courtesy of Lisa Park, MD.

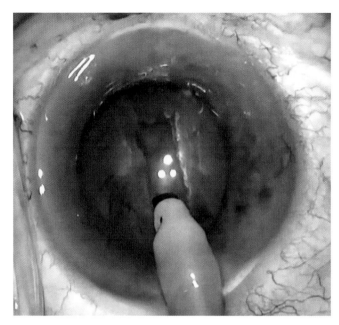

Figure 7-16 A central groove is sculpted under conditions of low vacuum. The ideal groove is deeper centrally to allow for effective cracking of the lens. *(Courtesy of Lisa Park, MD.)*

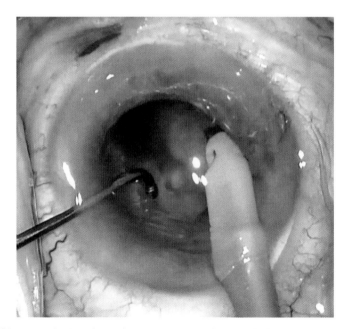

Figure 7-17 Photograph showing 2 instruments used to crack the crystalline lens. These instruments may include the phaco tip and a second instrument through a side port, as shown here. A nucleus cracker or 2 spatulas may also be used to separate the 2 hemispheres. *(Courtesy of Lisa Park, MD.)*

The surgeon can then engage a quadrant using the phaco tip and a segment removal setting. After adequate vacuum is attained, the nuclear quadrant is pulled toward the center of the capsular bag and emulsified. Each quadrant is sequentially removed in the same manner.

Gimbel HV. Divide and conquer nucleofractis phacoemulsification: development and variations. *J Cataract Refract Surg.* 1991;17(3):281–291.

Shepherd JR. In situ fracture. *J Cataract Refract Surg.* 1990;16(4):436–440.

Chopping techniques

The *horizontal phaco chop* technique, originally described by Kunihiro Nagahara, does not entail creation of a central groove but instead makes use of the natural fault lines in the lens nucleus for creation of a fracture plane. After burying the phaco tip in the center of the nucleus by using high vacuum, the surgeon inserts a chopping instrument under the anterior capsule flap, deeply engages the endonucleus in the periphery, and draws it toward the phaco tip, thereby cracking the nucleus into 2 pieces (Video 7-4). This technique requires the surgeon to place the chopper under the capsular rim and around the equatorial nucleus. The phaco tip is then buried in 1 of the nuclear halves, and the surgeon uses the chopping instrument in the same fashion to create multiple small wedges of nucleus for emulsification.

 VIDEO 7-4 Horizontal phaco chop technique. *Courtesy of Lisa Park, MD.*

Paul Koch and L. E. Katzen modified this procedure by sculpting a central groove and then cracking the nucleus into 2 pieces. The resulting heminuclei are then chopped into smaller pieces. This technique, known as *stop and chop,* affords the surgeon more room to manipulate the nuclear pieces in the capsular bag.

Vertical chopping techniques have also been described. After the center of the nucleus is impaled with the phaco tip using high vacuum, the surgeon buries a chopper with a sharp tip within the nucleus, just adjacent to the phaco tip. The phaco tip lifts while the chopper depresses, and the surgeon separates the instruments to complete the chop, which occurs along natural fault lines in the nucleus (Video 7-5).

 VIDEO 7-5 Vertical chop technique. *Courtesy of Lisa Park, MD.*

In practice, either the vertical or the horizontal chopping technique can be used with almost any other strategy for disassembly of the nucleus. Chopping is not effective for soft nuclei, such as pure posterior subcapsular cataracts. Other techniques, such as hydrodelineation and aspiration with minimal phaco power, may be more appropriate in these cases.

Chang DF. *Phaco Chop and Advanced Phaco Techniques: Strategies for Complicated Cataracts.* Thorofare, NJ: Slack; 2013.

Koch PS, Katzen LE. Stop and chop phacoemulsification. *J Cataract Refract Surg.* 1994;20(5): 566–570.

Steinert RF, ed. *Cataract Surgery.* 3rd ed. Philadelphia: Saunders; 2010.

Irrigation and Aspiration

Once phacoemulsification of the nucleus has been completed, a plate of soft epinucleus or transitional cortex may rest on the posterior capsule. The surgeon can use the phaco needle to accomplish I/A without ultrasound; reduced vacuum and flow settings can be employed to aspirate this material from the capsular fornix or posterior capsule.

The I/A system can also be used to remove peripheral cortical material by use of either coaxial or bimanual I/A. With coaxial cortical removal, the port is rotated toward the equator of the lens capsule. The cortical material should be engaged under low vacuum and stripped to the center of the inflated capsular bag. The surgeon rotates the port so that it is fully visible, and the cortex can be aspirated under greater vacuum. This procedure is repeated until all of the cortex is removed. If the surgeon finds it difficult to reach the subincisional cortex, a 45°, right-angled (90°), or U-shaped (180°) aspiration cannula may be useful.

The I/A functions may also be separated using a bimanual technique in which the aspiration port is introduced through the paracentesis incision while irrigation through a second side port maintains the chamber. The instruments may be interchanged as needed (Video 7-6). An advantage of this technique is that it allows the surgeon to more easily reach the subincisional cortex. A disadvantage is that the anterior chamber may become unstable if aspiration outpaces inflow of fluid through the separate handpiece.

VIDEO 7-6   Bimanual irrigation and aspiration of cortex.
Courtesy of Lisa Park, MD.

Cortex resistant to aspiration can be separated from the capsular bag with OVD (ie, viscodissection) to allow easier access with the I/A handpiece. Another strategy is to postpone removal of residual cortex until after implantation of the IOL. The IOL can be rotated within the capsular bag so that the haptics will further loosen the cortex. The surgeon must weigh the benefits of attempting to remove small amounts of residual cortex against the risk of damaging the posterior capsule. Very small amounts of retained fine cortical strands may easily be resorbed postoperatively.

The surgeon may then polish the posterior and/or anterior capsule surface to remove residual lens epithelial cells, which contribute to development of postoperative capsular opacification. Polishing can be accomplished with gentle aspiration using a sandblasted tip with an abrasive surface or a silicone tip. The surgeon must take care to avoid posterior capsule rupture during this maneuver.

Mathey CF, Kohnen TB, Ensikat HJ, Koch HR. Polishing methods for the lens capsule: histology and scanning electron microscopy. *J Cataract Refract Surg.* 1994;20(1): 64–69.

Nishi O. Removal of lens epithelial cells by ultrasound in endocapsular cataract surgery. *Ophthalmic Surg.* 1987;18(8):577–580.

Insertion of the IOL

In uncomplicated cataract surgery, the surgeon's goal is generally to place an IOL into the capsular bag. The surgeon must determine whether the support structures within the eye are adequate to maintain IOL centration and stability. With posterior capsule rupture, sufficient anterior capsule support may allow a PCIOL to be safely placed in the ciliary sulcus. Complete lack of capsular support warrants placement of an anterior chamber or a sutured posterior chamber lens.

In all cases, an OVD is used to fill the capsular bag or expand the ciliary sulcus, stabilize the anterior chamber during IOL insertion, and protect the corneal endothelium from contact with the IOL. The phaco incision must be large enough to accommodate the IOL and inserter; if necessary, the incision may be enlarged after removal of the cataract. For a more detailed discussion of the different types of IOLs that are currently available, see the section IOLs: Historical Perspectives and Lens Modifications, later in this chapter.

Foldable 1-piece IOLs

A foldable 1-piece IOL is loaded into an injector cartridge that has been prefilled with OVD. The cartridge is inserted into a handpiece, which is operated using a manual plunger or screw mechanism. Preloaded IOL injector systems and automated inserters are also now available. The tip of the injector is then introduced into the corneal wound and the IOL inserted, with the first haptic placed carefully into the capsular bag under direct visualization. The trailing haptic is flexed and placed into position, or "dialed in," by rotating it clockwise with slight posterior pressure utilizing either the tip of the injector or a second instrument such as a hook, so that the second haptic slides under the anterior capsule (Video 7-7).

 VIDEO 7-7 Injection of a 1-piece intraocular lens.
Courtesy of Lisa Park, MD.

Foldable 3-piece IOLs

Foldable 3-piece IOLs are generally made of an acrylic optic with polypropylene haptics. These lenses can be placed either into the capsular bag or into the ciliary sulcus using an injector or they can be folded in half and placed through the incision using implant forceps. The optic and trailing haptic are positioned using forceps or by dialing the lens, as described in the preceding section.

Polymethyl methacrylate IOLs

Polymethyl methacrylate (PMMA) IOLs are not foldable and may be safely inserted with standard, fine-tip, smooth forceps. The phaco incision must be widened to accommodate the size of the lens, and the IOL is advanced by first placing the leading haptic into position and then rotating the optic and trailing haptic into place.

Scleral- or iris-fixated posterior chamber IOLs

Several techniques have been described for securing a PCIOL behind the iris when capsular support is inadequate. If the lens is to be sutured to the sclera, polypropylene sutures should be used instead of nylon sutures, because nylon degrades over time and lens dislocation may result. Transscleral polypropylene sutures may be used to secure the IOL haptics in the ciliary sulcus, or the haptics may be sutured to the overlying iris. Alternative techniques have been described whereby the PCIOL haptics are secured via a scleral tunnel, with or without the use of surgical glue.

A scleral-fixated PCIOL is most valuable as an alternative to an anterior chamber IOL (ACIOL) in situations where an angle-supported lens might be problematic, such as when peripheral anterior synechiae are present or there is significant corneal endothelial compromise. Scleral-fixation techniques are more difficult than those used in standard implantation and are associated with a greater risk of complications such as vitreous hemorrhage, lens dislocation, lens tilt, or late endophthalmitis.

Agarwal A, Jacob S, Kumar DA, Agarwal A, Narasimhan S, Agarwal A. Handshake technique for glued intrascleral haptic fixation of a posterior chamber intraocular lens. *J Cataract Refract Surg.* 2013;39(3):317–322.

Anterior chamber IOLs

Modern flexible ACIOLs with 4-point fixation are supported by the anterior chamber angle and considered acceptable for use when implantation in the posterior chamber is not feasible. To determine the appropriate length of the ACIOL, it is common practice to use 1 mm plus the horizontal diameter of the limbus, as measured externally with a caliper ("white to white").

A typical phaco incision must be enlarged with the keratome or with corneal scissors to enable insertion of an ACIOL. The pupil is generally constricted pharmacologically before IOL implantation, and all vitreous should be removed from the anterior chamber. At least one peripheral iridectomy is performed to avoid pupillary block. The anterior chamber depth is stabilized, and the corneal endothelium protected with an OVD. A lens glide may be inserted across the anterior chamber into the distal angle to isolate the iris from the advancing IOL haptic. The surgeon then inserts the IOL, placing its leading haptic into the angle while observing the iris for any indication of distortion. If a glide has been used, it is removed as the IOL is stabilized with forceps. The posterior lip of the incision is gently retracted to allow placement of the trailing haptic in the angle (Video 7-8). Careful inspection should confirm the proper insertion. The pupil will peak toward any area of iris "tuck," and the IOL should be repositioned until the pupil is round and the optic is centered. The surgeon can adjust the ACIOL's position by using a hook to flex the optic toward either angle.

 VIDEO 7-8 Placement of an anterior chamber intraocular lens. *Courtesy of Lisa Park, MD.*

Donaldson KE, Gorscak JJ, Budenz DL, Feuer WJ, Benz MS, Forster RK. Anterior chamber and sutured posterior chamber intraocular lenses in eyes with poor capsular support. *J Cataract Refract Surg.* 2005;31(5):903–909.

Osher RH, Snyder ME, Cionni RJ. Modification of the Siepser slip-knot technique. *J Cataract Refract Surg.* 2005;31(6):1098–1100.

After IOL Insertion

After removing the cataract and inserting the IOL, the surgeon should remove the OVD from the anterior segment to minimize the risk of an increase in postoperative IOP. In an uncomplicated case with the IOL in the capsular bag, the OVD may be removed by inserting the I/A tip behind the optic or pushing the optic posteriorly to prolapse the OVD and allow its aspiration from the anterior chamber. In the setting of capsular rupture or sulcus IOL placement, removal of viscoelastic should be performed with minimal manipulation of the IOL to avoid destabilization.

To produce a slightly firm eye, balanced salt solution is instilled via the paracentesis incision, to re-form the anterior chamber. The main incision is then examined for adequate closure. If the incision leaks, both sides and/or the roof of the corneal tunnel incision can be hydrated with balanced salt solution injected via a syringe with a blunt 25- to 30-gauge irrigating tip. Hydration of the corneal incision causes temporary stromal swelling and increases the wound apposition between the roof and the floor of the tunnel. This anterior–posterior reapproximation, rather than apposition of the external corneal edges, is the critical anatomical feature that determines good wound closure.

With the continuing evolution of techniques for self-sealing incisions and the use of foldable IOLs, many surgeons elect not to suture the incision at the conclusion of a routine case. Long-term results have shown that the small incisions used in modern cataract surgery heal quickly, are relatively stable, and induce minimal astigmatism.

If there is wound leakage, however, the surgeon must be ready to use additional means of closure, including placement of a 10-0 nylon suture that can be removed postoperatively at the slit lamp. Incisions may also be closed with corneal sealants such as adhesives and glues.

IOLs: Historical Perspectives and Lens Modifications

Historical Perspectives

Before 1949, cataract surgery resulted in aphakia, and patients were destined (unless they had high myopia) to wear high-hyperopic spectacles, which were heavy and caused image magnification and distortion of peripheral vision. When they became available, scleral contact lenses and eventually corneal contact lenses were used instead.

The development of modern IOL implantation began in 1949. Harold Ridley, an English ophthalmologist, observed that PMMA fragments from airplane cockpit windshields were well tolerated in the anterior segment of the eyes of injured World War II pilots. After performing an ECCE on a 45-year-old woman, Ridley placed a disc-shaped PMMA lens into the posterior chamber of her eye (Fig 7-18).

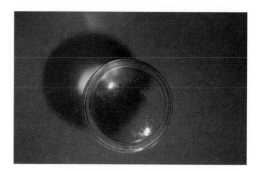

Figure 7-18 Photograph of the original Ridley lens, which was first implanted by Harold Ridley in November 1949. *(Courtesy of Robert C. Drews, MD.)*

Ridley's lens corrected aphakic vision, but a high incidence of postoperative complications such as glaucoma, uveitis, and dislocation caused him to abandon his design. Though frustrated in his attempts, Ridley showed foresight in 3 important areas. First, he constructed his original lens of PMMA in a biconvex design. Second, he used extracapsular surgery for implantation of the lens. Third, he placed the lens in the posterior chamber. Ridley set the stage for a period of advances in cataract surgery that continues to this day, and he received a knighthood for his contributions.

Extracapsular cataract surgery in the 1950s was crude by modern standards and was generally associated with retained lens cortex, which caused fibrosis and adhesions between iris and capsule. ICCE eliminated residual cortical material and became the preferred procedure. Because ICCE was more commonly performed in the early days of lens implantation, IOLs of that period featured optics with loops, struts, or holes for the sutures required for fixation to the iris for support (Fig 7-19).

The anterior chamber angle was an alternate site for IOL support. The first ACIOLs, created by Joaquin Barraquer, Benedetto Strampelli, and others, were crude and ultimately required explantation because of severe inflammatory reactions. Fitting the length of the lens to the width of the anterior chamber was difficult. The IOL length was selected by estimating the anterior chamber width on the basis of the horizontal corneal diameter. Because such estimation is inexact even with modern instruments, complications arose. Oversized lenses and closed-loop IOLs caused pupillary distortion and contributed to development of uveitis-glaucoma-hyphema (UGH) syndrome. ACIOLs that were too short would spin, decenter, and come into contact with the corneal endothelium.

Complications associated with rigid ACIOLs spurred the development of flexible, open-loop ACIOLs with 4-point fixation. These modifications have dramatically improved clinical outcomes and allowed ACIOLs to remain an acceptable treatment option for cases with compromised capsular support or for secondary IOL insertion (Fig 7-20).

Posterior Chamber IOLs and Other Lens Modifications

With advances in cataract surgery technology, the desire to place the IOL in the lens capsule spurred research into posterior chamber lens implantation. Steven Shearing modified a flexible version of a 3-piece IOL with closed loops by opening the loops and inserting the haptics into the capsular bag for posterior chamber placement. Subsequent modifications

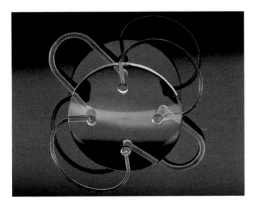

Figure 7-19 Original iris-fixated lens designed by Fyodorov, as made in the United States; 2 looped haptics were placed posterior to the iris, and the optic and 2 opposing loops were placed anterior to the iris. *(Courtesy of Robert C. Drews, MD.)*

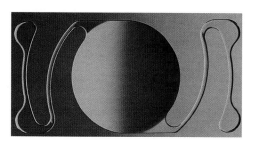

Figure 7-20 Kelman anterior chamber intraocular lens (IOL) with flexible 4-point fixation. *(Courtesy of Robert C. Drews, MD.)*

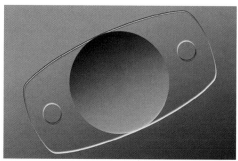

Figure 7-21 Mazzocco plate lens. *(Courtesy of STAAR Surgical.)*

of this lens by Shearing, Jerry Pierce, and Robert Sinskey allowed ECCE with PCIOL implantation to become the standard for modern cataract surgery.

Thomas Mazzocco is generally given credit for developing the foldable IOL (Fig 7-21). His plate-style lens design influenced the design of modern phakic refractive IOLs (see BCSC Section 13, *Refractive Surgery*). Foldable versions of the Shearing-style lens soon followed (Fig 7-22). The obvious advantage of the foldable-lens design is that it allows implantation of the IOL through a small incision. The availability of a small-incision lens influenced many ECCE surgeons' decision to adopt phacoemulsification as their primary technique.

Currently, most IOLs are manufactured from either silicone or acrylic materials. Although both silicone and acrylic are suitable for the majority of patients, silicone IOLs have caused problems in patients who undergo subsequent vitrectomy with silicone oil injection. When cataract surgery is to be performed in a patient who is likely to later require vitreoretinal surgery (eg, a patient with high myopia, proliferative diabetic retinopathy, retinal detachment in the fellow eye, uveitis, or any disease process that may lead to vitreous hemorrhage), an IOL material other than silicone is preferred.

IOL optic geometry has evolved from the earlier plano-convex models to the newer biconvex design. Numerous changes in the shape of the posterior IOL surface and edge design were advanced to reduce late opacification of the posterior lens capsule and to facilitate laser capsulotomy (Fig 7-23). Aspheric platforms to minimize spherical aberrations from the cornea have also been introduced.

Other lens modifications include the incorporation of UV-absorbing chromophores into the IOL material to protect the retina from UV radiation. Blue-blocking IOLs attenuate blue-wavelength light (400–460 nm). Proponents of these IOLs contend that they protect the eye, particularly the macula, from blue-light exposure; however, opponents claim that there is no evidence of benefit from blue-blocking IOLs, and they are concerned that these lenses might create problems with scotopic vision.

Most recently, next-generation or "premium" IOLs have been developed with the goal of addressing presbyopia and astigmatism without the aid of spectacles. These specialized

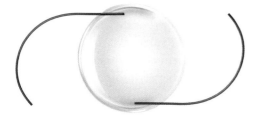

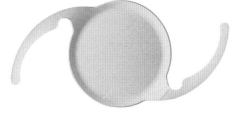

Figure 7-22 Modern 3-piece posterior chamber IOL. *(Courtesy of Bausch + Lomb Surgical.)*

Figure 7-23 Modern single-piece foldable posterior chamber IOL. *(Courtesy of Abbott.)*

designs include multifocal, accommodating, toric, and phakic IOLs. Toric IOLs are discussed in the section Modification of Preexisting Astigmatism, later in this chapter.

Mainster MA, Turner PL. Blue-blocking IOLs decrease photoreception without providing significant photoprotection. *Surv Ophthalmol.* 2010;55(3):272–289.

Tzelikis PF, Akaishi L, Trindade FC, Boteon JE. Spherical aberration and contrast sensitivity in eyes implanted with aspheric and spherical intraocular lenses: a comparative study. *Am J Ophthalmol.* 2008;145(5):827–833.

Multifocal IOLs

The original concept of the multifocal IOL was based on the principle that the pupil tends to constrict for near tasks; thus, the central portion of the lens was designed for near vision and the outer portion for distance vision. A drawback of the original design was that distance correction was not optimal when bright light constricted the pupil. Present versions of these lenses address this problem by having alternating zones for near and distance correction. A combination of geometric optics and diffraction optics can also achieve a multifocal effect. Multiple multifocal lenses have been approved for use in the United States (Fig 7-24).

The advantage of these lenses is an increased range of focus with reduced dependence on spectacles. Disadvantages include a reduction in contrast sensitivity and best-corrected visual acuity (also called *corrected distance visual acuity*) and the presence of glare and halos (see also BCSC Section 3, *Clinical Optics*). The cataract surgeon should spend a sufficient amount of "chair time" counseling patients receiving multifocal IOLs about the intended postoperative visual outcome and limitations; use of a specialized consent process is recommended. Multifocal IOLs require accurate biometry and IOL power calculations,

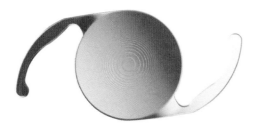

Figure 7-24 Multifocal IOL. See also Figure 6-12 in BCSC Section 3, *Clinical Optics*. *(Courtesy of Alcon.)*

and they may work best when implanted bilaterally and in patients with minimal astigmatism. Patients with hyperopia may be less bothered by some of the visual aberrations associated with these lenses than patients with myopia. The surgeon should be prepared to manage residual postoperative refractive errors with refractive surgery, spectacle or contact lens correction, and possible IOL exchange, preferably performed before capsular fibrosis increases the difficulty of explantation.

Cionni RJ, Osher RH, Snyder ME, Nordlund ML. Visual outcome comparison of unilateral versus bilateral implantation of apodized diffractive multifocal intraocular lenses after cataract extraction: prospective 6-month study. *J Cataract Refract Surg.* 2009;35(6): 1033–1039.

Cochener B, Lafuma A, Khoshnood B, Courouve L, Berdeaux G. Comparison of outcomes with multifocal intraocular lenses: a meta-analysis. *Clin Ophthalmol.* 2011;5:45–56.

Rocha KM, Chalita MR, Souza CE, et al. Postoperative wavefront analysis and contrast sensitivity of a multifocal apodized diffractive IOL (ReSTOR) and three monofocal IOLs. *J Refract Surg.* 2005;21(6):S808–S812.

Zhang F, Sugar A, Jacobsen G, Collins M. Visual function and patient satisfaction: comparison between bilateral diffractive multifocal intraocular lenses and monovision pseudophakia. *J Cataract Refract Surg.* 2011;37(3):446–453.

Accommodating and pseudoaccommodating lenses

In 1996, accommodating and pseudoaccommodating IOLs were introduced. These lenses incorporate various mechanisms designed to move the IOL during accommodative effort through either a single- or dual-optic design (Fig 7-25). Whether these lenses work predominantly by IOL movement or by another mechanism has been an area of debate.

Dhital A, Spalton DJ, Gala KB. Comparison of near vision, intraocular lens movement, and depth of focus with accommodating and monofocal intraocular lenses. *J Cataract Refract Surg.* 2013;39(12):1872–1878.

Menapace R, Findl O, Kriechbaum K, Leydolt-Koeppl C. Accommodating intraocular lenses: a critical review of present and future concepts. *Graefes Arch Clin Exp Ophthalmol.* 2007; 245(4):473–489.

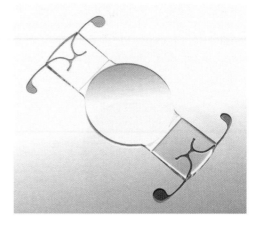

Figure 7-25 Accommodating IOL. *(Courtesy of Bausch + Lomb.)*

Modification of Preexisting Astigmatism

Elimination of spherical refractive error using IOLs and meticulous implant calculations is certainly possible. Increasingly, correction of astigmatism during cataract surgery has become a priority for both patients and surgeons. Multiple intraoperative methods of astigmatism reduction are available.

Because a cataract can induce refractive astigmatism, it is important to compare the preoperative refractive cylinder with keratometry readings. Surgeons should consider that, in aging eyes, there tends to be a natural against-the-rule drift of corneal astigmatism as a result of flattening of the superior meridian.

If the refractive cylinder matches the power and axis obtained by keratometry, cataract-induced astigmatism is negligible, and the refractive cylinder can be considered for reduction through surgery. Surgical planning for refractive cataract surgery includes consideration of incision size and location. A small incision is unlikely to induce much, if any, corneal astigmatism. If a larger incision is required, placing it across the steeper meridian may reduce preoperative astigmatism. The surgeon may also consider use of peripheral corneal relaxing incisions, toric IOLs, and postoperative astigmatism reduction with photorefractive corneal surgery. (See BCSC Section 13, *Refractive Surgery.*)

Gills JP. *A Complete Guide to Astigmatism Management.* Thorofare, NJ: Slack; 2003.

Astigmatic Keratotomy

Astigmatic keratotomy (AK) is a technique dating to the era of refractive keratotomy. Within the cornea, paired incisions are placed at varying distances from the apex of the steepest corneal meridian so as to decrease the curvature of that meridian and increase the curvature of the meridian 90° away (a technique known as *coupling*). Glare from the incisional scar is a potential problem for the cataract surgical patient, for whom postoperative quality of vision is paramount. Any infection near the center of the cornea has serious consequences. For these reasons, AK has largely been supplanted by limbal relaxing incisions.

Limbal Relaxing Incisions

Limbal relaxing incisions (LRIs), which might more accurately be called peripheral corneal relaxing incisions, have been advocated as an effective method for reducing 0.50–3.00 diopters (D) of astigmatism.

The 6- and 12-o'clock meridians are marked with the patient sitting upright. Marks are made at the limbus with either a sterile skin marker or another technique, such as use of a 25-gauge needle in the corneal epithelium. The steep meridian is then identified with these landmarks or other natural landmarks, if they exist. An incision is made at the limbus circumferentially across the steep meridian. One or more incisions are made depending on the surgeon's choice of nomogram. Some surgeons place the cataract incision within the LRI; others prefer to use a separate location. Use of the femtosecond laser to make incisions prior to cataract surgery shows promise for increasing precision and reproducibility. LRIs may also be done postoperatively in an office setting.

Budak K, Freidman NJ, Koch DD. Limbal relaxing incisions with cataract surgery. *J Cataract Refract Surg.* 1998;24(4):503–508.

Nichamin LD. Opposite clear corneal incisions. *J Cataract Refract Surg.* 2001;27(1):7–8.

Palanker DV, Blumenkranz MS, Andersen D, et al. Femtosecond laser-assisted cataract surgery with integrated optical coherence tomography. *Sci Transl Med.* 2010;2(58):58ra85.

Toric IOLs

Toric IOLs are designed to correct astigmatism without corneal incisions, which helps avoid additional incisional complications. The disadvantages of toric IOLs relate to possible lens rotation away from the desired axis.

Careful preoperative corneal measurements and calculations using a toric calculator are essential. To determine the power of the toric IOL, the surgeon must accurately measure the amount of corneal astigmatism, as total refractive astigmatism may include a lenticular component.

Preoperatively, the surgeon marks the 0°, 90°, and 180° axes on the cornea with the patient in the upright position to take into account possible torsional rotation of the eye in the supine position. Either prior to the start of surgery or once the cataract has been removed, the surgeon marks the predetermined axis for lens alignment on the cornea, using the reference marks for accuracy. The IOL is then inserted and rotated carefully into position within the capsular bag.

Intraoperative wavefront aberrometry is an innovation that may assist in more accurate IOL selection and placement. This technology uses infrared (IR) light and interferometry both to obtain an aphakic refraction as soon as the cataract has been removed (while the patient is on the operating table) and to confirm proper alignment of a toric IOL. This process allows the surgeon either to rotate the lens to minimize astigmatism or to exchange it immediately if the power is not accurate.

Unintentional postoperative rotation may be more likely when the IOL is implanted in a larger capsular bag. Each degree of rotation reduces the effect of astigmatism correction by approximately 3% and may induce higher-order aberrations, although a minor misalignment may not be clinically appreciated. If necessary, a second procedure to rotate the lens to the correct axis should be done early in the postoperative period, before complete capsular fixation of the lens occurs.

Ahmed II, Rocha G, Slomovic AR, et al; Canadian Toric Study Group. Visual function and patient experience after bilateral implantation of toric intraocular lenses. *J Cataract Refract Surg.* 2010;36(4):609–616.

Holland E, Lane S, Horn JD, Ernest P, Arleo R, Miller KM. The AcrySof Toric intraocular lens in subjects with cataracts and corneal astigmatism: a randomized, subject-masked, parallel-group, 1-year study. *Ophthalmology.* 2010;117(11):2104–2111.

Huelle JO, Katz T, Druchkiv V, et al. First clinical results on the feasibility, quality and reproducibility of aberrometry-based intraoperative refraction during cataract surgery. *Br J Ophthalmol.* 2014;98(11):1484–1491.

Alternative Technologies for Cataract Extraction

Laser Photolysis

Since the advent of phacoemulsification, alternative technologies have been developed to facilitate cataract extraction. The first laser system was approved by the US Food and Drug Administration (FDA) in 2000. The Dodick Photolysis system, a Q-switched Nd:YAG system (A.R.C. Laser Corp, Salt Lake City, UT), generates laser shock waves at 200–400 ns that strike a titanium target at the end of the aspirating handpiece, thereby breaking up the lens nucleus.

Fluid-Based Phacolysis

In 2003, the AquaLase liquefaction device was introduced (Alcon, Ft Worth, TX). This system generates pulses of heated balanced salt solution for liquefaction and removal of lens material.

Femtosecond Laser Cataract Extraction

In 2010, the US FDA approved femtosecond lasers for cataract extraction. Well known to refractive surgeons, these Nd:glass lasers generate focused, ultrashort pulses (10^{-15} s) at a wavelength of 1053 nm (in the near-IR region), creating cavitation bubbles within the tissues in a process known as photodisruption. Femtosecond laser technology virtually eliminates collateral damage and can therefore be used to dissect tissue on a microscopic scale, enabling creation of corneal incisions and capsulotomies, as well as subsequent lens disassembly.

Currently, 4 femtosecond laser technology platforms for cataract surgery are commercially available in the United States: Catalys (Abbott Medical Optics, Santa Ana, CA), LenSx (Alcon Laboratories, Fort Worth, TX), Lensar (LENSAR, Orlando, FL), and Victus (Bausch + Lomb, Bridgewater, NJ).

Prior to surgery, parameters such as the location of wounds and arcuate incisions are entered into the system's computer. For the capsulotomy, the intended size and centration method are selected. For lens fragmentation, the systems offer a choice of segmentation in quadrants, sextants, or other geometric patterns.

After the eye is dilated, the patient is positioned and secured in the supine position. A suction ring is placed on the eye and filled with balanced salt solution. The ring is then connected to the laser lens unit. After the ring system is placed on the eye and "docking" has been confirmed, the system automatically measures the dimensions of the anterior chamber and the lens with 3-dimensional spectral-domain optical coherence tomography (SD-OCT) or Scheimpflug imaging, mapping the ocular surfaces and creating laser exclusion zones. The surgeon then activates the femtosecond laser by depressing the foot pedal. Focal photodisruption creates the previously determined capsulotomy, corneal incisions, and lens fragmentation grid patterns.

During lens fragmentation, the gas released from the cavitation bubbles creates a pneumodissection effect, which separates the crystalline lens along the natural lamellar structure, reducing the need for hydrodissection and occasionally creating cubes of softened lens. This part of the procedure takes approximately 30–60 seconds.

After the laser portion of the procedure is finished, the ring system is released and removed from the eye. Some surgeons instill additional dilating eyedrops at this point to address possible laser-induced miosis.

The patient is then positioned beneath the operating microscope for lens removal using phacoemulsification. The surgeon must first verify that the capsulotomy is complete and carefully remove the anterior capsule with forceps before proceeding with nucleus removal.

Complications related to femtosecond laser–assisted cataract surgery may include subconjunctival hemorrhage due to use of the suction ring; incomplete capsulotomy, which may lead to a radial capsular tear; and buildup of gas bubbles within the capsular bag, which could lead to posterior capsule rupture, particularly in the setting of aggressive hydrodissection.

Since the femtosecond laser was introduced into cataract surgery, its utility has been intensely debated within the ophthalmological community. Proponents of this approach extol its precision, reproducibility, and safety. Those who doubt its merits usually cite the higher costs involved and point out that similar results can be achieved by small-incision phacoemulsification as it is currently practiced.

Outcomes of Cataract Surgery

Contemporary cataract surgery has an excellent success rate in both improving visual acuity and enhancing subjective visual function. More than 90% of otherwise healthy eyes achieve a best-corrected visual acuity of 20/40 or better after surgery. The rate of achieving a postoperative visual acuity of 20/40 or better for all eyes has been reported to be 85%–89% when eyes with comorbid conditions such as diabetic retinopathy, glaucoma, and age-related macular degeneration are included.

Visual acuity is only one measure of the functional success of cataract surgery. Research tools have been developed to assess how cataract progression and cataract surgery affect visual function (see Chapter 6). Prospective studies using these tools show that patients who undergo cataract surgery have significant improvement in many quality-of-life parameters, including performance of community and home activities, number of falls, mental health, driving ability, and life satisfaction.

Gray CS, Karimova G, Hildreth AJ, Crabtree L, Allen D, O'Connell JE. Recovery of visual and functional disability following cataract surgery in older people: Sunderland Cataract Study. *J Cataract Refract Surg.* 2006;32(1):60–66.

Harwood RH, Foss AJ, Osborn F, Gregson RM, Zaman A, Masud T. Falls and health status in elderly women following first eye cataract surgery: a randomised controlled trial. *Br J Ophthalmol.* 2005;89(1):53–59.

Ishii K, Kabata T, Oshika T. The impact of cataract surgery on cognitive impairment and depressive mental status in elderly patients. *Am J Ophthalmol.* 2008;146(3):404–409.

CHAPTER 8

Complications of Cataract Surgery

Complications of cataract surgery vary in timing as well as scope. Undesirable consequences of surgery may occur intraoperatively or postoperatively. Many large-scale peer-reviewed studies of cataract surgery complications contain data from large-incision extracapsular surgery or from procedures performed with earlier phacoemulsification technology. Studies show that the incidence of severe adverse events after cataract surgery, including endophthalmitis, suprachoroidal hemorrhage, and retinal detachment, has declined over the past 2 decades.

Fortunately, complications resulting in loss of vision are rare with modern surgical techniques and technology in the hands of experienced cataract surgeons. The most common serious *intraoperative* complication of phacoemulsification is posterior capsule rupture (reported in 1.5%–3.5% of cases). Common *postoperative* complications include posterior capsule opacification, corneal edema (reported in 0.03%–5.18% of cases), clinically apparent cystoid macular edema (CME) (1.2%–3.5% of cases), and retained lens fragments (0.45%–1.70% of cases). The incidence of retinal detachment in the first postoperative year averages approximately 0.7%; that of endophthalmitis, 0.04%–0.20%; and that of intraocular lens (IOL) dislocation, 0.19%–1.10%.

American Academy of Ophthalmology Cataract/Anterior Segment Panel. Preferred Practice Pattern Guidelines. *Cataract in the Adult Eye*. San Francisco: American Academy of Ophthalmology; 2011. Available at www.aao.org/ppp.

Greenberg PB, Tseng VL, Wu WC, et al. Prevalence and predictors of ocular complications associated with cataract surgery in United States veterans. *Ophthalmology.* 2011;118(3): 507–514.

Schmier JK, Halpern MT, Covert DW, Lau EC, Robin AL. Evaluation of Medicare costs of endophthalmitis among patients after cataract surgery. *Ophthalmology.* 2007;114(6): 1094–1099.

Stein JD. Serious adverse events after cataract surgery. *Curr Opin Ophthalmol.* 2012;23(3): 219–225.

Stein JD, Grossman DS, Mundy KM, Sugar A, Sloan FA. Severe adverse events after cataract surgery among Medicare beneficiaries. *Ophthalmology.* 2011;118(9):1716–1723.

Steinert RF, ed. *Cataract Surgery.* 3rd ed. Philadelphia: Saunders; 2010.

Corneal Complications

Corneal Edema

Stromal and/or epithelial edema may occur in the immediate postoperative period. The incidence is higher in eyes with preexisting corneal endothelial dysfunction such as Fuchs dystrophy. Edema is usually caused by a combination of mechanical trauma, prolonged surgery, chemical injury, inflammation, or elevated intraocular pressure (IOP), resulting in acute endothelial decompensation with an increase in corneal thickness (Table 8-1).

Table 8-1 Principal Causes of Corneal Edema After Cataract Surgery

Surgical trauma
   Mechanical energy from phacoemulsification
   Instruments
   Intraocular lens (IOL)
   Irrigating solutions
   Lens fragments
   Prior or prolonged intraocular surgery

Corneal endothelial disease
   Fuchs dystrophy
   Low endothelial cell density

Chemical injury
   Toxic anterior segment syndrome
   Preservatives in intraocular solutions
   Residual toxic chemicals on instruments (eg, detergents, dried solutions)
   Improper concentrations of intraocular solutions (eg, antibiotics, anesthetics, irrigating solutions)
      Osmotic damage
      Direct toxicity

IOL related
   IOL–endothelial touch
   Uveitis-glaucoma-hyphema syndrome
   Rigid anterior chamber IOL (chronic inflammation?)

Endothelial contact
   Flat chamber centrally
      Wound leak
      Ciliary block (aqueous misdirection)
      Suprachoroidal effusion or hemorrhage
   Flat chamber peripherally
      Pupillary block
      Iris bombé
   Vitreous touch

Descemet membrane detachment

Late trauma from retained foreign material
   Nuclear fragments
   Particulate matter

Elevated intraocular pressure

Inflammation

Membranous ingrowth
   Epithelial or fibrous ingrowth
   Endothelial proliferation

Brown-McLean syndrome

Adapted with permission from Steinert RF. *Cataract Surgery.* 3rd ed. Philadelphia: Saunders; 2010:596.

Toxic substances inadvertently introduced into the anterior chamber can cause acute endothelial dysfunction with diffuse corneal edema referred to as *toxic anterior segment syndrome* (*TASS;* discussed later in this chapter). Late postoperative focal corneal edema may occur because of small nuclear fragments retained in the anterior chamber angle. These fragments may be noticed on initial postoperative examinations, or they may be identified up to years later if they migrate into the anterior chamber from a secluded location in the posterior chamber.

The ophthalmologist must thoroughly examine the eye to identify factors that may cause or exacerbate edema. If epithelial edema is present in the face of a compact stroma immediately after surgery, it is likely due to elevated IOP with an intact endothelium. Lowering IOP medically or via aqueous release from the paracentesis site often results in rapid resolution of epithelial edema in these cases. As a rule, if the corneal periphery is clear, the corneal edema will resolve with time. Edema from surgical trauma generally resolves completely within 4–6 weeks of surgery. Corneal edema that persists after 3 months usually does not clear. Significant chronic corneal edema from loss of endothelial cells results in bullous keratopathy (Fig 8-1), which is associated with reduced vision, ocular irritation, foreign-body sensation, epiphora, and occasionally infectious keratitis.

In its early stages, corneal edema after cataract surgery can be managed with topical hyperosmotic agents, corticosteroids, and/or aqueous suppressants, if indicated. A bandage (therapeutic) contact lens may be used, if necessary. Over time, subepithelial scarring may develop, resulting in a decrease in bullae formation and discomfort. Decreased vision, recurrent keratitis, and pain are possible indications for endothelial or penetrating keratoplasty. Endothelial keratoplasty has been very successful in restoring clear corneas and improving vision. Bullae and pain associated with bullous keratopathy may be alleviated with phototherapeutic keratectomy, cautery of Bowman membrane, anterior stromal micropuncture, or corneal crosslinking (not approved by the US Food and Drug Administration). For the eye with little or no visual potential, when comfort is the primary goal, a Gundersen conjunctival flap or an amniotic membrane graft is an option; neither of

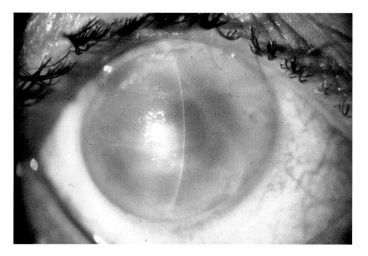

Figure 8-1 Pseudophakic bullous keratopathy. *(Courtesy of Karla J. Johns, MD.)*

these carries the greater risks of endothelial or penetrating keratoplasty. (See also BCSC Section 8, *External Disease and Cornea.*)

Brown-McLean syndrome

Brown-McLean syndrome is a clinical condition of unknown etiology that occurs following cataract surgery and is characterized by peripheral corneal edema with a clear central cornea. The condition occurs most frequently following intracapsular cataract surgery, but it has also been reported following extracapsular surgery and phacoemulsification. The edema usually starts inferiorly and progresses circumferentially; the central 5–7-mm zone of the cornea is typically not involved. Central cornea guttae frequently appear, and punctate brown pigment on the endothelium often underlies the edematous areas. In rare cases, Brown-McLean syndrome progresses to clinically significant central corneal edema.

Vitreocorneal adherence and persistent corneal edema

Vitreocorneal touch or adherence may contribute to persistent corneal edema after cataract surgery complicated by vitreous prolapse. Removing all vitreous from the anterior chamber during complicated cataract surgery decreases the risk of corneal edema and retinal detachment. If vitreous prolapse with corneal touch or incarceration in the wound is recognized postoperatively and corneal edema or CME develops, an anterior vitrectomy or Nd:YAG laser vitreolysis may be indicated. In more advanced cases with prolonged corneal edema, penetrating or endothelial keratoplasty combined with vitrectomy may be indicated.

Incision and Wound Complications

Proper incision construction and closure are critical in reducing intraoperative and postoperative complications. Scleral, limbal, or corneal wound strength is only 10% of normal tissue strength at 1 week, increasing to only 40% by 8 weeks and 75%–80% of its original strength by 2 years. There is concern that the increased use of sutureless clear corneal incisions may be responsible for an increased incidence of postoperative wound leakage and subsequent greater risk of endophthalmitis.

Signs of wound leakage include decreased vision, hypotony, corneal striae, shallow anterior chamber, hyphema, choroidal folds, choroidal effusion, macular edema, and optic nerve edema. A Seidel test, ultrasound biomicroscopy, or anterior segment optical coherence tomography (OCT) may help diagnose or confirm subtle cases. Management of wound leaks depends on their etiology, timing, and severity. Small leaks in the early postoperative period may be asymptomatic and self-limited. Medical treatment may include prophylactic topical antibiotics, cycloplegia, aqueous inhibitors, patching, decreasing or stopping corticosteroid therapy, or a collagen shield or bandage contact lens. In more serious cases with persistent shallowing of the anterior chamber, iris prolapse, prolonged hypotony, choroidal effusion, or macular edema, surgical repair is indicated. Suturing the wound is usually sufficient, but an amniotic membrane graft or tissue adhesives such as cyanoacrylate or hydrogel glue may be used.

A wound leak under a conjunctival flap may lead to an inadvertent filtering bleb. Over time, the fistula may epithelialize, become resistant to medical management, and require surgical intervention. Efforts to promote wound healing and cicatrization of the bleb include cryotherapy, diathermy, chemical cauterization with trichloroacetic acid, or injection of an autologous blood patch. In chronic cases, it may be necessary to excise the bleb/conjunctiva and search for a fistula, which should be scraped free of invading epithelium or excised and covered, if necessary, with a scleral patch graft followed by resuturing of the wound. Tenon capsule and conjunctiva should be used to cover the exposed sclera.

Thermal wound burns

Thermal injury to the incision may result in whitening of the corneal tissue, contraction, and wound gape. During phacoemulsification, heat may be transferred from the needle to the cornea because of inadequate cooling of the phaco tip. This can result from an insufficient inflow of coaxial irrigation fluid or from occlusion of outflow at the phaco tip or aspiration line by an ophthalmic viscosurgical device (OVD) or lens material. This complication is more common with dispersive OVD and increased lens density. Bimanual small-incision surgery raises the risk, as the phaco needle is in direct contact with the cornea without an irrigating jacket.

Friction produces heat and thereby causes the corneal collagen to contract at a temperature of 60°C or higher, subsequently distorting the incision. If the distortion is significant, wound gape may occur with associated leakage. These incisions are not usually self-sealing, and they require suturing, a sliding scleral flap, or patch grafts for adequate closure.

Wound dehiscence or rupture

Postoperative wound dehiscence may be spontaneous or secondary to trauma. The severity depends on the size and integrity of the wound and the degree of healing, which may be affected by the use of corticosteroids or the presence of systemic disease that alters collagen metabolism. The trend toward smaller incisions has decreased the occurrence of wound dehiscence. Traumatic wound rupture is often accompanied by extrusion of intraocular contents and almost always requires surgical repair.

Descemet Membrane Detachment

Descemet membrane detachment results in stromal swelling and epithelial bullae localized in the area of detachment. This complication can occur when an instrument or IOL is introduced through the incision or when fluid or an OVD is inadvertently injected between the Descemet membrane and the corneal stroma. Small detachments may resolve spontaneously. Otherwise, they may be reattached with air or an expansile gas (eg, sulfur hexafluoride [SF_6] or perfluoropropane [C_3F_8]) tamponade in the anterior chamber. Larger detachments can be sutured back into place under gas or an OVD. These cases should be referred to a surgeon familiar with these techniques.

Induced Astigmatism

Localized change in corneal curvature may result from corneal burns produced by the phaco tip or, more commonly, from surgical incisions. Most well-constructed peripheral corneal, limbal, or scleral incisions less than 3 mm in length will induce less than 1.00 D of astigmatism, usually flattening in the axis of the incision. Larger incisions closer to the corneal apex or those that require suture closure are more likely to induce astigmatism. Tight radial sutures may cause steepened corneal curvature in the axis of the suture. The astigmatism induced by larger sutured incisions, such as those used in intracapsular cataract extraction (ICCE), extracapsular cataract extraction (ECCE), or secondary IOL implantation, may decrease by several diopters over time as the sutures dissolve or relax, making suture removal unnecessary. If removal is needed to modulate astigmatism, it is preferable to wait 6–8 weeks postoperatively. Sutures may be cut at the slit lamp with a blade or lysed by an argon or diode laser. If more than 1 suture is to be removed, it is preferable to cut adjacent sutures in a series of visits rather than all at once. Removal of too many sutures too early in the postoperative period may result in either significant corneal flattening in the axis of the incision or wound dehiscence.

Corneal Melting

Keratolysis, or sterile melting of the cornea, may occur following cataract extraction. It is most frequently associated with preexisting tear film abnormalities resulting from keratoconjunctivitis sicca (KCS), Sjögren syndrome, or autoimmune diseases such as rheumatoid arthritis. Keratitis may be exacerbated by the chemical or mechanical stress of surgery or the topical medications used perioperatively. The frequent perioperative use of nonpreserved topical lubricants, punctal plug placement, or lateral tarsorrhaphy performed at the time of surgery may be considered to lessen the morbidity in eyes with preexisting tear film abnormalities.

Stromal melting has been reported with the postoperative use of topical diclofenac and other nonsteroidal anti-inflammatory drugs (NSAIDs). The melting may be due in part to the epithelial toxicity and hypoesthesia that these drugs can induce. Stromal melting is more likely to occur in patients with KCS, systemic autoimmune disease, or collagen vascular disease.

Persistent epithelial defects accompanied by stromal dissolution require intensive treatment with nonpreserved topical lubricants. Use of topical medications, particularly preserved medications, should be minimized to reduce their toxic effect on the corneal epithelium. Additional treatment modalities to encourage epithelialization and to arrest stromal melting include punctal occlusion, bandage contact lenses, tarsorrhaphy, autologous serum eyedrops, collagenase inhibitors such as acetylcysteine 10% or hydroxyprogesterone 1%, and systemic matrix metalloproteinase inhibitors such as doxycycline. The prophylactic use of topical antibiotics must be monitored closely. After a week's application, many topical antibiotics begin to cause secondary toxic effects that may inhibit epithelial healing. If the disease continues to progress despite medical therapy, an amniotic membrane graft or lamellar or penetrating keratoplasty should be considered. Corneal melting may recur even with grafted tissue. For the treatment of any underlying autoimmune disease, systemic immunosuppressive therapy may be necessary.

Other Anterior Segment Complications

Epithelial or Fibrous Ingrowth

Epithelial ingrowth (or *downgrowth*) is a rare complication of intraocular surgery. This condition is characterized by the growth of epithelium intraocularly following trauma or a surgical incision and by proliferation over the corneal endothelium, trabecular meshwork, and/or iris surfaces. Epithelial cells introduced into the anterior chamber during surgery may adhere to intraocular structures and proliferate as a cellular mass or membrane. Alternatively, a sheet of epithelium from the ocular surface may grow through a wound or incision. Signs of epithelial ingrowth include elevated IOP, clumps of cells floating in the anterior chamber, a grayish retrocorneal membrane (usually with overlying corneal edema), an abnormal iris surface, and pupillary distortion. The elevated IOP may be due to outflow obstruction caused by growth of the epithelial membrane over the trabecular meshwork or by epithelial cells clogging the meshwork. Argon laser burns applied to the membrane on the iris surface will appear white if epithelial cells are present, which helps confirm the diagnosis.

Fibrous ingrowth is more prevalent than epithelial ingrowth. Fibrovascular tissue, rather than epithelial cells alone, proliferates from a penetrating wound. Fibrous ingrowth progresses more slowly than epithelial ingrowth and may be self-limited. It is a common cause of corneal graft failure and may result in formation of peripheral anterior synechiae (PAS) and secondary angle-closure glaucoma.

Risk factors for both epithelial and fibrous ingrowth include trauma, prolonged inflammation, wound dehiscence, delayed wound closure, vitreous incarceration, and Descemet membrane tears. No treatment for these conditions has been found to be uniformly successful. Many surgical procedures, including membrane excision and fistula repair, have been suggested. Local application of cryotherapy or of 5-fluorouracil has been reported to be effective. Medical therapy for secondary glaucoma may be indicated. However, the IOP is often difficult to control, and filtering procedures or tube shunt implantation may be necessary.

Toxic Anterior Segment Syndrome

Toxic anterior segment syndrome (TASS) is an acute sterile postoperative inflammation. The symptoms and signs of TASS may mimic those of infectious endophthalmitis and include photophobia, severe reduction in visual acuity, corneal edema, and marked anterior chamber reaction, occasionally with hypopyon. TASS presents within hours of surgery, whereas acute infectious endophthalmitis typically develops 2–7 days postoperatively. Other potentially distinguishing features of TASS include diffuse, limbus-to-limbus corneal edema; anterior chamber fibrinous exudate; a dilated, irregular, or nonreactive pupil; and elevated IOP. The pathologic changes are limited to the anterior chamber. Pain is typically much milder than that experienced with an infection. If endophthalmitis is suspected, diagnostic and therapeutic interventions (described later in this chapter) should be undertaken. Treatment of TASS consists of use of intensive topical corticosteroids until the inflammation subsides. A brief course of systemic corticosteroids may be beneficial. Frequent follow-up is necessary to monitor IOP and to reassess for signs of bacterial infection.

TASS is thought to be caused by the inadvertent introduction of a substance toxic to the corneal endothelium or uvea. Subconjunctival antibiotic injections and topical ophthalmic ointments applied with patching have been reported to enter the anterior chamber through corneoscleral incisions. Skin cleansers containing chlorhexidine gluconate have been reported to cause irreversible corneal edema and opacification if they come into contact with the endothelium. Clusters of TASS due to irrigation fluids tainted with bacterial endotoxin have been reported. Other possible causes of TASS include improperly cleaned surgical instruments; surgical glove residue or talc on instruments or IOLs; use of a denatured OVD; substitution of sterile water for balanced salt solution; or the intraocular use of inappropriate irrigating solutions, antibiotics, or anesthetics. All solutions used intracamerally should ideally be free of stabilizers and preservatives and buffered to physiologic osmolarity and pH. The risk of TASS is higher with reusable irrigation/aspiration (I/A) handpieces, cannulas, or irrigation tubing, as residue of detergents, enzymatic cleaners, or OVD may be present. The risk of TASS can be reduced by careful cleaning, rinsing, and air-drying of reusable cannulas; by use of disposable instrumentation; and by avoiding the intraocular use of any nonphysiologic or preserved solutions.

Bodnar Z, Clouser S, Mamalis N. Toxic anterior segment syndrome: update on the most common causes. *J Cataract Refract Surg.* 2012;38(11):1902–1910.

Mamalis N. Toxic anterior segment syndrome (TASS). *Focal Points: Clinical Modules for Ophthalmologists.* San Francisco: American Academy of Ophthalmology; 2009, module 10.

Mamalis N, Edelhauser HF, Dawson DG, Chew J, LeBoyer RM, Werner L. Toxic anterior segment syndrome. *J Cataract Refract Surg.* 2006;32(2):324–333.

Shallow or Flat Anterior Chamber

Intraoperative

During ECCE or phacoemulsification, the anterior chamber may become shallow because of inadequate infusion, leakage through an oversized incision, external pressure on the globe, "positive vitreous pressure," fluid misdirection syndrome, suprachoroidal effusion, or suprachoroidal hemorrhage. If the reason for loss of normal chamber depth is not apparent, the surgeon should first reduce aspiration, raise the infusion bottle height, and check the incision. If the incision is too large, the surgeon may partially suture it in order to keep the chamber formed. External pressure on the globe can be relieved by readjusting the surgical drapes or the eyelid speculum. "Positive vitreous pressure," or forward displacement of the lens–iris diaphragm, occurs more commonly in obese or thick-necked patients, in patients with pulmonary disease such as chronic obstructive pulmonary disease (COPD), and in patients experiencing a level of anxiety or discomfort that may lead them to squeeze their eyelids or perform a Valsalva maneuver. Placing obese patients in a reverse Trendelenburg position may be useful. Intravenous mannitol can be used to reduce the vitreous volume and deepen the anterior chamber in selected cases.

If the reason for the loss of anterior chamber depth or elevated IOP is unknown, the surgeon should check the red reflex to evaluate the possibility of a suprachoroidal hemorrhage or effusion. In these situations, the eye typically becomes very firm, and the patient becomes agitated and reports having pain. To confirm this diagnosis, the surgeon should examine the fundus with an indirect ophthalmoscope or fundus lens. If the hemorrhage or effusion is significant, the incisions should be closed and the operation postponed until the pressure has decreased. (See the section Suprachoroidal Effusion or Hemorrhage, later in this chapter, and BCSC Section 12, *Retina and Vitreous.*)

During phacoemulsification or irrigation/aspiration, the anterior chamber may become shallow and the lens or posterior capsule may bulge anteriorly because of *posterior fluid misdirection syndrome.* Irrigation fluid infused into the anterior chamber may be misdirected into the vitreous cavity through intact zonular fibers or through a zonular or capsular tear, causing an increase in the vitreous volume with subsequent forward displacement of the lens and shallowing of the anterior chamber. The fluid may accumulate in the retrolental space or dissect posteriorly along the vitreoretinal interface. If gentle posterior pressure on the lens or reinflation of the capsular bag with OVD does not alleviate the situation, intravenous mannitol infusion and waiting at least 20 minutes may allow the anterior chamber to deepen. If suprachoroidal effusion or hemorrhage has been ruled out, the surgeon can insert a 20- to 23-gauge needle through the pars plana into the vitreous by direct visualization, gently aspirate fluid vitreous, and deepen the anterior chamber with irrigation fluid or OVD. Alternatively, vitreous aspiration may be performed with a cutting/aspirating pars plana vitrectomy tip inserted through a sclerotomy 3.5 mm behind the limbus, combined with infusion of balanced salt solution or injection of additional OVD into the anterior chamber.

Postoperative

A flat anterior chamber during the postoperative period may cause permanent damage to ocular structures. Prolonged apposition of the iris to angle structures can result in PAS formation and chronic angle-closure glaucoma. Following either ICCE or ECCE, iridovitreal or iridocapsular synechiae can also lead to pupillary block. Corneal contact with vitreous or an IOL can result in endothelial cell loss and chronic corneal edema.

Postoperative shallow or flat anterior chambers can be classified according to their etiology and level of IOP. Causes include a leaking incision, choroidal detachment, pupillary block, ciliary block, capsular block, and suprachoroidal hemorrhage.

Cases associated with ocular hypotension (IOP below 10 mm Hg) are usually secondary to leakage of aqueous at the incision site or to choroidal or ciliary body detachment. Patients may be asymptomatic, especially if a leaking incision is plugged by iris incarceration, allowing re-formation of the anterior chamber. Even without iris incarceration, slow or intermittent leaks may coexist with a formed anterior chamber. Carefully comparing the chamber depth of the surgical eye with that of the fellow eye may help the surgeon identify these cases. (For a discussion of evaluation and management of an incisional leak, see the section Incision and Wound Complications, earlier in this chapter.)

In cases of prolonged hypotony, an associated ciliochoroidal detachment may develop that can resolve spontaneously after incision closure. Surgical exploration with re-formation of the anterior chamber and repair of the incision is indicated if no improvement occurs within 24–48 hours, if obvious wound gape is present, if the iris is prolapsed out of the incision, or if intraocular structures such as the IOL are in contact with the corneal endothelium.

Late hypotony without obvious leakage from the incision is uncommon after cataract surgery. It may result from retinal detachment, cyclodialysis, filtering bleb formation, or persistent uveitis.

Cases of a shallow anterior chamber with normal or high IOP are usually the result of pupillary block, ciliary block, capsular block, or suprachoroidal hemorrhage. Pupillary block that occurs in the early postoperative period may follow a resolved incision leak.

Postoperative uveitis with iridovitreal or iridocapsular synechiae may cause relatively late pupillary block. Failure to perform a peripheral iridectomy after placement of an anterior chamber IOL (ACIOL) may also be associated with early or late postoperative pupillary block. If initial attempts at pupillary dilation fail to deepen the anterior chamber and lower the pressure, a laser peripheral iridotomy is usually effective. Ciliary block glaucoma, capsular block, and suprachoroidal hemorrhage are discussed later in this chapter.

Elevated Intraocular Pressure

A mild, self-limited rise in IOP is common following cataract surgery. However, a significant and sustained elevation may require timely management.

OVD retained in the eye after cataract surgery is frequently responsible for early postoperative IOP elevation, which peaks 4–6 hours after surgery. The large molecules of the viscoelastic material can impair aqueous outflow through the trabecular meshwork. Even when all apparent OVD is removed from the anterior chamber, residual OVD, particularly dispersive agents, can lodge in the posterior chamber or behind the lens implant. All types of OVDs, but in particular the higher-viscosity agents, may cause the pressure to rise. IOP elevation usually does not last more than a few days and is amenable to medical treatment. The clinician may quickly manage marked IOP elevation in the early postoperative period by applying gentle pressure on the posterior lip of a preexisting paracentesis incision to release a small amount of aqueous humor. Topical and/or systemic pressure-lowering agents should also be administered, as IOP reduction after aqueous release is short-lived, with the IOP likely to rise again within 1–2 hours of the decompression.

Elevated IOP without angle closure after cataract surgery may be caused by hyphema, TASS, endophthalmitis, retained lens material (phacolytic or phacoanaphylactic reactions), uveitis, iris pigment release, preexisting glaucoma, corticosteroid use, vitreous in the anterior chamber, ghost cell glaucoma, or α-chymotrypsin use. Angle-closure glaucoma may be due to pupillary block, ciliary block, epithelial ingrowth, neovascular glaucoma, or PAS. Treating the underlying cause of the IOP elevation should be curative.

Intraoperative Floppy Iris Syndrome

Intraoperative floppy iris syndrome (IFIS) is the intraoperative triad of iris billowing and floppiness, iris prolapse into the incisions, and progressive pupillary miosis. Studies have shown that IFIS, especially when unexpected, results in a higher rate of surgical complications, including iris trauma, posterior capsule rupture, and vitreous loss. IFIS was originally associated with either the current or prior use of tamsulosin, a selective α_{1a}-adrenergic antagonist. Since then, IFIS has been reported with the use of other selective and nonselective α-adrenergic antagonists, such as doxazosin, terazosin, alfuzosin, and silodosin. It may also occur following the use of some antipsychotic agents, such as chlorpromazine, or other drugs and supplements with α-adrenergic antagonist activity (Table 8-2). Drugs that are selective α_{1a}-adrenergic antagonists seem to have a greater effect on the iris dilator muscle than do nonselective drugs.

Tamsulosin is most commonly used to treat lower urinary tract symptoms associated with benign prostatic hypertrophy. It is also used to treat patients with renal stones and occasionally to treat women with urinary retention. Doxazosin, terazosin, prazosin, and

Table 8-2 Medications Associated With Intraoperative Floppy Iris Syndrome

Selective α_{1a}-adrenergic antagonists
Tamsulosin (Flomax)
Silodosin (Rapaflo)
Tamsulosin and dutasteride (Jalyn)

Nonselective α_1-adrenergic antagonists
Alfuzosin (Uroxatrol)
Doxazosin (Cardura)
Prazosin (Minipress)
Terazosin (Hytrin)

Other drugs with α-adrenergic antagonist activity
Chlorpromazine (Thorazine)
Donepezil (Aricept)
Labetalol (Normodyne, Trandate)
Mianserin
Naftopidil
Rispiridone (Risperdal)
Zuclopenthixol

labetalol (which is both an α-adrenergic antagonist and a β-adrenergic antagonist) are used to treat hypertension. IFIS may occur in patients who have had no apparent exposure to α-adrenergic antagonists, and it has been reported more commonly in patients with hypertension but not diabetes mellitus.

IFIS may be mild, moderate, or severe. Patients taking tamsulosin experience these degrees of severity in approximately equal numbers. There is no correlation with adrenergic antagonist dosage or duration of therapy, and discontinuing the medication preoperatively seems to have no effect on the degree of IFIS.

All preoperative patients should be questioned about their use of α-adrenergic antagonists. Since 2005, the US Food and Drug Administration (FDA) has required that these medications be labeled with a precautionary statement about IFIS and cataract surgery.

The following interventions have been proposed to reduce the intraoperative effects of IFIS:

- use of preoperative atropine
- intracameral injection of α-adrenergic agonists, such as phenylephrine or epinephrine
- careful attention to incision location and construction to reduce wound leak
- use of iris hooks or pupil expansion rings for stabilization
- use of bimanual microincision surgical techniques
- employment of highly retentive OVDs to "viscodilate" the pupil and maintain a concave iris near the incisions
- discontinuation of fluid inflow prior to withdrawal of instruments to prevent fluid and iris egress
- use of low-flow settings to minimize anterior chamber turbulence and eliminate a higher pressure gradient posterior to the iris

Many surgeons employ intracameral irrigation with 0.5–1.0 mL of buffered, preservative-free lidocaine 0.75% mixed with preservative-free epinephrine 1:4000 or phenylephrine 1.5%. Because these solutions must be compounded, there is a risk of mixing errors and subsequent TASS. Additive-free epinephrine is currently not available in the United States, but epinephrine stabilized with bisulfite has been used successfully when diluted in a ratio of at least 1:4 with balanced salt solution. A commercial solution of unpreserved ketorolac and phenylephrine used as an additive to the irrigation solution is now available in the United States. Despite these interventions, significant miosis and/or iris prolapse still occurs intraoperatively in some patients.

American Society of Cataract and Refractive Surgery (ASCRS). ASCRS issues clinical alert on intracameral alpha agonists. March 13, 2013. Available at http://eyeworld.org/article.php?sid=6762. Accessed November 2, 2015.

Bell CM, Hatch WV, Fischer HD, et al. Association between tamsulosin and serious ophthalmic adverse events in older men following cataract surgery. *JAMA.* 2009;301(19):1991–1996.

Chang DF. Intraoperative floppy iris syndrome. *Focal Points: Clinical Modules for Ophthalmologists.* San Francisco: American Academy of Ophthalmology; 2010, module 11.

Chang DF, Campbell JR. Intraoperative floppy iris syndrome associated with tamsulosin. *J Cataract Refract Surg.* 2005;31(4):664–673.

Chatziralli IP, Sergentanis TN. Risk factors for intraoperative floppy iris syndrome: a meta-analysis. *Ophthalmology.* 2011;118(4):730–735.

Lens–Iris Diaphragm Retropulsion Syndrome

Lens–iris diaphragm retropulsion syndrome (LIDRS) during cataract extraction is characterized by posterior displacement of the lens–iris diaphragm with a marked deepening of the anterior chamber, posterior iris bowing, and pupil dilation. It is more common in highly myopic eyes and in eyes that have undergone previous vitrectomy. LIDRS is due to a high level of infusion pressure in the anterior chamber with a reverse pupillary block and may cause stress on the zonular apparatus and considerable patient discomfort under topical anesthesia. Also, because of the excessively deep anterior chamber, surgery may be more difficult. Lifting the iris off the anterior capsule is usually sufficient to break the pupillary block and restore normal anterior chamber depth.

Cionni RJ, Barros MG, Osher RH. Management of lens-iris diaphragm retropulsion syndrome during phacoemulsification. *J Cataract Refract Surg.* 2004;30(5):953–956.

Iridodialysis and Iris Trauma

Iridodialysis, the tearing of the iris at its root or insertion, may occur at the time of insertion of the phaco tip or IOL if iris tissue is engaged. Traction on the iris root due to aspiration of iris tissue during phacoemulsification can cause a tear and subsequent hyphema. If the iridodialysis is small or insignificant, it can be left alone. More extensive iridodialysis that could cause optical problems or that could be cosmetically significant may require surgical reattachment.

Chronic mydriasis or iris damage from surgery or trauma may cause excessive glare, particularly if the pupillary light response is inadequate or if the edge of the IOL is not covered. Suturing an iris defect, performing pupillary cerclage, or implanting artificial iris devices may alleviate symptoms or address a patient's cosmetic concerns. An iris-colored contact lens may be considered as a nonsurgical alternative.

Cyclodialysis

Cyclodialysis, the separation of the ciliary body from its insertion at the scleral spur, may occur as a result of trauma or surgical manipulation of intraocular tissue. Gonioscopic observation shows a deep-angle recess with a gap between the sclera and the ciliary body. Repair of a cyclodialysis cleft is often indicated if hypotony results. Closure may be achieved with argon laser photocoagulation at the site of cyclodialysis. If this is ineffective, it may be necessary to reattach the ciliary body with sutures.

Ciliary Block Glaucoma

Ciliary block glaucoma (also known as *malignant glaucoma, aqueous misdirection,* or *vitreous block*) was classically thought to be caused by anterior rotation of the ciliary body and posterior misdirection of aqueous into the vitreous body. More recently, the condition has been described as a ciliolenticular block induced by anterior movement of the lens–iris diaphragm, poor vitreous fluid conductivity, and choroidal expansion. These factors cause the central and peripheral portions of the anterior chamber to become very shallow and lead to a secondary elevation of IOP as a consequence of angle obstruction. Ciliary block glaucoma occurs most commonly after intraocular surgery in eyes with prior angle-closure glaucoma, but it can also occur in small eyes with open angles. It must be differentiated from pupillary block glaucoma, capsular block, suprachoroidal hemorrhage, and choroidal detachment.

IOP may be elevated despite the presence of a patent iridectomy or iridotomy. Thus, ciliary block glaucoma, unlike pupillary block, is not relieved by iridectomy but requires either intense medical therapy or more aggressive surgical therapy.

Medical treatment consists of cycloplegia with atropine and aggressive aqueous suppression with β-adrenergic antagonists, α-adrenergic agonists, and/or oral or topical carbonic anhydrase inhibitors, as well as hyperosmotic agents (such as oral glycerin or intravenous mannitol). Miotics should be avoided because they can make ciliary block glaucoma worse by exacerbating the anterior displacement of the lens–iris diaphragm. Medical therapy may be successful in 50% of these cases.

Surgical intervention consists of Nd:YAG laser iridozonulohyaloidotomy and, occasionally, vitrectomy to disrupt the anterior vitreous face and vitreous–ciliary body interface so as to establish, in effect, a unicameral eye with an open channel for aqueous to circulate into the anterior chamber. (See also BCSC Section 10, *Glaucoma.*)

Kaplowitz K, Yung E, Flynn R, Tsai JC. Current concepts in the treatment of vitreous block, also known as aqueous misdirection. *Surv Ophthalmol.* 2015;60(3):229–241.

Lundy DM. Ciliary block glaucoma. *Focal Points: Clinical Modules for Ophthalmologists.* San Francisco: American Academy of Ophthalmology; 1999, module 3.

Varma DK, Belovay GW, Tam DY, Ahmed II. Malignant glaucoma after cataract surgery. *J Cataract Refract Surg.* 2014;40(11):1843–1849.

Postoperative Uveitis

Following cataract extraction, nearly all eyes exhibit some degree of intraocular inflammation. With uncomplicated cataract surgery and the use of postoperative topical corticosteroids and/or NSAIDs, most eyes should be free of inflammation by 3–4 weeks postoperatively. Complicated cases requiring manipulation of intraocular tissues (eg, iris sphincterotomy, iridectomy, or repair), involving vitreous loss or prolapse, or requiring sulcus fixation of an IOL may have a more prolonged recovery. Increased inflammation may also be seen in children; in patients with diabetes mellitus; in patients who have had previous surgery, pseudoexfoliation syndrome, or pigment dispersion syndrome; and with long-term miotic use.

Low-grade inflammation lasting more than 4 weeks raises the possibility of chronic infection, retained lens fragments, or other causes of chronic inflammation. IOL malposition is an important cause of chronic inflammation if the lens comes in contact with the iris, ciliary body, or angle structures. An IOL designed for capsular bag placement may cause inflammation if placed in the ciliary sulcus. Retained lens material may be an insidious cause of chronic low-grade inflammation or corneal edema (see the following section). The presence of hypopyon or vitritis should prompt intervention to determine the source of the inflammation and to rule out an infectious etiology.

The surgeon should also investigate the possibility of microbial endophthalmitis in patients who have persistent uveitis without a previous history of inflammation. Chronic uveitis following cataract surgery has been reported in association with low-grade infections with bacterial pathogens, including *Propionibacterium acnes* and *Staphylococcus epidermidis*. Such patients may have an unremarkable early postoperative course and lack the classic findings of acute endophthalmitis. Weeks or months after surgery, however, they develop chronic uveitis that is variably responsive to topical corticosteroids. This condition is usually associated with granulomatous keratic precipitates and, less commonly, with hypopyon. A localized focus of infection sequestered within the capsular bag may occasionally be observed. Diagnosis requires a high level of clinical suspicion, coupled with examination and cultures of appropriate specimens of aqueous, vitreous, and (where applicable) retained lens material that may harbor a nidus of infection. Appropriate intravitreal antibiotic therapy is indicated. If this treatment fails, the clinician may need to search for and remove any visible focus of infection in order to sterilize the eye. In some cases, total removal of the residual capsule and IOL is necessary.

Patients with preexisting uveitis may have excessive postoperative inflammation but generally do well with small-incision cataract surgery with IOL implantation in the capsular bag. Some surgeons prefer acrylic IOL material over silicone in patients with preexisting uveitis or a risk of chronic inflammation.

Management of chronic uveitis is directed toward the cause. Surgery is used for correction of mechanical issues with IOL malposition, vitreous incarceration, or retained lens fragments. If no obvious etiology can be found, prolonged use of topical or subconjunctival corticosteroids is indicated, with continued efforts to identify a cause.

Van Gelder RN, Leveque TK. Cataract surgery in the setting of uveitis. *Curr Opin Ophthalmol.* 2009;20(1):42–45.

Retained Lens Material

During cataract extraction, lens material may remain in the anterior chamber angle or in the posterior chamber behind the iris, or it may migrate into the vitreous cavity if zonular dehiscence or posterior capsule rupture occurs. Retained lens material in the aqueous chamber is thought to occur more frequently with phacoemulsification than with ECCE; the reported postoperative prevalence is 0.45%–1.70%, but the actual rates may be higher because of unrecognized cases. Intraocular turbulence during phacoemulsification may force small lens fragments to lodge in the angle or behind the iris, out of sight of the surgeon. Dispersive OVD may trap and retain more lens fragments than cohesive OVD. Retained lens material may be seen in the inferior anterior chamber during the first postoperative slit-lamp examination, or it may emerge months or even years later from a hidden position in the posterior chamber.

Patients with retained lens material present with varying degrees of inflammation, depending on the size of the lens fragment, the type of lens material, the amount of time elapsed since surgery, and the patient's individual response. The clinical signs of retained lens material may include uveitis, elevated IOP, corneal edema, and vitreous opacities.

Retained cortical lens material or capsular fragments do not necessarily require surgical intervention. In general, cortical material is better tolerated and more likely to reabsorb over time than is nuclear material, which, even in small amounts, persists longer and is more likely to incite a significant inflammatory reaction, corneal edema, or elevated IOP.

Inflammation should be controlled with corticosteroid and nonsteroidal anti-inflammatory drops. Elevated IOP can be treated with hypotensive drops or oral carbonic anhydrase inhibitors. Surgical intervention may be necessary to remove residual lens material in the following situations:

- presence of a large or visually significant amount of lens material
- increased inflammation not readily controlled with topical medications
- medically unresponsive elevated IOP resulting from inflammation
- corneal edema
- associated retinal detachment or retinal tears
- associated endophthalmitis

For retained lens fragments in the anterior chamber with an intact posterior capsule, simple I/A or viscoexpression of the residual material may be performed through the original phacoemulsification incision.

The reported incidence of intravitreal retained lens fragments is between 0.1% and 1.6%. If lens material has migrated into the vitreous cavity through a defect in the zonular fibers or posterior capsule, referral to a vitreoretinal surgeon for pars plana vitrectomy and removal of the lens material is indicated. The vitreoretinal surgeon can delay intervention for more than a week after the cataract surgery, if necessary, without jeopardizing the successful outcome. A meta-analysis of vitrectomy for retained posterior lens fragments found that surgery performed within 1–2 weeks resulted in better vision and a lower likelihood of retinal detachment, glaucoma, and chronic inflammation in comparison to delayed surgery.

Merani R, Hunyor AP, Playfair TJ, et al. Pars plana vitrectomy for the management of retained lens material after cataract surgery. *Am J Ophthalmol.* 2007;144(3):364–370.

Vanner EA, Stewart MW. Vitrectomy timing for retained lens fragments after surgery for age-related cataracts: a systematic review and meta-analysis. *Am J Ophthalmol.* 2011;152(3): 345–357.

Capsular Rupture

If posterior capsule rupture occurs during surgery, lens material may enter the posterior chamber. The surgeon should reduce fluid inflow and stabilize the anterior segment. Evaluation of the location and size of the tear will determine the appropriate response. A small rupture in the posterior capsule during emulsification of the nucleus can be managed by alteration of the surgical technique. The surgeon can compartmentalize the vitreous with OVD and use low-flow, low-vacuum settings to remove the remaining nuclear and cortical material. Full occlusion of the aspiration port and minimal phaco power reduce the risk of aspiration of vitreous or further damage to the capsule.

If a small rent appears in the posterior capsule during aspiration of the cortex and the vitreous face remains intact, the surgeon should attempt to remove the residual cortex without expanding the tear. Using low-flow I/A helps avoid disruption of the vitreous face. Some surgeons prefer a manual dry-aspiration technique. This approach involves using a cannula attached to a handheld syringe to remove the residual cortex after a capsular rupture, thereby avoiding any pressure from irrigation. After the anterior chamber is stabilized with the use of an OVD, capsulorrhexis forceps may be employed to convert the tear in the posterior capsule into a round posterior capsulorrhexis that will resist extending equatorially.

If most of the nucleus remains and the capsular tear is large, further attempts at phacoemulsification should be abandoned. To extract the remaining nuclear fragments mechanically, the surgeon should enlarge the incision and remove the nucleus with a lens loop or spoon in a manner that minimizes vitreous traction and further damage to the capsule. Insertion of a second instrument or lens glide behind the nuclear remnant may help prevent the remnant from being dislocated into the vitreous. Alternatively, OVD can be introduced posterior to the fragment in an effort to float it anteriorly, or the nucleus can be elevated into the anterior chamber with an instrument or nuclear spear. Retrieval of nuclear fragments from the deep vitreous is not recommended.

If vitreous prolapse occurs, it is best to remove all vitreous from the anterior chamber during the initial surgery. Doing so will facilitate the removal of residual cortex and the subsequent placement of an IOL. In addition, a vitrectomy can reduce the chance of vitreoretinal traction or vitreous adherence to the IOL, the iris, or the incision. Vitreous loss during cataract surgery is associated with an increased risk of retinal detachment, CME, and endophthalmitis.

The vitreous may be stained with unpreserved or washed triamcinolone for better visualization. The surgeon should avoid manually externalizing and cutting vitreous through the incision. A coaxial anterior vitrectomy can be performed through the main incision site, but it may be preferable to perform a 2-port anterior vitrectomy with separate infusion and aspirating/cutting instruments inserted through new, properly sized limbal incisions. Alternatively, the aspiration/cutting instrument may be placed through a pars plana incision while irrigation is continued through the limbus or cornea. This directs flow posteriorly and reduces the amount of vitreous that migrates into the anterior segment, thereby decreasing vitreoretinal traction.

If posterior capsule support for intracapsular placement of the IOL is inadequate, the surgeon should attempt to preserve the anterior capsule and capsulorrhexis to enable capture of the IOL optic in the capsular bag with the haptics placed in the ciliary sulcus. A 3-piece IOL with a total diameter greater than 12.5 mm may be inserted into the ciliary sulcus with or without optic capture. A single-piece acrylic IOL is not suitable for the ciliary sulcus because of the possible development of uveitis-glaucoma-hyphema (UGH) syndrome. If capsular integrity is insufficient, the surgeon may substitute an anterior chamber lens. A posterior chamber IOL (PCIOL) may also be used in the absence of capsular support by suturing the haptics to the iris or by fixation of the haptics to the sclera through the ciliary sulcus. If significant lens material remains in the posterior chamber, it should be approached within 1–2 weeks via a pars plana vitrectomy performed by a vitreoretinal surgeon.

Steps for managing posteriorly dislocated lens fragments include the following:

- Maintain a normotensive globe and prevent anterior chamber collapse.
- Avoid intraoperative vitreous traction.
- Compartmentalize the lens and vitreous with OVD.
- Attempt retrieval of the lens fragments only if they are visible and easily accessible.
- Using either a biaxial limbal or pars plana approach, perform an anterior vitrectomy until no vitreous is seen anterior to the capsule.
- Insert an IOL only when safe and indicated—preferably a posterior chamber lens placed in the ciliary sulcus or fixated to iris or sclera, or an anterior chamber lens with prophylactic peripheral iridotomy.
- Adjust the lens power appropriately for the position and type of IOL used.
- Perform a watertight incision closure and remove the OVD.
- Arrange a prompt referral to a vitreoretinal surgeon for removal of posteriorly dislocated lens fragments.
- Disclose and discuss all surgical complications with the patient.

Arbisser LB. Anterior vitrectomy for the anterior segment surgeon. *Focal Points: Clinical Modules for Ophthalmologists.* San Francisco: American Academy of Ophthalmology; 2009, module 2.

Fishkind WJ. The torn posterior capsule: prevention, recognition, and management. *Focal Points: Clinical Modules for Ophthalmologists.* San Francisco: American Academy of Ophthalmology; 1999, module 4.

Kaynak S, Celik L, Kocak N, Oner FH, Kaynak T, Cingil G. Staining of vitreous with triamcinolone acetonide in retained lens surgery with phacofragmentation. *J Cataract Refract Surg.* 2006;32(1):56–59.

Vitreous Prolapse in the Anterior Chamber

In cases with vitreous prolapse, the surgeon should attempt to remove all of the vitreous in the anterior chamber to reduce the likelihood of long-term complications. Vitreous in the anterior chamber may lead to chronic intraocular inflammation, corneal edema, glaucoma, and CME. The pupil may be distorted by vitreous adherent to the incision. Inflammation, symptoms of glare due to an exposed IOL edge, and patient dissatisfaction with the appearance of the iris may prompt intervention. In symptomatic patients, Nd:YAG laser vitreolysis or anterior vitrectomy may be considered if the response to topical anti-inflammatory therapy is inadequate. If the vitreous extends through the incision to the ocular surface, a vitrectomy should be performed. The exposed vitreous may act as a wick, enabling bacteria to enter the eye and increasing the risk of endophthalmitis. In cases of suspected corneal compromise, a posterior vitrectomy approach may be preferable to an anterior approach to reduce the surgical trauma to the cornea.

Complications of IOL Implantation

Decentration and Dislocation

The reported incidence of symptomatic subluxation or dislocation of an IOL after uncomplicated cataract surgery is 0.19%–3.00%. The dislocated IOL may be either inside the capsule (intracapsular) or outside it (extracapsular) (Fig 8-2). The most common cause of intracapsular IOL dislocation is zonular degradation associated with pseudoexfoliation syndrome. Insufficient zonular support may also be associated with trauma, previous vitreoretinal surgery, capsular contraction, retinitis pigmentosa, high myopia, uveitis, or congenital conditions that affect zonular integrity. Asymmetric bag/sulcus haptic positions (ie, 1 haptic in the capsular bag and 1 in the sulcus) aggravated by capsular fibrosis and contraction may tilt or decenter an IOL. The most common cause of extracapsular IOL dislocation is sulcus placement of an inadequately sized IOL. Extracapsular dislocation may also occur in the setting of a decentered or oversized capsulorrhexis, localized zonular defects, capsular defects, or IOL haptic damage.

Decentration can cause unwanted glare and reflections or multiple images if the edge of the lens is within the pupillary space. If an aspheric, multifocal, or accommodating lens is decentered, the lens's desired effect is diminished. Decentration of an aspheric lens with negative spherical aberration (used to counteract the positive spherical aberration of the aging cornea) results in greater higher orders of aberration compared with a decentered

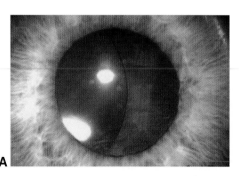
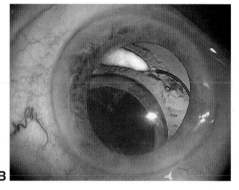

A   **B**

Figure 8-2 Intraocular lens (IOL) dislocation. **A,** Extracapsular (out-of-the-bag) dislocation. **B,** Intracapsular (in-the-bag) dislocation. *(Part A reprinted from Dorey MW, Condon GP. Management of dislocated intraocular lenses.* Focal Points: Clinical Modules for Ophthalmologists. *San Francisco: American Academy of Ophthalmology; 2009, module 9:2. Part B reprinted with permission from Gimbel HV, Condon GP, Kohnen T, Olson RJ, Halkiadakis I. Late in-the-bag intraocular lens dislocation: incidence, prevention, and management. J Cataract Refract Surg. 2005;31(11):2193–2204. © 2005, with permission from Elsevier.)*

spherical lens. Decentration of any PCIOL may lead to pupillary capture or any component of UGH syndrome due to contact with uveal tissue. Minor decentration may be treated with miotics to constrict the pupil over the IOL optic or with cycloplegics to reduce iris chafing by the IOL optic or haptics in cases of pigment dispersion or recurrent hyphema. Laser pupilloplasty may be used to realign the pupillary aperture with the IOL optical center. This procedure may be particularly useful with multifocal lenses. More-severe cases of IOL decentration are managed with IOL repositioning, stabilization with sutures, or exchange.

An IOL designed for intracapsular fixation is prone to decentration or dislocation when 1 or both haptics are placed in the sulcus. Occasionally, a lens decentered in the sulcus or in the capsular bag with a posterior capsule rent may be stabilized by prolapsing the optic through an intact capsulorrhexis. An extracapsular decentered IOL may be rotated and repositioned into a stable axis if there is sufficient support. Many extracapsular and selected intracapsular 3-piece IOL dislocations can be managed with peripheral iris suture fixation using a McCannel suture or Siepser slipknot technique with a nonabsorbable monofilament suture, such as 9-0 or 10-0 polypropylene (Fig 8-3). Iris fixation has some advantages over scleral fixation, including a decreased risk of late suture erosion or breakage, IOL tilting, intraocular hemorrhage, and endophthalmitis. Disadvantages include possible posterior iris pigment chafing, pupil distortion, pseudophakodonesis, and hyphema. Current 1-piece uniplanar acrylic IOLs are not suitable for sulcus or iris fixation because of possible development of UGH syndrome.

Irregular capsular fibrosis may gradually decenter an IOL placed in the capsular bag. Deformation of the haptics may render simple rotation insufficient to center the IOL properly. In such cases, it may become necessary to move the IOL haptics into the ciliary sulcus or replace the lens. Haptics fixated in the capsular bag or sulcus can be either amputated and left in place or slipped out of a fibrous cocoon when removing the optic prior to implanting a new IOL.

Severe pseudophakodonesis or intracapsular (in-the-bag) dislocation of an IOL due to zonular loss may be managed with haptic fixation to the sclera. Many different ab externo and ab interno approaches and suture configurations have been described (Fig 8-4). A concurrent anterior vitrectomy is often necessary. Iris retractors may be used for better visualization or to stabilize the haptics during suturing. Sutures through the scleral wall should be covered by a flap to prevent erosion through the conjunctiva. The scleral flap can be created through a conjunctival incision or a tunnel incision dissected posteriorly from the limbus. If dislocation of the IOL is complete, pars plana vitrectomy techniques are required to retrieve the lens or lens-capsule complex and elevate it safely into the anterior segment, where it can then be suture fixated to the iris or sclera through an anterior approach. Alternatively, the IOL haptics may be externalized through the sulcus, inserted into prepared scleral tunnels, and fixated with tissue adhesive. In some cases, the implant may be removed altogether and replaced with either an ACIOL or a transscleral or iris-fixated PCIOL. Suture breakage and subluxation of scleral-fixated sutured IOLs occurring 3–9 years after implantation with 10-0 polypropylene fixation sutures have been reported. Double-fixation techniques and thicker 9-0 polypropylene or 8-0 Gore-Tex sutures (off-label use) are currently recommended for scleral fixation of IOLs. Other complications of sutured IOLs include vitreous or suprachoroidal hemorrhage, lens tilting, CME, retinal

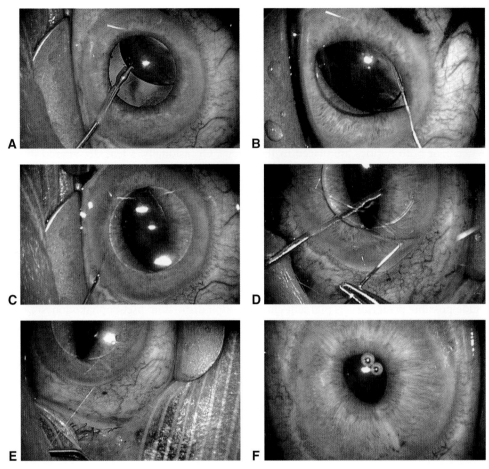

Figure 8-3 Peripheral iris suture fixation technique for IOL dislocation out of the capsular bag. **A,** Grasping and rotation of the IOL with microsurgical forceps. **B,** Iris hooks are used to bring the optic above the iris plane. **C,** Optic capture by the pupil is completed through the addition of acetylcholine to induce miosis. **D,** The needle has been passed through a paracentesis incision, then through the iris and behind the haptic, and then back out through the iris and distal clear cornea. **E,** A Siepser sliding knot is used to secure the haptic to the peripheral iris. **F,** After both haptics are secured, the optic is prolapsed back into the posterior chamber. The sutures are minimally visible at the 5- and 10-o'clock positions. *(Reprinted with permission from Condon GP. Following a posterior capsular rent, the sulcus-fixated intraocular lens has become decentered. How should I proceed? In: Chang DF, ed.* Curbside Consultation in Cataract Surgery. *Thorofare, NJ: Slack; 2007:227–232.)*

tears or detachment, suture erosion, and infection. (See also BCSC Section 12, *Retina and Vitreous.*)

An ACIOL may be associated with decentration, iris tucking, UGH syndrome, corneal edema, or pseudophakodonesis, which would prompt repositioning of the lens or IOL exchange with either a differently sized flexible ACIOL or, preferably, a PCIOL. An ACIOL associated with pseudophakic bullous keratopathy is treated by endothelial or penetrating keratoplasty, usually in combination with IOL exchange.

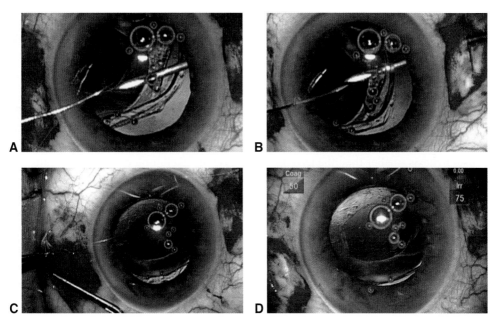

Figure 8-4 Ab externo scleral fixation technique. **A,** A partial-thickness scleral groove is made 1.0–1.5 mm posterior to the limbus. A hollow 26-gauge needle is inserted through the scleral groove behind the iris plane and over the haptic into the pupillary zone. A preplaced 9-0 poly-propylene suture on a long needle is placed through a corneal paracentesis tract in the oppo-site direction. This needle can fit into the hollow 26-gauge needle and can then be retrieved back through the original scleral groove site. **B,** The 26-gauge needle is inserted again into the scleral groove approximately 1 mm away from the original pass site; it is then inserted behind the iris plane beneath the haptic/capsule complex and up again into the pupillary zone. A simi-larly preplaced 9-0 polypropylene suture on a long needle is placed and the suture retrieved in an identical fashion through the original scleral groove site. **C,** The knot is tied but not yet locked. **D,** The other haptic is secured in a similar process. The optic is centered, and the knots are locked and then buried in the scleral grooves. *(Reprinted from Masket S. Cataract surgical problem: February consultation #1. J Cataract Refract Surg. 2008;34(2):185. © February 2008, with permission from Elsevier.)*

If an iris-supported lens becomes dislocated or associated with corneal edema or UGH syndrome, it should be surgically exchanged. If further surgery is contraindicated, repositioning of a partially dislocated lens by pharmacologic manipulation of the pupil and patient positioning may be successful.

Chang DF. Siepser slipknot for McCannel iris-suture fixation of subluxated intraocular lenses. *J Cataract Refract Surg.* 2004;30(6):1170–1176.

Dorey MW, Condon GP. Management of dislocated intraocular lenses. *Focal Points: Clinical Modules for Ophthalmologists.* San Francisco: American Academy of Ophthalmology; 2009, module 9.

Gimbel HV, Condon GP, Kohnen T, Olson RJ, Halkiadakis I. Late in-the-bag intraocular lens dislocation: incidence, prevention, and management. *J Cataract Refract Surg.* 2005;31(11): 2193–2204.

Hannush SB. Sutured posterior chamber intraocular lenses. *Focal Points: Clinical Modules for Ophthalmologists.* San Francisco: American Academy of Ophthalmology; 2006, module 9.

Pupillary Capture

Postoperative pupillary capture of the IOL optic can occur for various reasons, such as formation of synechiae between the iris and underlying posterior capsule, improper placement of the IOL haptics, shallowing of the anterior chamber, or anterior displacement of the PCIOL optic. The last of these is associated with placement of nonangulated IOLs in the ciliary sulcus, upside-down placement of an angulated IOL so that the IOL vaults anteriorly, excessive Soemmering ring formation, or asymmetric capsule contraction. Placement of a posteriorly angulated PCIOL in the capsular bag and creation of an anterior capsulorrhexis smaller than the lens optic decrease the likelihood of pupillary capture.

Pupillary capture may be simply a cosmetic concern. If the condition is chronic and the patient is asymptomatic, it can be left untreated. Occasionally, pupillary capture can cause glare, photophobia, chronic uveitis, unintended myopia, or monocular diplopia, which requires surgical repositioning of the lens. In an acute pupillary capture, pharmacologic manipulation of the pupil with the patient in the supine position is sometimes successful in freeing the optic. If conservative management fails, surgical intervention may be required in order to free the iris, lyse synechiae, manage capsule contraction or residual lens proliferation, and reposition the lens (Figs 8-5, 8-6).

Capsular Block Syndrome

Capsular block syndrome (CBS) is caused by the intracapsular accumulation of liquefied material posterior to the nucleus or IOL and subsequent occlusion of the anterior capsulotomy. CBS can occur intraoperatively during hydrodissection of the nucleus and may lead to posterior capsule blowout, especially in eyes with preexisting capsule defects or posterior polar cataract. Early postoperative CBS may occur when residual OVD becomes trapped within the capsular bag, between the posterior capsule and the posterior surface of the IOL. This may cause a myopic shift in the refractive error as a result of anterior displacement of the lens optic. Anterior displacement of the iris diaphragm with shallowing of the anterior chamber may also occur, which must be differentiated from a ciliary block mechanism. If left untreated, CBS may lead to posterior synechiae and secondary

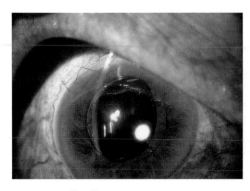

Figure 8-5 Pupillary capture. *(Courtesy of Karla J. Johns, MD.)*

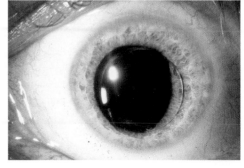

Figure 8-6 Pupillary capture by an angulated posterior chamber IOL in a patient who was assaulted 2 months after lens implantation surgery. *(Courtesy of Steven I. Rosenfeld, MD.)*

glaucoma. Nd:YAG laser anterior capsulotomy peripheral to the optic or posterior capsulotomy results in release of the trapped fluid, with resultant posterior movement of the IOL optic to its intended position, deepening of the anterior chamber, and resolution of the myopic shift.

Late postoperative CBS may occur years after surgery with the accumulation of a turbid or milky fluid between the posterior capsule and the IOL that is consistent with the by-products of trapped, residual lens epithelial cells. The patient may be asymptomatic, and myopic shift is uncommon in these cases. Simple laser posterior capsulotomy usually resolves this condition without complications.

> Miyake K, Ota I, Ichihashi S, Miyake S, Tanaka Y, Terasaki H. New classification of capsular block syndrome. *J Cataract Refract Surg* 1998;24(9):1230–1234.

Uveitis-Glaucoma-Hyphema Syndrome

Uveitis-glaucoma-hyphema (UGH) syndrome was first described in the context of rigid or closed-loop ACIOLs. It may also develop in patients with posterior chamber lenses, owing to contact between lens haptics and uveal tissue in the posterior chamber. The classic triad or individual components of the syndrome may occur as a result of inappropriate IOL sizing, contact between the implant and vascular structures or the corneal endothelium, or defects in implant manufacturing. Uveitis, glaucoma, and/or hyphema may respond to treatment with cycloplegics and topical anti-inflammatory or ocular hypotensive medications. If medical therapy does not sufficiently address the findings or if inflammation threatens either retinal or corneal function, IOL removal must be considered. This procedure may be complicated because of inflammatory scars, particularly in the anterior chamber angle or posterior to the iris. If such scarring is present, the surgeon may need to amputate the haptics from the optic and remove the lens piecemeal, rotating the haptic material out of the synechial tunnels to minimize trauma to the eye. In some cases, it is safer to leave portions of the haptics in place. Early lens explantation may reduce the risk of corneal decompensation and CME.

Pseudophakic Bullous Keratopathy

Certain IOL designs, particularly iris-clip lenses (iris-fixated lenses with the optic anterior to the iris) and closed-loop flexible anterior chamber lenses, were associated with an increased risk of corneal decompensation. Iris-clip lenses have been shown to contact the corneal endothelium during eye movement. Endothelial cell loss associated with closed-loop ACIOLs is thought to be due to chronic inflammation and contact between the lens and peripheral corneal endothelial cells. Thus, these two lens types are no longer in clinical use. Patients with underlying corneal endothelial dysfunction such as Fuchs corneal dystrophy have an increased risk of postoperative corneal edema.

Unexpected Refractive Results

Cataract surgery and IOL implantation afford an important opportunity to provide patients with desirable refractive outcomes. See Chapter 7 in this volume and BCSC Section 13, *Refractive Surgery,* for a discussion of cataract surgery as a refractive procedure.

Unintended postoperative refractive errors may be the result of a preoperative error in measurement of axial length or in keratometry readings. Choosing the correct IOL power is more difficult in patients undergoing simultaneous penetrating keratoplasty, in patients with silicone oil in the vitreous cavity, and in patients who have had prior refractive surgery (see Chapter 6). The surgeon's failure to confirm the proper IOL at the time of surgery may result in implantation of the incorrect lens. Unexpected postoperative refractive results may occur because of the inversion of an angulated IOL or placement of the lens in the sulcus when it was calculated for placement in the capsular bag, either of which results in anterior displacement and changes the effective power of the IOL. The clinician should rule out or treat other causes of an anterior or posterior shift in the IOL position, such as posterior capsule rupture, capsular block, or ciliary block. Mislabeling or manufacturing defects are rarely the cause of these problems. Incorrect lens power should be suspected early in the postoperative course when the visual acuity is less than expected and is confirmed by refraction. Medical-record documentation of the source of the error and full disclosure to the patient are necessary.

If the magnitude of the postoperative refractive error produces symptomatic ametropia, anisometropia, or dissatisfaction on the part of the patient, the surgeon can consider several options:

- overrefraction for glasses or contact-lens wear
- IOL exchange
- insertion of a piggyback IOL
- a secondary keratorefractive procedure

IOL Glare, Dysphotopsia, and Opacification

In addition to lens decentration and capsular opacification, glare can result when the diameter of the IOL optic is smaller than the diameter of the scotopic pupil. Optics with a square-edge design and multifocal IOLs are more likely to produce glare and halos, even when well centered. Spherical aberration may cause some degree of distortion or glare under scotopic conditions when the pupil is dilated, even if the iris covers the edge of the lens optic. Aspheric IOLs may reduce some of these phenomena and improve contrast sensitivity. Spherical aberration of the cornea changes with age and corneal refractive surgery, and various aspheric IOLs can be matched to the degree of corneal asphericity.

Positive dysphotopsia is described as glare, streaks, flashes, arcs, or halos of light in the midperiphery. It is more common with truncated square-edge IOLs and those manufactured from higher-index materials. *Negative dysphotopsia* is described as an arcuate dark or dim crescent-shaped region, usually in the temporal visual field. It occurs in the setting of a PCIOL centered in the capsular bag with the anterior capsule edge overlapping the lens optic. Though reported with most styles of PCIOLs, negative dysphotopsia is more common with smaller, square-edge optic designs. Temporal light rays may interact with the nasal lens edge and anterior capsule, causing a shadow (penumbra) on the nasal retina in susceptible eyes. This effect is more common with a miotic or nasally located pupil and is relieved with dilation or by blocking light from the temporal side. Although symptoms are common in the early postoperative period, they improve over time in most patients, presumably as the capsule contracts or opacifies in the periphery. Initially, observation is advised. For patients with prolonged symptoms and compromised vision, surgery may be necessary. Repositioning of the optic anterior to the capsulorrhexis by reverse optic capture through the capsulorrhexis (with the haptics in the capsular bag) or sulcus fixation of an appropriate PCIOL with a larger optic with rounded edges may be successful in most cases. Implantation of a piggyback IOL or an anterior capsulectomy has been successful in some cases.

Several types of IOLs have developed opacities or discoloration, either immediately after implantation or progressively over years. There are many different causes, which vary with the IOL manufacturer, material, and storage, as well as surgical adjuvants and associated patient conditions. Five general processes of IOL opacification have been identified:

- deposits or precipitates on the surface of or in the IOL optic (such as calcium deposits on silicone IOLs in asteroid hyalosis)
- influx of water in hydrophobic optic material (glistenings)
- staining of the IOL by capsular dyes or medications
- IOL coating by substances such as ophthalmic ointment or silicone oil
- progressive degradation of the IOL material (such as snowflake degeneration in polymethyl methacrylate [PMMA] IOLs)

Calcium deposition within or on the surface of hydrophilic acrylic lenses can produce significant visual symptoms, and IOL explantation may be required. Calcium deposits on silicone lenses have been reported in eyes with asteroid hyalosis, usually after posterior capsulotomy.

Glistenings are fluid-filled microvacuoles that form within an IOL optic when it is in an aqueous environment. They are observed within all types of IOL material but are associated primarily with certain hydrophobic acrylic IOLs. Glistening formation and intensity increase with time. Although their appearance may be striking on slit-lamp examination, glistenings have not been shown to affect best-corrected visual acuity. Although studies have documented a negative effect on contrast sensitivity at high spatial frequency, IOL explantation for glistenings is rarely reported.

Interlenticular opacifications have been noted between piggybacked PCIOLs, especially in cases when both are made of hydrophobic acrylic material and placed in the capsular bag. Using IOLs made of 2 different materials, enlarging the capsulorrhexis, and placing 1 lens in the capsular bag and 1 in the sulcus may reduce the incidence.

Patients with diffractive or refractive multifocal IOLs are more likely to experience glare, decreased contrast sensitivity, or loss of desired multifocality with minor IOL decentration, altered pupil diameter or position, or posterior capsule opacity. A pseudoaccommodating lens may vault anteriorly (a condition known as Z syndrome) due to misplaced haptics or asymmetric capsular contraction. This syndrome can often be managed by posterior capsulotomy, but the lens may need to be surgically repositioned or explanted.

Toric IOLs must be located on a precise axis for maximal astigmatic correction. These lenses may need to be repositioned if they are placed improperly or rotate postoperatively. Toric IOL rotation is more common in highly myopic eyes when the lens is oriented in the vertical meridian.

Colin J, Praud D, Touboul D, Schweitzer C. Incidence of glistenings with the latest generation of yellow-tinted hydrophobic acrylic intraocular lenses. *J Cataract Refract Surg.* 2012;38(7): 1140–1146.

Espandar L, Mukherjee N, Werner L, Mamalis N, Kim T. Diagnosis and management of opacified silicone intraocular lenses in patients with asteroid hyalosis. *J Cataract Refract Surg.* 2015;41(1):222–225.

Holladay JT, Zhao H, Reisin CR. Negative dysphotopsia: the enigmatic penumbra. *J Cataract Refract Surg.* 2012;38(7):1251–1265.

Jin H, Limberger IJ, Ehmer A, Guo H, Auffarth GU. Impact of axis misalignment of toric intraocular lenses on refractive outcomes after cataract surgery. *J Cataract Refract Surg.* 2010;36(12):2061–2072.

Masket S, Fram NR. Pseudophakic negative dysphotopsia: Surgical management and new theory of etiology. *J Cataract Refract Surg.* 2011;37(7):1199–1207.

Werner L. Causes of intraocular lens opacification or discoloration. *J Cataract Refract Surg.* 2007;33(4):713–726.

Werner L. Glistenings and surface light scattering in intraocular lenses. *J Cataract Refract Surg.* 2010;36(8):1398–1420.

Capsular Opacification and Contraction

Posterior Capsule Opacification

The most common late complication of cataract surgery by means of ECCE or phacoemulsification is posterior capsule opacification (PCO). In addition, contracture of a continuous curvilinear capsulorrhexis may occlude the visual axis because of anterior capsule fibrosis and phimosis. Posterior or anterior capsule opacification is amenable to treatment by intraocular peeling or polishing of the capsule or by means of Nd:YAG laser capsulotomy.

Capsular opacification stems from the continued viability of lens epithelial cells that remain after removal of the nucleus and cortex. Opaque secondary membranes are formed by proliferating lens epithelial cells, fibroblastic metaplasia, and collagen deposition. Lens epithelial cells proliferate in several patterns. Sequestration of nucleated bladder cells *(Wedl cells)* in a closed space between the adherent edges of the anterior and posterior capsule results in a doughnut-shaped configuration, referred to as a *Soemmering ring.* If the epithelial cells migrate out of the capsular bag, translucent globular masses resembling fish eggs *(Elschnig pearls)* form on the edge of the capsular opening. These pearls can fill the pupil or remain hidden behind the iris. Histologic examination shows that these "fish eggs" are nucleated bladder cells, identical to those proliferating within the capsule of a Soemmering ring but usually lacking a basement membrane. If the epithelial cells migrate across the anterior or posterior capsule, they may cause capsular wrinkling and opacification. Significantly, the lens epithelial cells are capable of undergoing metaplasia with conversion to myofibroblasts. These cells can produce a matrix of fibrous and basement membrane collagen. Contraction of this collagen matrix causes wrinkles in the posterior capsule, with resultant distortion of vision and glare.

The reported incidence of PCO varies widely but has been diminishing with current IOL design and placement. Older studies report that the frequency of Nd:YAG laser capsulotomy varies between 3% and 53% within 3 years of cataract surgery. More recent clinical series with a 3- to 5-year follow-up of cases with either hydrophobic acrylic or silicone square-edge design show PCO rates between 0% and 4.7%. Factors thought to influence this rate include the age of the patient, history of intraocular inflammation, presence of pseudoexfoliation syndrome, size of the anterior capsulorrhexis, quality of the cortical cleanup, capsular fixation of the implant, design of the lens implant (specifically, a reduction in incidence with posterior convex or a truncated square-edge optic design), modification of the lens surface, and time elapsed since surgery. There seems to be no difference in PCO rates with prolonged use of postoperative topical corticosteroids or NSAIDs. The presence of intraocular silicone oil may dramatically speed up the progression of PCO.

The IOL material has a modest effect on opacification rates. Hydrogel IOLs lead to the highest rate, followed by PMMA, then silicone; hydrophobic acrylic material IOLs lead to the lowest rate. However, the IOL design is now considered the dominant factor both in inhibiting posterior migration of lens epithelial cells and in influencing the rate of PCO. The truncated-edge design is associated with lower rates of PCO in both silicone and acrylic IOLs, although these lenses may increase the incidence of undesirable optical reflections and positive dysphotopsias.

Cheng JW, Wei RL, Cai JP, et al. Efficacy of different intraocular lens materials and optic edge designs in preventing posterior capsular opacification: a meta-analysis. *Am J Ophthalmol.* 2007;143(3):428–436.

Dewey S. Posterior capsule opacification. *Curr Opin Ophthalmol.* 2006;17(1):45–53.

Rönbeck M, Zetterström C, Wejde G, Kugelberg M. Comparison of posterior capsule opacification development with 3 intraocular lens types: five-year prospective study. *J Cataract Refract Surg.* 2009;35(11):1935–1940.

Sacu S, Menapace R, Findl L, Kiss B, Buehl W, Georgopoulos M. Long-term efficacy of adding a sharp posterior edge to a three-piece silicone intraocular lens on capsule opacification: five-year results of a randomized study. *Am J Ophthalmol.* 2005;139(4):696–703.

Anterior Capsule Fibrosis and Phimosis

Capsular fibrosis is associated with clouding of the anterior capsule. If a substantial portion of the IOL optic is covered by the opaque anterior capsule, including portions exposed through the undilated pupil, the patient may become symptomatic. Symptoms may include glare, especially at night due to physiologic mydriasis in darkness, or a perception that vision has become cloudy or hazy.

The term *capsular phimosis* is used to describe the postoperative contraction of the anterior capsule opening as a result of circumferential fibrosis. Phimosis produces symptoms similar to and often more pronounced than those of fibrosis itself and may cause stress on the zonular fibers or decentration of an IOL optic. Anterior capsule contraction and fibrosis occur more frequently with smaller capsulorrhexis openings, in patients with underlying pseudoexfoliation syndrome, and in other situations with abnormal or asymmetric zonular support (eg, penetrating or blunt trauma, Marfan syndrome, or surgical trauma). Anterior capsule contraction may contribute to late pseudophakodonesis or in-the-bag IOL subluxation due to stress on the zonular apparatus. Anterior capsule polishing to remove residual lens epithelial cells may help reduce anterior capsule contraction but not PCO.

Capsular phimosis can be treated with several radial Nd:YAG anterior capsulotomies to release the annular contraction, reduce the traction on the zonular fibers, and enlarge the anterior capsule opening (Fig 8-7). This procedure is performed in a fashion similar to Nd:YAG laser posterior capsulotomy, with care taken to not defocus too far posteriorly and damage the underlying IOL with laser pitting. In general, the anterior capsule tissue or a fibrotic ring is tougher and thus requires more laser power than does the posterior capsule.

Nd:YAG Laser Capsulotomy

Use of the Nd:YAG laser is now a standard procedure for the treatment of secondary opacification of the posterior capsule or contraction of the anterior capsule. Alternatively, intraocular surgical cleaning of the capsule may be performed during the course of concurrent anterior segment surgery if it is desirable to maintain an intact posterior capsule. If possible, posterior capsulotomy should be delayed until there is adequate apposition and fusion of the anterior and posterior capsule peripheral to the lens optic to reduce the possibility of vitreous prolapse around the IOL and into the anterior chamber. Otherwise, an ideal time to perform posterior capsulotomy for treatment of symptomatic posterior capsule opacity has not been established.

Indications

The following are indications for Nd:YAG capsulotomy:

- visual acuity symptomatically decreased as a result of PCO
- a hazy posterior capsule preventing the clear view of the ocular fundus required for diagnostic or therapeutic purposes

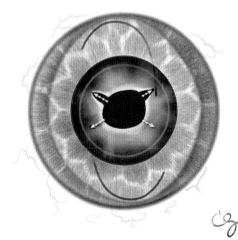

Figure 8-7 Nd:YAG laser anterior capsulotomy. Multiple radial anterior capsulotomies can relieve anterior capsule phimosis and traction on the zonular fibers. *(Illustration by Christine Gralapp.)*

- monocular diplopia, a Maddox rod–like effect, or glare caused by wrinkling of the posterior capsule or by encroachment of a partially opened posterior capsule into the visual axis
- contraction of anterior capsulotomy (capsular phimosis), causing encroachment on the visual axis, excessive traction on the zonular fibers, or alteration of the lens optic position
- capsular block syndrome

Contraindications

The following are contraindications for Nd:YAG laser capsulotomy:

- inadequate visualization of the posterior capsule
- a patient who is unable to remain still or hold fixation during the procedure (use of a contact lens or retrobulbar anesthesia may enhance the feasibility of a capsulotomy in such patients)
- active intraocular inflammation, uncontrolled glaucoma, high risk of retinal detachment, and suspected CME are all relative contraindications

Procedure

Observation of the posterior capsule through an undilated pupil can help the surgeon pinpoint the location of the visual axis. The center of the visual axis is the desired site for the opening, which is usually adequate at 3–4 mm in diameter. In some circumstances, larger-diameter openings may be required for more complete visualization of the fundus. Dilation is not always necessary for the procedure but may be helpful if a larger opening in the posterior capsule is desired. When viewing the posterior capsule, the surgeon should note *before* dilation any specific landmarks near the visual axis, because the location of the visual axis may not be obvious through the dilated pupil.

A high-plus-powered anterior segment laser lens, used with topical anesthesia, improves ocular stability and enlarges the cone angle of the beam, reducing the depth of focus. The smaller focus diameter facilitates the laser pulse puncture of the capsule, and structures in front of and behind the point of focus are less likely to be damaged.

Capsulotomy can be performed in a spiral (Fig 8-8A), cruciate (Fig 8-8B), or inverted-D-shaped pattern, beginning in the periphery to reduce the likelihood of central optic pitting until ideal energy levels and focus have been established. Occasional IOL dislocation into the vitreous following capsulotomy has been reported, particularly with silicone plate-haptic lenses. Constructing the capsulotomy in a spiraling circular pattern, rather than in a cruciate pattern, creates an opening that is less likely to extend radially, reducing the risk of dislocation. Also, the diameter of the capsulotomy should not exceed that of the IOL optic.

If minimal laser energy is applied, the anterior vitreous face may remain intact. A ruptured anterior vitreous face will usually not result in anterior chamber prolapse by the barrier effect of a PCIOL, although vitreous strands occasionally migrate around the lens and through the pupil.

Any PCIOL can be damaged by laser energy, but the threshold for lens damage appears to be lower for silicone than for other materials. The laser pulse should be focused

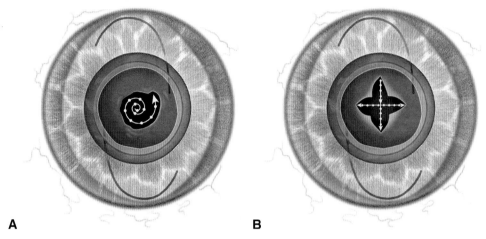

A   **B**

Figure 8-8 Nd:YAG laser posterior capsulotomy. **A,** A spiral pattern *(arrow)* may reduce the risk of radial tears. **B,** A cruciate pattern *(arrows)* or an inverted-D-shaped pattern (not shown) with an inferior flap hinge allows for initial punctures in the periphery and may help reduce the risk of central IOL laser damage. *(Illustration by Christine Gralapp.)*

just behind the posterior capsule; pulses too far behind the IOL will be ineffective. The safest approach is to focus the laser beam slightly behind the posterior surface of the capsule for the initial application and then move anteriorly for subsequent applications, until the desired puncture is achieved.

In cases of anterior capsule contraction, multiple relaxing incisions of the fibrotic ring relieve the contracting force and create a larger optical opening (see Fig 8-7).

The success rate of Nd:YAG laser posterior capsulotomy exceeds 95%. Occasionally, the Nd:YAG laser is insufficient to address exceptionally dense fibrosis, which may require surgical manipulation with a discission knife, vitrectomy handpiece, or scissors.

In addition to capsulotomy, the Nd:YAG laser can be used for vitreolysis, synechialysis, iris cystotomy, iridotomy, anterior hyaloidotomy for ciliary block, removal of precipitates and membranes from an IOL surface, and fragmentation of retained cortical material.

Complications

Complications of Nd:YAG laser capsulotomy include transient or long-term elevated IOP, retinal detachment, CME, hyphema, damage to or dislocation of the IOL, corneal edema, and corneal abrasions (from the focusing contact lens for the laser surgery). Transient elevation of IOP occurs in a significant number of patients, with pressure levels peaking 2–3 hours after surgery. This elevation is likely due to obstruction of the outflow pathways by debris scattered by the laser treatment. It is more common in eyes with vitreous prolapse, those without in-the-bag fixation of the IOL, or those with preexisting glaucoma. Such elevation responds quickly to topical glaucoma medications, which can be continued for 3–5 days following the procedure. For any type of laser capsular surgery, many surgeons prescribe prophylactic preoperative and postoperative ocular hypotensive medications (α-adrenergic agonist or β-blocker drops), as well as either topical corticosteroids or NSAIDs to reduce the risk of postprocedure IOP spikes, inflammation, and CME.

Nd:YAG laser capsulotomy may increase the risk of retinal detachment; the reported incidence is 0%–3.6%. Approximately 50%–75% of the retinal detachments following cataract extraction occur within 1 year of surgery or within 6 months of capsulotomy, often in association with a posterior vitreous detachment (PVD). In many cases, it is difficult to ascertain whether the retinal detachment is related to the capsulotomy or to the cataract surgery itself or whether it is simply a consequence of a naturally occurring PVD. Axial myopia, male sex, young age, trauma, vitreous prolapse, a family history of retinal detachment, and preexisting vitreoretinal pathology are factors that increase the risk of retinal detachment following Nd:YAG capsulotomy. All patients at increased risk of retinal detachment should be instructed to promptly report any new symptoms suggesting a PVD or retinal tear.

CME can occur following Nd:YAG capsulotomy. In patients with a history of CME, or in high-risk patients such as those with diabetic retinopathy, the prophylactic use of topical corticosteroids or NSAIDs may be beneficial.

American Academy of Ophthalmology Cataract/Anterior Segment Panel. Preferred Practice Pattern Guidelines. *Cataract in the Adult Eye.* San Francisco: American Academy of Ophthalmology; 2011. Available at www.aao.org/ppp.

Jahn CE, Richter J, Jahn AH, Kremer G, Kron M. Pseudophakic retinal detachment after uneventful phacoemulsification and subsequent neodymium: YAG capsulotomy for capsule opacification. *J Cataract Refract Surg.* 2003;29(5):925–929.

Olsen G, Olson RJ. Update on a long-term, prospective study of capsulotomy and retinal detachment rates after cataract surgery. *J Cataract Refract Surg.* 2000;26(7):1017–1021.

Tuft SJ, Minassian D, Sullivan P. Risk factors for retinal detachment after cataract surgery: a case-control study. *Ophthalmology.* 2006;113(4):650–656.

Hemorrhage

Systemic Anticoagulation

A large, prospective cohort study did not show an increased risk of hemorrhagic complications in patients on anticoagulant or antiplatelet therapy during cataract surgery. In addition, no increase in the risk of medical complications was observed when such therapy was temporarily discontinued for surgery. This result contrasts with earlier reports suggesting that anticoagulation increases the risk of suprachoroidal effusion and hemorrhage, and with more recent reports that cessation of anticoagulation therapy carries significant risks of thromboembolic complications. In general, patients undergoing cataract surgery with topical or sub-Tenon anesthesia do not require cessation of anticoagulant therapy. If the surgeon is considering discontinuation of anticoagulants, consultation with the patient's primary care physician is recommended.

Katz J, Feldman MA, Bass EB, et al; Study of Medical Testing for Cataract Surgery Team. Risks and benefits of anticoagulant and antiplatelet medication use before cataract surgery. *Ophthalmology.* 2003;110(9):1784–1788.

Kobayashi H. Evaluation of the need to discontinue antiplatelet and anticoagulant medications before cataract surgery. *J Cataract Refract Surg.* 2010;36(7):1115–1119.

Retrobulbar Hemorrhage

Retrobulbar hemorrhages are more common with retrobulbar anesthetic injections than with peribulbar injections, and they may vary in intensity. These hemorrhages have become rare with the declining use of retrobulbar injections for cataract surgery. Reports estimate the incidence of significant retrobulbar hemorrhage after retrobulbar injection to be 0.44%–0.74%.

Venous retrobulbar hemorrhages are usually self-limited and tend to spread slowly. They often do not require treatment. *Arterial retrobulbar hemorrhages* occur more rapidly and are associated with taut orbital swelling, marked proptosis, elevated IOP, reduced mobility of the globe, inability to separate the eyelids, and massive ecchymosis of the eyelids and conjunctiva. This type of retrobulbar hemorrhage causes an increase in orbital volume and associated orbital pressure, which can restrict the vascular supply to the globe. Large orbital vessels may be occluded. Tamponade of the smaller vessels in the optic nerve may occur, resulting in severe vision loss from anterior ischemic optic neuropathy and subsequent optic atrophy, despite the absence of obvious retinal vascular occlusion.

Ophthalmologists can often make the diagnosis of retrobulbar hemorrhage by observing the rapid onset of eyelid and conjunctival ecchymosis and tightening of the orbit. The diagnosis can be confirmed by tonometry revealing elevated IOP. Direct ophthalmoscopy may reveal pulsation or occlusion of the central retinal artery in severe cases.

Treatment of acute retrobulbar hemorrhage consists of maneuvers to lower the intraocular and orbital pressure as quickly as possible. These may include digital massage, intravenous osmotic agents, aqueous suppressants, lateral canthotomy and cantholysis, localized conjunctival peritomy (to allow egress of blood), and occasionally anterior chamber paracentesis. The planned surgery should be postponed until the IOP and mobility of the globe and eyelids are normal. To reduce the risk of a recurrent retrobulbar hemorrhage, it may be advisable to use another form of anesthesia for the second attempt at surgery.

In addition to retrobulbar hemorrhage, potential complications of retrobulbar injections include central retinal artery occlusion, ischemic optic neuropathy, toxic neuropathy or myopathy, diplopia, ptosis, and inadvertent subdural injections with possible CNS depression and apnea. Ischemic complications are more common if epinephrine is used in the anesthetic. (See BCSC Section 1, *Update on General Medicine,* and Section 6, *Pediatric Ophthalmology and Strabismus.*)

Davis DB 2nd, Mandel MR. Efficacy and complication rate of 16,224 consecutive peribulbar blocks. A prospective multicenter study. *J Cataract Refract Surg.* 1994;20(3):327–337.

Dutton JJ, Hasan SA, Edelhauser HF, Kim T, Springs CL, Broocker G. Anesthesia for intraocular surgery. *Surv Ophthalmol.* 2001;46(2):172–184.

Morgan CM, Schatz H, Vine AK, et al. Ocular complications associated with retrobulbar injections. *Ophthalmology.* 1988;95(5):660–665.

Hyphema

Hyphema in the immediate postoperative period usually originates from the incision or the iris. It is commonly mild and resolves spontaneously. The risk of hyphema is greater in patients with pseudoexfoliation syndrome, anterior segment neovascularization, Fuchs heterochromic uveitis, or vascular tufts at the pupillary margin. Resolution may take longer if vitreous is mixed with the blood. The two major complications from prolonged hyphema are elevated IOP and corneal blood staining. IOP should be monitored closely and initially treated medically, although it may be difficult to control if the blood is mixed with the OVD used during the procedure. Surgical evacuation is occasionally necessary.

Hyphema occurring months to years after surgery is usually the result of incision vascularization or erosion of vascular tissue in the iris or ciliary body by an IOL haptic or optic edge. Argon laser photocoagulation of the bleeding vessel, often performed through a goniolens, may stop the bleeding or prevent rebleeding. To reduce the risk of continued or recurrent bleeding, antiplatelet or anticoagulation therapy may be withheld, if medically possible, until the hyphema resolves. Occasionally, it is necessary to reposition or exchange an IOL that comes in contact with iris or angle structures and results in recurrent intraocular hemorrhage.

Suprachoroidal Effusion or Hemorrhage

Suprachoroidal effusion with or without suprachoroidal hemorrhage usually occurs intraoperatively, but may also occur later in cases with prolonged postoperative hypotony. Suprachoroidal effusion typically presents as a forward prolapse of ocular structures, including iris, lens diaphragm, and vitreous, generally accompanied by a change in the red reflex. Clinically, suprachoroidal effusion may be difficult to differentiate from suprachoroidal hemorrhage. Patient agitation and pain followed by an extremely firm globe suggest suprachoroidal hemorrhage. Both complications are more common in the presence of associated hypertension, arteriosclerotic cardiovascular disease, tachycardia, obesity, high myopia, glaucoma, advanced age, nanophthalmos, choroidal hemangioma associated with Sturge-Weber syndrome, or chronic ocular inflammation. Fortunately, both suprachoroidal effusion and suprachoroidal hemorrhage are much less likely with small-incision phacoemulsification than with larger-incision surgery because the relatively closed system formed by the small, self-sealing incisions and the relatively tight fit of the phaco tip in the incision prevents prolonged hypotony and reduces intraoperative fluctuations in IOP.

Suprachoroidal effusion may be a precursor to suprachoroidal hemorrhage. Exudation of fluid from choroidal vasculature ultimately stretches veins or arteries that supply the choroid after coursing through the sclera. If suprachoroidal hemorrhage occurs in this situation, it is presumably a result of disruption of one or more of these taut blood vessels. Alternatively, suprachoroidal hemorrhage may represent a spontaneous rupture of choroidal vasculature, particularly in patients with underlying systemic vascular disease. (See also BCSC Section 12, *Retina and Vitreous.*)

Expulsive Suprachoroidal Hemorrhage

Expulsive suprachoroidal hemorrhage, a rare but serious condition, generally occurs intraoperatively. The hemorrhage usually presents as a sudden increase in IOP accompanied by acute onset of pain and the following:

- darkening of the red reflex
- incision gape
- iris prolapse
- expulsion of the lens, vitreous, and bright red blood

The instant this condition is recognized, the surgeon must close the incision with sutures or digital pressure. Prolapsed vitreous should be excised and uveal tissue, reposited. After the wound is securely closed, the surgeon may consider posterior sclerotomies to allow the escape of suprachoroidal blood to decompress the globe, enable repositioning of prolapsed intraocular tissue, and facilitate permanent closure of the cataract incision. Drainage of suprachoroidal blood may be achieved by performing sclerotomies in one or more quadrants, 5–7 mm posterior to the limbus. Elevated IOP serves both to stop bleeding and to expel suprachoroidal blood. Once there is optimal clearance of blood from the suprachoroidal space, the sclerotomies may be left open to allow further drainage postoperatively. It may be necessary to repeat the drainage procedure 7 days or more after an expulsive hemorrhage in cases of residual suprachoroidal blood that threatens ocular integrity or vision. These procedures may lower dangerously elevated IOPs and restore appropriate anatomical relationships within the eye, but they carry some risk that bleeding will recur.

If the incision can be closed without posterior sclerotomies, more rapid tamponade of the bleeding vessel can be achieved. Most surgeons would then terminate the operation and observe for 7–14 days to allow clotting and liquefaction of the hemorrhage, while managing elevated IOP medically. Referral to a vitreoretinal surgeon for management and subsequent drainage of choroidal hemorrhage should be considered. The patient needs to be informed of the guarded prognosis for restoration of vision.

Delayed Suprachoroidal Hemorrhage

Delayed suprachoroidal hemorrhage may occur in the early postoperative period, presenting with sudden onset of pain, loss of vision, and shallowing of the anterior chamber. Predisposing factors for postoperative choroidal hemorrhage or effusion include prolonged hypotony, wound leak, unrecognized scleral perforation, trauma, uveitis, cyclodialysis, and excessive filtration. This condition is far more common after glaucoma filtering procedures than routine cataract surgery and may also arise following laser photocoagulation or cryotherapy. If the incision remains intact and the IOP can be controlled medically, limited suprachoroidal hemorrhage may be observed and frequently will resolve spontaneously. If the incision is not intact, surgical revision may be sufficient to allow the hemorrhage to resolve. Medical management consists of systemic corticosteroids, topical and oral ocular hypotensive agents for elevated IOP, topical cycloplegia, and close observation. Surgical drainage of the suprachoroidal space is indicated if there is a flat anterior chamber, medically uncontrolled glaucoma, or persistent or adherent (kissing) choroidal detachments.

Endophthalmitis

Endophthalmitis is a rare but dreaded complication of cataract surgery that may lead to severe loss of vision or loss of the eye. Early diagnosis and prompt treatment are essential for achieving a satisfactory outcome. Recent large retrospective studies of the incidence of endophthalmitis after cataract surgery reveal rates between 0.04% and 0.20%. Some studies, particularly with older data, reveal higher rates. A comprehensive review of

440,000 consecutive cataract surgeries performed in Canada from 2002 to 2006 revealed an incidence of 0.14%. Factors that increase the risk of infection include diabetes mellitus, older age, male gender, complicated or prolonged surgery, vitreous loss, posterior capsule rupture, wound leaks, and possibly the use of clear corneal incisions.

Infectious endophthalmitis may present in an acute form or in a more indolent or chronic form; the latter is associated with organisms of lower pathogenicity. The symptoms of endophthalmitis include mild to severe ocular pain, vision loss, floaters, and photophobia. The hallmark of endophthalmitis is vitreous inflammation, but other signs include eyelid or periorbital edema, ciliary injection, chemosis, anterior chamber inflammation, hypopyon, decreased visual acuity, corneal edema, and retinal hemorrhages (Fig 8-9). Most cases present within 3–10 days of surgery, with a median of 6 days, as reported in the Endophthalmitis Vitrectomy Study (EVS). A significant percentage (22%) of cases presented 2–6 weeks after surgery. The most common bacterial causes in that study were gram-positive coagulase-negative *Staphylococcus epidermidis* (70%), *Staphylococcus aureus* (9.9%), *Streptococcus* species (9.0%), other gram-positive bacteria (3.1%), *Enterococcus* species (2.2%), and gram-negative bacteria (5.9%). Most infections are caused by organisms similar to the patients' own periocular bacterial flora. Drug-resistant strains are becoming more common.

To reduce the risk of infection, preoperative 10% povidone-iodine skin prep, povidone-iodine 5% drops, careful eyelid and eyelash draping, and sterile technique should be utilized. This method is the most effective and least expensive way to reduce the incidence of postoperative endophthalmitis. Meticulous attention to watertight incision closure is also important in preventing endophthalmitis, particularly when clear corneal incisions are employed.

Prophylactic preoperative and postoperative topical antibiotics are usually prescribed for cataract surgery, although there are no randomized clinical studies to support this practice.

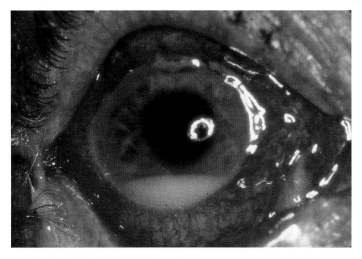

Figure 8-9   Endophthalmitis. *(Courtesy of Karla J. Johns, MD.)*

In 2006, the Endophthalmitis Study Group of the European Society of Cataract and Refractive Surgeons (ESCRS) reported a decrease in endophthalmitis rates from 0.34% to 0.07% in patients given intracameral cefuroxime 1 mg at the conclusion of surgery in comparison to patients given topical levofloxacin alone. The high incidence of infection in the control group confounded the results. The ESCRS also reported a 4.92-fold increase in endophthalmitis when intracameral cefuroxime was not used and a 5.88-fold increase in risk with the use of clear corneal incisions instead of scleral tunnels. Other studies have also supported the use of an intracameral bolus of antibiotic at the conclusion of surgery. Although the practice is not universally accepted, many surgeons use an intracameral antibiotic such as vancomycin, moxifloxacin, or a broad-spectrum cephalosporin. Given the difficulty of obtaining commercially available, preservative-free antibiotics in doses appropriate for intracameral prophylaxis, surgeons must weigh these results against the risk of TASS from dilutional errors or preservative toxicity.

Diagnosis

Acute endophthalmitis, defined as occurring within 6 weeks of surgery, typically develops 3–10 days postoperatively and runs a fulminant course. Early diagnosis is extremely important, as delay of treatment can substantially alter the visual prognosis.

Chronic endophthalmitis, in contrast, may develop weeks or months after surgery. It may be characterized by chronic iridocyclitis or granulomatous uveitis and is often associated with decreased vision, little or no pain, and the presence of a nidus of the infectious agent within the eye. The most common causes are *P acnes, S epidermidis,* and fungi. (See also BCSC Section 9, *Intraocular Inflammation and Uveitis,* and Section 12, *Retina and Vitreous.*)

Acute infectious endophthalmitis must be differentiated from TASS (discussed earlier in this chapter). The clinical presentation is often diagnostic, but occasionally the clinician may be able to diagnose sterile endophthalmitis only by excluding possible infectious causes by means of appropriate aqueous and vitreous cultures.

Treatment

The recommended approach to the diagnosis and management of postoperative endophthalmitis is based on the results of the EVS. As soon as a clinical diagnosis of endophthalmitis is suspected, assessment of visual acuity will help direct management decisions. Needle biopsy for anterior chamber and vitreous samples for culture and Gram stain will help determine the appropriate antibiotic selection. Fortified topical antibiotics may be started if doing so does not delay referral to a vitreoretinal specialist. Immediate pars plana vitrectomy and antibiotic injections are indicated when the patient's visual acuity has been reduced to light perception.

When the visual acuity is hand motions or better, a less-invasive anterior chamber and vitreous biopsy for cultures with subsequent intravitreal injection of antibiotics may be sufficient. To expedite the delivery of antibiotics, this procedure can be performed in the office under sterile conditions. Because clinical features do not distinguish between gram-positive and gram-negative organisms, the mainstay of treatment for both remains broad-spectrum intravitreal antibiotics. Currently, vancomycin 1 mg and ceftazidime 2.25 mg or amikacin 0.4 mg are preferred. Fortified topical or subconjunctival antibiotics are administered in the period following intravitreal antibiotic injection while waiting for culture results. Topical cycloplegic and corticosteroid drops are advised. Intravenous or oral antibiotics have shown little benefit, although bactericidal aqueous and intravitreal concentrations of parenteral fourth-generation fluoroquinolones have been documented. Although intravitreal corticosteroids are frequently used because of their theoretical role in reducing inflammation and scarring, their benefit has yet to be demonstrated in a controlled study.

Chronic or delayed-onset endophthalmitis is also best treated with vitreous biopsy and intraocular antibiotics. However, due to sequestration of infectious material in the capsular bag or vitreous, a vitrectomy and posterior capsulectomy or even IOL exchange is often necessary to remove the nidus of infection. See BCSC Section 12, *Retina and Vitreous,* for additional discussion.

Doft BH. Managing infectious endophthalmitis: results of the Endophthalmitis Vitrectomy Study. *Focal Points: Clinical Modules for Ophthalmologists.* San Francisco: American Academy of Ophthalmology; 1997, module 3.

Endophthalmitis Study Group, European Society of Cataract and Refractive Surgeons (ESCRS). Prophylaxis of postoperative endophthalmitis following cataract surgery: results of the ESCRS multicenter study and identification of risk factors. *J Cataract Refract Surg.* 2007; 33(6):978–988.

Hatch WV, Cernat G, Wong D, Devenyi R, Bell CM. Risk factors for acute endophthalmitis after cataract surgery: a population-based study. *Ophthalmology.* 2009;116(3):425–430.

Lundström M, Wejde G, Stenevi U, Thorburn W, Montan P. Endophthalmitis after cataract surgery: a nationwide prospective study evaluating incidence in relation to incision type and location. *Ophthalmology.* 2007;114(5):866–870.

Nentwich MM, Ta CN, Kreutzer TC, et al. Incidence of postoperative endophthalmitis from 1990 to 2009 using povidone-iodine but no intracameral antibiotics at a single academic institution. *J Cataract Refract Surg.* 2015;41(1):58–66.

Packer M, Chang DF, Dewey SH, et al. Prevention, diagnosis, and management of acute postoperative bacterial endophthalmitis. *J Cataract Refract Surg.* 2011;37(9):1699–1714.

Retinal Complications

Cystoid Macular Edema

Cystoid macular edema (CME) after cataract surgery, also known as *Irvine-Gass syndrome,* is a common cause of postoperative decreased vision. Although the pathogenesis of CME is unknown, the final common pathway appears to be increased perifoveal capillary permeability with accumulation of fluid in the inner nuclear and outer plexiform layers. CME is often associated with intraocular inflammation and may be mediated through the release of prostaglandins and leukotrienes.

CME may be recognized by an otherwise unexplained reduction in vision, by the characteristic petaloid appearance of cystic spaces in the macula on ophthalmoscopy or fluorescein angiography (Fig 8-10A), or by cystic areas of low reflectivity and retinal thickening on spectral-domain optical coherence tomography (SD-OCT) (Fig 8-10B). Angiographic evidence of CME occurs in 40%–70% of eyes following ICCE and in

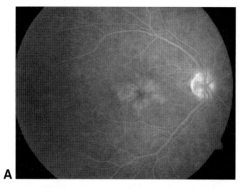
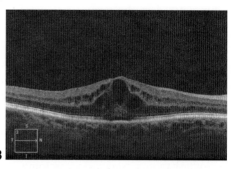

A   B

Figure 8-10 Cystoid macular edema (CME). **A,** Fluorescein angiogram demonstrates late pooling of dye in a petaloid pattern in the macula and staining of the optic nerve head. **B,** Spectral-domain optical coherence tomography (SD-OCT) scan shows diffuse retinal thickening with cystic areas of low reflectivity predominantly in the inner nuclear and outer plexiform layers. *(Courtesy of Thomas L. Beardsley, MD.)*

approximately 1%–19% of eyes following ECCE via nucleus expression or phacoemulsification. OCT studies may detect postoperative macular thickening in up to 41% of eyes following phacoemulsification. Most of the affected patients are asymptomatic, although there may be some loss of contrast sensitivity even in the absence of reduced Snellen visual acuity.

If the diagnosis of clinically significant CME is based on vision loss to the 20/40 level or worse, the incidence is 2%–10% following intracapsular surgery and 1%–2% following extracapsular surgery with an intact posterior capsule. The risk of clinical CME after small-incision phacoemulsification with an intact posterior capsule is believed to be even lower (0.10%–2.35%). However, patients with angiographic CME after phacoemulsification score significantly lower in logMAR (logarithm of minimum angle of resolution) visual acuity than do patients with no CME, even though their Snellen visual acuities remain better than 20/40.

The peak incidence of both angiographic and clinical CME occurs 6–10 weeks after surgery. Spontaneous resolution occurs in approximately 95% of uncomplicated cases, usually within 3–12 months. In rare cases, CME may develop many years after surgery, especially in association with delayed postoperative rupture of the anterior vitreous face. CME has also been associated with the use of topical epinephrine and dipivefrin for the treatment of aphakic glaucoma. Prostaglandin analogues have been associated with reversible CME in eyes that have undergone recent intraocular surgery, although a cause-and-effect relationship has not been established. The risk is believed to be greater in the absence of an intact posterior capsule.

Preoperative risk factors for CME include coexisting uveitis, preexisting epiretinal membrane, vitreomacular traction, diabetes mellitus and diabetic retinopathy, previous retinal vein occlusion, retinitis pigmentosa, and previous occurrence of CME. Surgical and postoperative risk factors include posterior capsule rupture, vitreous loss, iris prolapse, prolonged surgical time, improper IOL positioning, retained lens fragments, poorly controlled postoperative inflammation, and transient or prolonged hypotony.

The risk of CME may be reduced with postoperative prophylactic use of topical corticosteroids and/or NSAID drops. A meta-analysis of randomized clinical trials found that topical NSAIDs alone or in combination with corticosteroids reduced the odds of developing CME in the first 3 months after cataract surgery. A recent American Academy of Ophthalmology report found that topical NSAIDs after cataract surgery are effective in reducing the incidence of CME detected by angiography or OCT and hasten the visual recovery in the short term. There is a lack of level 1 evidence supporting the long-term benefit of NSAID therapy when applied alone or in combination with corticosteroid therapy to prevent vision loss from CME at 3 months or more after cataract surgery. Furthermore, although use of NSAIDs before surgery may increase the speed of visual recovery in the first several postoperative weeks, there is no evidence that this practice affects long-term visual outcomes.

Medical treatment of chronic postoperative CME typically begins with a course of anti-inflammatory drugs such as topical corticosteroids, NSAIDs, or both. Controlled clinical studies have not identified a superior regimen. However, a prospective randomized clinical trial for treatment of chronic CME found that combination therapy with ketorolac 0.5% and prednisolone acetate 1.0% four times a day was more effective than either drug alone in improving visual acuity. Topical anti-inflammatory therapy may take 3–6 months to resolve chronic CME, and the condition may recur after cessation of therapy. If topical medications fail, sub-Tenon steroid injection or intravitreal injections of corticosteroids alone or via a sustained drug-delivery system may be effective. In refractory cases, systemic carbonic anhydrase inhibitors may be beneficial. Intravitreal vascular endothelial growth factor (VEGF) inhibitors have been used with success in chronic CME cases that do not respond to conventional treatment.

Surgical therapy may be indicated when an inciting source of chronic CME can be defined and the edema fails to respond to medical therapy. Any retained lens fragments should be removed. Nd:YAG laser vitreolysis or vitrectomy can be used to remove vitreous adhering to the cataract incision in order to relieve iris deformity or vitreomacular traction. If the IOL is malpositioned and contributing to chronic uveitis, repositioning or exchange may be helpful. For further discussion of CME, see BCSC Section 12, *Retina and Vitreous*.

Guo S, Patel S, Baumrind B, et al. Management of pseudophakic cystoid macular edema. *Surv Ophthalmol.* 2015;60(2):123–137.

Henderson BA, Kim JY, Ament CS, Ferrufino-Ponce ZK, Grabowska A, Cremers SL. Clinical pseudophakic cystoid macular edema. Risk factors for development and duration after treatment. *J Cataract Refract Surg.* 2007;33(8):1550–1558.

Kessel L, Tendal B, Jørgensen KJ, et al. Post-cataract prevention of inflammation and macular edema by steroid and nonsteroidal anti-inflammatory eye drops: a systematic review. *Ophthalmology.* 2014;121(10):1915–1924.

Kim SJ, Schoenberger SD, Thorne JE, Ehlers JP, Yeh S, Bakri SJ. Topical nonsteroidal anti-inflammatory drugs and cataract surgery. A report by the American Academy of Ophthalmology. *Ophthalmology.* 2015;122(11):2159–2168.

Wielders LHP, Lambermont VA, Schouten JS, et al. Prevention of cystoid macular edema after cataract surgery in nondiabetic and diabetic patients: a systematic review and meta-analysis. *Am J Ophthalmol.* 2015;160(5):968–981.e33.

Retinal Light Toxicity

Prolonged exposure to the illuminating filament of the operating microscope can result in an increased risk of CME or a burn to the retinal pigment epithelium (RPE). The risk of an RPE burn is particularly high during cataract surgery, when the filtering effects of the natural lens (cataract) are removed, exposing the vulnerable RPE to unfiltered blue light and near-ultraviolet (near-UV) radiation. If a burn occurs, a central or paracentral scotoma may result. Minimizing retinal exposure to the operating microscope light, filtering light wavelengths below 515 nm, and, when possible, using pupillary shields and oblique lighting reduce the risk of this complication.

US Food and Drug Administration (FDA). Retinal photic injuries from operating microscopes during cataract surgery: FDA Public Health Advisory. FDA website. October 16, 1995. Available at www.fda.gov/MedicalDevices/Safety/AlertsandNotices/PublicHealthNotifications /ucm062683.htm. Accessed October 26, 2015.

Retinal Detachment

Rhegmatogenous retinal detachment (RRD) is an uncommon but serious complication of cataract surgery. The incidence of pseudophakic RRD has been reported at 0.2%–3.6%, depending on follow-up time and patient demographics. RRD occurs most frequently within 1 year of cataract surgery or 6 months following posterior capsulotomy. During the first postoperative year following phacoemulsification, the incidence of RRD ranges from 0.6% to 1.7%, with an average of 0.7%. The cumulative risk for pseudophakic RRD increases with time. For all age and gender groups, eyes that have undergone cataract surgery have a fourfold-higher risk of RRD when compared with fellow phakic eyes. The incidence of RRD was 2 times higher following ICCE than ECCE and has continued to decline since the adoption of small-incision phacoemulsification surgery.

Most acute RRDs are subsequent to a PVD. Uncomplicated cataract surgery and laser posterior capsulotomy are risk factors for RRD in part because these procedures are risk factors for earlier onset of PVD. Myopic eyes have a much higher risk of RRD whether pseudophakic or phakic, and this risk rises with each additional millimeter of axial length. Predisposing risk factors for RRD include axial myopia (6- to 10-times-greater risk with axial length >25 mm), younger age (4-times-greater risk with age <60 years), male gender, lattice degeneration of the retina, a previous retinal tear or detachment in the surgical eye, a history of retinal detachment in the fellow eye, or a family history of retinal detachment.

The presence of an intact posterior capsule reduces the incidence of RRD. Conversely, the risk of postoperative RRD after cataract surgery complicated by posterior capsule rupture is increased at least tenfold. Some studies have reported that Nd:YAG laser posterior capsulotomy may increase the risk for RRD by 3.9–4.9 times, whereas other studies found no evidence of increased risk caused by capsulotomy. The rate of RRD after uncomplicated Nd:YAG capsulotomy without vitreous prolapse may be equal to the spontaneous rate in a matched pseudophakic population. Neither the size of the capsulotomy nor the total energy delivered is thought to increase risk.

The successful repair of retinal detachment is not influenced by the presence or absence of either an ACIOL or a PCIOL. Pars plana vitrectomy with or without a scleral buckle is the most commonly used procedure for repair of RRD; the success rate is approximately 85% with one operation and ultimately 98% with multiple procedures. (See also BCSC Section 12, *Retina and Vitreous.*)

Arya AV, Emerson JW, Engelbert M, Hagedorn CL, Adelman RA. Surgical management of pseudophakic retinal detachments: a meta-analysis. *Ophthalmology.* 2006;113(10): 1724–1733.

Bjerrum SS, Mikkelsen KL, La Cour M. Risk of pseudophakic retinal detachment in 202,226 patients using the fellow nonoperated eye as reference. *Ophthalmology.* 2013;120(12): 2573–2579.

Boberg-Ans G, Henning V, Villumsen J, La Cour M. Longterm incidence of rhegmatogenous retinal detachment and survival in a defined population undergoing standardized phacoemulsification surgery. *Acta Ophthalmol Scand.* 2006;84(5):613–618.

Clark A, Morlet N, Ng JQ, Preen DB, Semmens JB. Risk for retinal detachment after phacoemulsification: a whole-population study of cataract surgery outcomes. *Arch Ophthalmol.* 2012;130(7):882–888.

Neuhann IM, Neuhann TF, Heimann H, Schmickler S, Gerl RH, Foerster MH. Retinal detachment after phacoemulsification in high myopia: analysis of 2356 cases. *J Cataract Refract Surg.* 2008;34(10):1644–1657.

Tuft SJ, Minassian D, Sullivan P. Risk factors for retinal detachment after cataract surgery: a case-control study. *Ophthalmology.* 2006;113(4):650–656.

Preparing for Cataract Surgery in Special Situations

▶ *This chapter includes related videos, which can be accessed by scanning the QR codes provided in the text or going to www.aao.org/bcscvideo_section11.*

A complete discussion of the indications for and technique of cataract surgery in the pediatric age group is presented in BCSC Section 6, *Pediatric Ophthalmology and Strabismus*.

Psychosocial Considerations

Claustrophobia

Patients with claustrophobia find it helpful to be told about the operating room and sterile-draping requirement prior to their surgery. The medical team can make accommodations for the patient who becomes anxious and extremely uncomfortable when confined to a small space or when the patient's head is covered by a surgical drape. The anesthetist can titrate intravenous sedation and hold the patient's hand to provide comfort and reassurance during surgery. When feasible, the surgeon can supplement topical or local ocular anesthesia with a "vocal local," providing soothing support to the patient. Options for reducing the sensation of claustrophobia and avoiding retention of carbon dioxide under the drape include placing a suction catheter under the drape, tenting open the side of the drape, or placing an elevated Mayo stand over the patient's torso. General anesthesia is chosen when a patient cannot tolerate the aforementioned measures to address claustrophobia.

Neurocognitive and Neurodevelopmental Disorders

When dementia or other central nervous system impairment interferes with a patient's ability to communicate symptoms of cataract, the patient's functional deficit must be evaluated by other methods, such as discussion with a caregiver or family member about the patient's capacity to carry out activities of daily living. The surgeon may have to rely on objective findings such as degradation of the red reflex, slit-lamp abnormalities, and view of the retina, rather than subjective measurements of visual acuity, to estimate the degree of visual impairment resulting from the cataract. The patient's ability to tolerate sedation and draping throughout surgery must be appraised, and general anesthesia should be considered for the patient who cannot cooperate. In certain instances when general anesthesia is required, the surgeon may consider immediate sequential bilateral cataract surgery. Improving the view of the fundus to monitor and treat retinal disease, as well as the potential for vision rehabilitation and better quality of life, remains the foundation of the decision to proceed with cataract extraction in these situations.

Patient Communication During Eye Surgery

Reviewing the mechanics of the surgical experience is beneficial for all patients preoperatively and especially for those who have hearing loss or who do not speak the same language as the surgical team. Patients may wear their hearing aid in the ear opposite to the eye having surgery, both to allow communication and to avoid water damage to the hearing aid ipsilateral to the surgical site. The surgeon, anesthetist, and patient should determine how best to communicate with one another in the operating room. For example, simple hand signals between the patient and the anesthetist are effective. If the patient is very anxious and cannot communicate adequately, general anesthesia should be considered instead of topical or local anesthesia.

Systemic Considerations

Medical Status

Medical evaluation by the patient's primary care physician may be part of the preoperative planning process. Conditions such as hypertension and diabetes mellitus should be stabilized. Because patients are required to fast prior to surgery, insulin or oral hypoglycemic medication often requires adjustment in diabetic patients. Procedures on these patients should be performed as early in the day as possible to minimize large fluctuations in blood glucose levels.

In patients with lung disease, pulmonary function should be optimized prior to and during surgery; patients may be permitted to bring their inhalers into the operating room. Patients with lung disease may be prone to coughing, which can damage ocular structures during surgery and threaten wound security. Coughing should be controlled judiciously with medication and the patient instructed to warn the surgeon of any need to cough. With small-incision surgery, the risk of such intraoperative complications can be reduced and wound security enhanced. Patients with chronic obstructive pulmonary disease (COPD), bronchitis, congestive heart failure, or obesity benefit from being placed in the reverse Trendelenburg position to reduce venous congestion in the head and neck and lessen the risk of vitreous loss and choroidal hemorrhage.

Ocular inflammation such as scleritis and uveitis associated with connective tissue or inflammatory diseases should be controlled preoperatively to minimize the risk of scleral or corneal necrosis. The ophthalmologist can work in conjunction with the other physicians involved in the patient's care to gauge therapy with systemic corticosteroid and immunosuppressive agents.

For patients with severe arthritis, it can be difficult to lie comfortably during surgery. Usually, the surgical table can be adjusted and pillows added to provide sufficient comfort without interfering with surgical access to the eye. A patient who has ankylosing spondylitis with cervical immobility presents an extreme challenge in surgical positioning (Fig 9-1). If no systemic medical contraindications exist and if adequate access cannot be attained otherwise, the surgeon should consider general anesthesia.

For a more complete discussion of ocular surgery in patients with systemic disease, see BCSC Section 1, *Update on General Medicine.*

Anticoagulation Therapy or Bleeding Disorders

Clear corneal cataract surgery performed with topical anesthesia in patients receiving anticoagulation therapy is not associated with an increased incidence of vision-threatening hemorrhagic complications. Minor bleeding problems, such as eyelid ecchymosis, hyphema, and subconjunctival hemorrhage, are more common with anticoagulant use, but these are transient and self-limited. If a retrobulbar block is used, the risk of retrobulbar hemorrhage is 3 times higher when the patient has been taking anticoagulants. The surgeon should weigh the systemic risks of discontinuing therapy with the surgical risks of continuing anticoagulation or antiplatelet therapy. When warfarin is continued, the international normalized ratio (INR) should be maintained within the therapeutic range.

If anticoagulation therapy is to be discontinued or adjusted for surgery, coordination with the prescribing physician is recommended. Discontinuation of anticoagulation is recommended in patients who have previously experienced a suprachoroidal hemorrhage because these patients are predisposed to recurrent bleeding. Restoring normal coagulation usually requires 3–5 days after stopping warfarin, and restoring platelet function requires

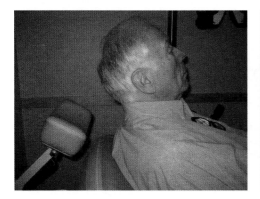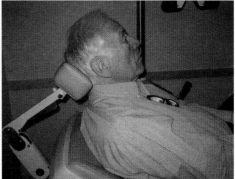

Figure 9-1 Inflammatory systemic disease. Individuals with ankylosing spondylitis, such as the patient shown in these photos, often have cervical immobility. Evaluating patients in the office examination chair allows the surgeon to anticipate accommodations necessary for carrying out surgery safely and comfortably for both patient and surgeon in the operating room. This patient requires adjustment of the headrest to provide adequate support of his head and neck. *(Courtesy of Lisa Rosenberg, MD.)*

Table 9-1 Anticoagulant and Antiplatelet Medications Approved by the US Food and Drug Administration*

Anticoagulants	Antiplatelet Agents
Apixaban (Eliquis)	Anagrelide (Agrylin)
Dabigatran (Pradaxa)	Aspirin/dipyridamole (Aggrenox)
Rivaroxaban (Xarelto)	Cilostazol (Pletal)
Warfarin (Coumadin)	Clopidogrel (Plavix)
	Dipyridamole (Persantine)
	Prasugrel (Effient)
	Ticagrelor (Brilinta)
	Ticlopidine (Ticlid)
	Vorapaxar (Zontivity)

*Approved as of 2015.

10–21 days after stopping antiplatelet therapy. The clinician should ask the patient about the use of all medications, including nonprescription items that may contain aspirin, vitamin E, or vitamin K, which could affect coagulation status. Table 9-1 presents a list of anticoagulant and antiplatelet agents approved by the US Food and Drug Administration.

In the absence of hypotony or hemorrhagic complications, anticoagulation therapy may be safely resumed following the first postoperative visit. Assessment of the patient's coagulation profile prior to surgery should be considered for systemic conditions that might alter clotting ability. For further discussion of ocular hemorrhage, see the discussion of hemorrhage in Chapter 8.

Benzimra JD, Johnston RL, Jaycock P, et al. The Cataract National Dataset electronic multicentre audit of 55,567 operations: antiplatelet and anticoagulant medications. *Eye.* 2009;23(1):10–16.

Grzybowski A, Ascaso FJ, Kupidura-Majewski K, Packer M. Continuation of anticoagulant and antiplatelet therapy during phacoemulsification cataract surgery. *Curr Opin Ophthalmol.* 2015;26(1):28–33.

Jonas JB, Pakdaman B, Sauder G. Cataract surgery under systemic anticoagulant therapy with coumarin. *Eur J Ophthalmol.* 2006;16(1):30–32.

Morris A, Elder MJ. Warfarin therapy and cataract surgery. *Clin Experiment Ophthalmol.* 2000;28(6):419–422.

External Ocular Abnormalities

Blepharitis and Acne Rosacea

Blepharitis, which is particularly common in patients with acne rosacea, should be controlled before surgery in order to reduce the bacterial colony counts of the ocular surface. Uncontrolled blepharitis causing irritation and an unhealthy tear film may adversely affect the quality of the patient's vision after cataract surgery. Treatment of anterior blepharitis includes hot compresses and eyelid scrubs. The mainstay of therapy for meibomian gland dysfunction is systemic tetracycline, doxycycline, or minocycline, all of which saponify inspissated meibomian secretions. Although topical ointments poorly penetrate meibomian orifices, newer topical eyedrops such as azithromycin aim to reduce bacterial flora at the surface of the meibomian glands. For a detailed description of the signs and symptoms of blepharitis, see BCSC Section 8, *External Disease and Cornea*.

Novosad BD, Callegan MC. Severe bacterial endophthalmitis: towards improving clinical outcomes. *Expert Rev Ophthalmol.* 2010;5(5):689–698.

Packer M, Chang DF, Dewey SH, et al. Prevention, diagnosis, and management of acute postoperative bacterial endophthalmitis. *J Cataract Refract Surg.* 2011;37(9):1699–1714.

Wykoff CC, Parrott MB, Flynn HW Jr, Shi W, Miller D, Alfonso EC. Nosocomial acute-onset postoperative endophthalmitis at a university teaching hospital (2002–2009). *Am J Ophthalmol.* 2010;150(3):392–398.

Keratoconjunctivitis Sicca

Optimizing dry eye therapy prior to cataract surgery improves visual outcomes. This can be especially important in patients considering premium intraocular lenses (IOLs) such as toric and multifocal lenses. A variety of aqueous layer supportive treatments can be individualized for each surgical candidate; these treatments include topical preserved and nonpreserved liquid tear preparations, gels, and ointments; topical cyclosporine; and punctal plugs. (For a detailed discussion of dry eye therapy, see BCSC Section 8, *External Disease and Cornea*.) During the procedure, the surgeon can prevent desiccation of the corneal epithelium by frequently hydrating the area with irrigating solution or by coating the cornea with a topical ophthalmic viscosurgical device (OVD). Visual recovery may be delayed by exacerbation of the patient's dry eye condition.

Patients with dry eyes associated with collagen vascular disease, mucous membrane pemphigoid, rheumatoid arthritis, or Sjögren syndrome present a special challenge to the cataract surgeon. Close observation of these patients in the weeks following surgery is warranted to identify and treat toxic keratoconjunctivitis and corneal ulceration from collagenase activation by postoperative corticosteroid therapy. If prescribed, topical non-steroidal anti-inflammatory drugs (NSAIDs) should be used with caution because of the increased risk of corneal melting associated with their use in these patients. In extreme cases, persistent epithelial defects with stromal loss may require a bandage (therapeutic) contact lens, tarsorrhaphy, or amniotic membrane transplant.

Asai T, Nakagami T, Mochizuki M, Hata N, Tsuchiya T, Hotta Y. Three cases of corneal melting after instillation of a new nonsteroidal anti-inflammatory drug. *Cornea.* 2006; 25(2):224–227.

Mucous Membrane Pemphigoid

Eyes with mucous membrane pemphigoid are severely dry due to scarring of the meibomian glands and accessory lacrimal glands and occlusion of the lacrimal gland orifices. Corneal haze or opacification impairs the surgeon's view into the anterior segment during surgery. Extensive symblepharon or ankyloblepharon may limit positioning and exposure of the eye during surgery. The eyelid speculum must be positioned carefully to avoid traction and pressure on the globe.

Exposure Keratitis and Seventh Nerve Palsy

Patients with paralytic or mechanical eyelid abnormalities may have significant corneal dryness, which may be exacerbated by cataract surgery. Administration of topical anesthetics in the preoperative suite prior to surgery may desiccate the corneal epithelium. A peribulbar or retrobulbar block can cause a neurotrophic cornea for hours after surgery and may cause a large corneal abrasion unless a pressure patch is applied. Lubrication with antibiotic ointment may be necessary in the early postoperative period to facilitate healing of the epithelial surface and to control pain from an abrasion.

Corneal Conditions

Corneal Disease

The cornea has the most refractive power of any structure in the eye. Thus, prior to surgery, the surgeon should identify corneal abnormalities that might contribute to visual impairment and affect the degree of expected improvement in vision, including corneal scars, tear film abnormalities, and epithelial basement membrane dystrophy. An abnormal tear film should be addressed (see the sections Blepharitis and Acne Rosacea, and Keratoconjunctivitis Sicca, earlier in this chapter). Irregular astigmatism may degrade vision. Corneal topography is useful in diagnosing and quantifying irregular astigmatism resulting from a variety of corneal conditions. A trial gas-permeable contact lens can be used to mask an irregular astigmatism and help the clinician determine what effect astigmatism has on visual impairment.

Corneal irregularities affect the accuracy of keratometry and lead to erroneous lens power calculation. In an eye with epithelial basement membrane dystrophy, epithelial debridement may help produce a smoother corneal surface (Fig 9-2). After debridement,

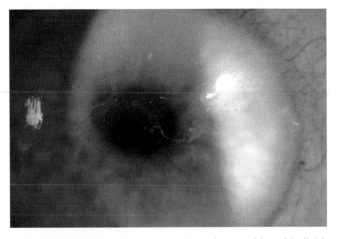

Figure 9-2 Irregular corneal astigmatism occurs in patients with epithelial basement membrane dystrophy. This corneal condition can further decrease vision in a patient with cataract-related visual impairment, in which case the visual improvement after cataract surgery might be less than expected. *(Courtesy of Christopher J. Rapuano, MD.)*

it is necessary to wait at least 6–8 weeks for the corneal surface to smooth and stabilize before repeating keratometry. Mild corneal stromal opacities in the presence of a pristine anterior refractive surface are unlikely to reduce vision.

In patients with a history of herpes simplex virus (HSV) infection, epithelial or stromal keratitis may be exacerbated after cataract surgery. Although the Herpetic Eye Disease Study (HEDS) did not specifically address HSV following surgery, it did show that prophylactic treatment with oral acyclovir, 400 mg, twice daily reduces the incidence of recurrent HSV keratitis. Because recurrent stromal keratitis may result in loss of visual acuity, many ophthalmologists use oral acyclovir, famciclovir, or valacyclovir perioperatively and observe the patient closely for recurrent keratitis postoperatively.

Wilhelmus KR, Beck RW, Moke PS, et al; Herpetic Eye Disease Study Group. Acyclovir for the prevention of recurrent herpes simplex virus eye disease. *N Engl J Med.* 1998;339(5): 300–306.

Cataract and Keratoplasty

When both cataract and corneal opacity contribute to a patient's vision loss, the surgeon has 3 options: (1) remove the cataract first; (2) repair the cornea first; or (3) combine the procedures. Removing the cataract first requires adequate visualization of the anterior segment; it may be possible in this circumstance to remove the cataract and monitor the patient for worsening corneal opacity. However, eyes that exhibit corneal endothelial dysfunction are at higher risk of corneal decompensation following cataract surgery. Signs and symptoms of corneal endothelial dysfunction are microcystic edema, stromal thickening, low cell count on specular microscopy, and/or diurnal fluctuations in vision with prolonged blurred vision upon waking. Keratoplasty should be performed in these eyes.

A penetrating keratoplasty (PKP) or an endothelial keratoplasty (EK) may be performed, either as primary surgery or as part of a combined procedure with cataract extraction (triple procedure). The advantages of performing keratoplasty as a stand-alone procedure include less postoperative inflammation and more reliable keratometry readings for future IOL power calculation. In patients who have primarily corneal endothelial disease, the advantages of EK over PKP include faster rehabilitation and more dependable keratometry readings with which to calculate IOL power, although a hyperopic shift from 0.50 D to 1.50 D may be encountered. IOL power calculation is less reliable for eyes that have undergone PKP than for those that have undergone EK.

A triple procedure (combined keratoplasty [PKP or EK], cataract extraction, and IOL implantation) may be chosen if both the cataract and the corneal disease are significant and the patient would benefit from concurrent treatment. The advantages of the triple procedure include a single visit to the operating room, which reduces the attendant perioperative surgical risks, and relatively rapid rehabilitation. The disadvantages of PKP with cataract surgery include less-predictable IOL calculation and a period of "open sky," or exposure of intraocular contents while the cataract is removed and the IOL is placed, prior to replacement of the corneal button.

The advantages of EK with cataract surgery include rapid corneal rehabilitation with greater likelihood of regular astigmatism and relative ease of regrafting. Disadvantages include possible damage to grafted corneal endothelium when the additional entry into the anterior chamber is made, as well as possible disruption of the graft. Cornea surgeons find EK easier to perform in the aphakic or pseudophakic eye than in the phakic eye. (For a detailed discussion of keratoplasty procedures, see BCSC Section 8, *External Disease and Cornea.*)

If the cataract is not the primary source of visual impairment, it may still be advisable to remove the cataract at the time of corneal surgery because of the eventual need for cataract removal, the possible progression of cataract due to prolonged postoperative corticosteroid therapy, and the risk of additional damage to the corneal endothelium during secondary surgery.

Cataract Following Keratoplasty

Cataract formation soon after keratoplasty may be caused by lens trauma during the transplantation procedure or by prolonged corticosteroid use to prevent graft rejection. Ideally, cataract surgery should be delayed until all PKP sutures are removed, the corneal contour and surface are stable, and accurate keratometry readings can be obtained for IOL power selection. The probability of graft survival 5 years after cataract surgery is at least 80%; nevertheless, a corneal graft may not survive even routine cataract surgery.

Before surgery, the surgeon should evaluate the corneal graft for thickening and anticipate reduced intraoperative clarity through the graft. A scleral tunnel approach is farther from the corneal transplant and minimizes endothelial trauma during surgery. The risk of postoperative graft failure is minimized by protecting the corneal endothelium with a dispersive OVD during surgery and by aggressively treating postoperative inflammation.

Selecting the IOL power before the cornea is fully healed can lead to implantation of an incorrectly powered IOL and symptomatic anisometropia. Posterior chamber lenses are preferred because they minimize contact between the optic and the corneal endothelium. If capsular support is inadequate for IOL placement in the capsular bag ("in-the-bag"), a posterior chamber lens sutured to the sclera or iris may be placed. If the additional manipulation required for a sutured lens poses a risk of excessive endothelial trauma, insertion of a flexible anterior chamber IOL is an option.

Cataract Following Refractive Surgery

Patients who have undergone corneal refractive surgery and later develop a visually significant cataract present several unique challenges. Measurement of corneal power after refractive surgery is problematic, requiring multiple instruments and/or formulas to try to determine the new corneal power. Also, accurate axial length measurement with optical biometry or similar techniques is required. In addition, advanced IOL calculations must be used to determine the appropriate IOL power. (For a detailed discussion of IOL power calculation, see Chapter 6 in this volume and BCSC Section 13, *Refractive Surgery.*) Irregular astigmatism resulting from a refractive surgical procedure may compromise the ultimate visual outcome after cataract removal (Fig 9-3). Because unanticipated postoperative refractive results may occur, the surgeon must thoroughly inform the patient about the limits of precision in lens power calculation and the possible requirement for postsurgical refractive correction to obtain optimal vision.

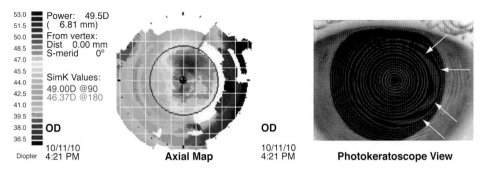

Figure 9-3 Accurate lens implant power is difficult to determine when the corneal surface is abnormal, as shown here by an irregular corneal topographic map *(left)* and distorted corneal rings *(right, arrows)*. *(Courtesy of Lisa Rosenberg, MD.)*

In general, postoperative hyperopia is more commonly encountered after cataract surgery in patients who have undergone previous refractive surgery. The corneal refractive incisions in eyes that have undergone radial keratotomy (RK) often swell after cataract surgery, thereby flattening the cornea and inducing hyperopia. Swelling may require more than 3 months to resolve. If a clear corneal incision is chosen, it should be placed between the RK incisions. Violating an old RK incision can destabilize the wound, causing it to pull apart. The presence of multiple deep RK incisions or unstable wounds increases the likelihood of anterior chamber shallowing during cataract surgery and makes final closure of the wound difficult. A scleral tunnel incision is preferable to reduce the likelihood of violating an RK incision, unless adequate clearance between RK incisions can be ensured with a clear corneal approach.

In eyes that have undergone laser in situ keratomileusis (LASIK), the surgeon should make the clear corneal cataract incisions posterior enough and avoid a long tunnel that could disrupt the LASIK flap. Corneal swelling after LASIK may require more than 1 month to resolve. Cataract surgery in eyes that have undergone photorefractive keratectomy (PRK) does not present the technical challenges of surgery in post-LASIK eyes.

Compromised Visualization of the Lens

Small Pupil

As discussed in Chapter 6, operating through a small pupil may increase the risk of intraoperative complications. Maximum pharmacologic pupil dilation should be noted in the preoperative evaluation so that the surgeon is adequately prepared for a small pupil. A small pupil that is minimally responsive to dilating agents may be widened intraoperatively using one of several techniques. Bimanually stretching the pupil with Kuglen or Lester hooks or tethering the iris with hooks (Fig 9-4) or pupil-expansion devices (Fig 9-5) breaks posterior synechiae and releases the pupillary sphincter. However, excessive manipulation of the iris with these instruments poses a risk of increased inflammation postoperatively. Also, the iris tends to be flaccid and floppy after manual stretching and release,

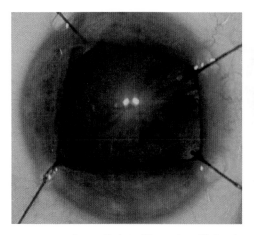

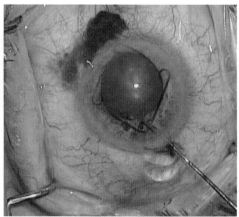

Figure 9-4 A pupil that dilates insufficiently to allow access to the lens may be widened with iris hooks. In this case, 4 hooks are placed to expose the lens for surgery. *(Courtesy of Lisa Rosenberg, MD.)*

Figure 9-5 A Malyugin ring is positioned at the pupillary margin circumferentially. *(Courtesy of Steven Vold, MD.)*

and it is more likely to be damaged by the phaco tip. Viscodilation with a high-viscosity OVD is another method for enlarging a pupil.

To enlarge a small pupil resulting from intraoperative floppy iris syndrome (IFIS), most surgeons prefer pupil expansion devices, because progressive miosis of the floppy iris tends to occur as the surgery proceeds unless the pupil is held open mechanically (Video 9-1). IFIS is a common cause of small pupils and is discussed in detail in Chapter 8.

 VIDEO 9-1 Malyugin ring insertion.
Courtesy of Boris Malyugin, MD, PhD.
Access all Section 11 videos at www.aao.org/bcscvideo_section11.

Poor Red Reflex

As discussed in Chapter 7, creation of a continuous curvilinear capsulorrhexis (CCC) is a key component of safe phacoemulsification. Conditions that cause an abnormal red reflex make it difficult for the surgeon to discriminate the capsular edge, thus increasing the risk of an incomplete or errant capsulorrhexis. In an eye with dense brunescent or cortical cataract, the capsule becomes subject to radial tears because of vaulting of the anterior capsule, which is due to increased lens thickness. Corneal scars not only compromise the surgeon's view of the capsule but also make intraocular manipulation treacherous. Staining the capsule with trypan blue aids visualization and makes manipulation of the capsule easier (Fig 9-6).

Prior to capsulotomy, anterior chamber fluid can be replaced with air, while a small amount of OVD is used to occlude the paracentesis site. Alternatively, a high-viscosity OVD can be instilled to fill approximately two-thirds of the anterior chamber. The surgeon then injects trypan blue through a 27-gauge blunt cannula, starting as far away from the paracentesis incision as possible to deliver the dye directly to the capsule. The dye is

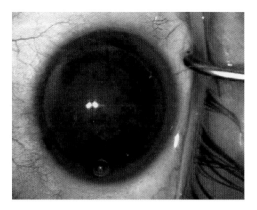

Figure 9-6 The anterior capsule is stained lightly blue by trypan blue, thereby aiding visualization of the capsule during creation of a capsulorrhexis. This technique is helpful in eyes with dense brunescent or cortical cataracts that interfere with the red reflex. *(Courtesy of Lisa Rosenberg, MD.)*

then rinsed out of the anterior chamber with balanced salt solution and replaced with a high-viscosity OVD, under which the stained anterior capsule is easily visible. The high-viscosity OVD exerts pressure on the anterior capsule, maintaining chamber depth and flattening the anterior capsule to prevent radial extension of the capsular tear. A CCC is then created (Video 9-2).

VIDEO 9-2 Capsule staining with trypan blue dye.
Courtesy of Lisa Park, MD.

Jacobs DS, Cox TA, Wagoner MD, Ariyasu RG, Karp CL; American Academy of Ophthalmology; Ophthalmic Technology Assessment Committee Anterior Segment Panel. Capsule staining as an adjunct to cataract surgery: a report from the American Academy of Ophthalmology. *Ophthalmology.* 2006;113(4):707–713.

Marques DM, Marques FF, Osher RH. Three-step technique for staining the anterior lens capsule with indocyanine green or trypan blue. *J Cataract Refract Surg.* 2004;30(1):13–16.

Altered Lens and Zonular Anatomy

Intumescent Cataract

An intumescent cataract is swollen and enlarged with cortical material that often envelops a hard nucleus floating within the capsular bag. This type of cataract presents specific challenges during phacoemulsification cataract surgery. Intumescent cataracts have weak zonular fibers and fragile capsules. Because intumescence creates positive pressure in the capsular bag, the initial incision in the capsule may extend peripherally (Video 9-3). The following steps can be performed to reduce the risk of such complications. The capsule should be stained with trypan blue and then the anterior chamber filled with high viscosity OVD (see the section Poor Red Reflex, earlier in this chapter). Prior to capsulotomy, the surgeon may place a 25- or 27-gauge needle attached to a syringe at the center of the anterior capsule. While suction is applied, the needle is used to pierce the anterior capsule and aspirate the milky cortex. This serves to decompress the lens to avoid radial extension of the CCC. Next, the use of a cystotome attached to the OVD syringe during creation of the CCC enables injection of additional OVD to clear away the milky egress. Caution is advised during phacoemulsification because the freely mobile lens makes segmentation challenging.

 VIDEO 9-3 Intumescent mature cataract.
Courtesy of Virgilio Centurion, MD, and Juan Carlos Caballero, MD.

Advanced Cataract

In the case of dense, brunescent cataracts, surgical manipulation increases the risk of iris trauma, zonular tearing, capsular rupture, vitreous loss, and the dropping of lens fragments into the posterior segment. The increased ultrasound energy required for phacoemulsification of dense lenses increases the risk of endothelial trauma and wound burn. Creation of a larger capsulorrhexis is helpful, as it allows the surgeon to perform the maneuvers that are necessary to minimize these complications. Thorough hydrodissection and hydrodelineation of the nucleus facilitate smooth rotation during phacoemulsification. When an initial groove is made in the hard nucleus, it is important that the surgeon make a deep and even pass so that the nucleus cracks without leaving interdigitations; such interdigitations interfere with removal and can lead to posterior capsule rupture. Viscodissection helps separate sticky cortical attachments that impede rotation. If the surgeon uses excessive mechanical force on a nucleus that does not freely rotate, zonular dialysis may result from transmittal of that force to the capsular bag. Mechanical segmentation techniques of nucleus disassembly, such as vertical and horizontal chopping, require less ultrasound energy and may induce less zonular stress than the "divide-and-conquer" method (discussed in Chapter 7). Familiarity with multiple techniques, and the ability to switch from one technique to another as the situation requires, enable the surgeon to minimize complications.

If phacoemulsification ceases to be an appropriate technique for lens removal, conversion to an extracapsular technique should be considered. The surgeon must decide whether to proceed through the corneal incision by enlarging it to permit passage of the cataract and lens implant. Alternatively, the corneal wound can be closed and a new, larger corneoscleral incision created in the superior portion of the eye. The corneoscleral incision may be more stable, inducing less astigmatism postoperatively compared with a large corneal wound.

Iris Coloboma and Corectopia

Zonular dehiscence or absence commonly occurs in the area of iris coloboma (Fig 9-7A) or a misshapen pupil. Pharmacologic dilation reveals the extent of zonular abnormality. Iris hooks can be used intraoperatively to pull a flaccid iris out of the way. A capsular tension ring (CTR) that incorporates a coloboma diaphragm (Fig 9-7B) not only helps stabilize the capsular bag but also serves as an artificial iris diaphragm. The surgeon also has the option of repairing the coloboma with a suture at the conclusion of the case.

Posterior Polar Cataract

A weak or absent area of posterior lens capsule in the region of a posterior polar opacity places the eye at increased risk of capsular rupture during surgery. To minimize the

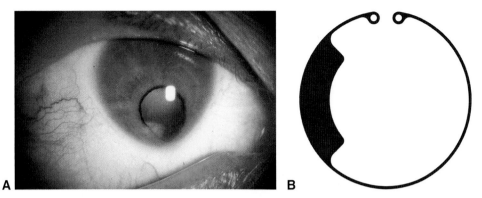

Figure 9-7 **A,** Coloboma of the iris with nuclear cataract. Absent or abnormal zonular fibers correlate with the area of the iris defect. Preoperative evaluation to identify associated posterior segment abnormalities is important in determining visual potential. **B,** Capsular tension ring with coloboma diaphragm. *Note:* This device is not approved by the US Food and Drug Administration; compassionate use available. *(Part A courtesy of Robert S. Feder, MD; part B courtesy of Morcher GmbH, Stuttgart, Germany.)*

likelihood of this complication, the surgeon should avoid creating excessive pressure within the capsular bag or placing excessive pressure on the posterior capsule. Complete hydrodissection is avoided because of possible tearing of the capsule directly under the opacity. Instead, small volumes of fluid are directed around the cortex up to but not across the opacity. Next, gentle hydrodelineation is performed, leaving a generous amount of epinuclear bowl in which to mobilize the nucleus and protect the capsule. Anterior chamber depth should be maintained and fluctuations in IOP controlled by low irrigation and aspiration.

After the nucleus is removed, OVD is used for viscodissection of the epinucleus from the capsular bag. The posterior polar opacity is removed last; viscodissection can be performed for this step as well. If the central portion of the posterior capsule is missing, filling the capsular bag with OVD before removing the irrigating phaco handpiece from the eye stabilizes the chamber for lens insertion. Alternatively, if the posterior polar opacity is very adherent, it can be left in place, assessed for its impact on vision postoperatively, and treated by laser capsulotomy if indicated. After the IOL is placed in the capsular bag in uncomplicated surgery, the surgeon should take care to minimize movement of the bag with slow and gentle OVD removal.

Zonular Dehiscence With Lens Subluxation or Dislocation

Common causes of zonular incompetence include pseudoexfoliation syndrome (Fig 9-8), ocular trauma, prior vitrectomy, prior trabeculectomy, and high myopia. Marfan syndrome, Ehlers-Danlos syndrome, homocystinuria, hyperlysinemia, and Weill-Marchesani syndrome are less-common sources of inadequate zonular support. Iridodonesis detected at the slit lamp may be the initial finding that signals zonular weakness or absence. If the entire lens becomes dislocated into the posterior segment, surgical removal of the lens may not be required unless uveitis develops. In some cases, the remaining zonular fibers may tether the lens within the anterior vitreous such that when the patient sits upright at the slit lamp, the lens seems accessible for extraction. However, when the patient is supine

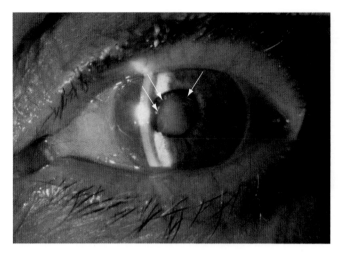

Figure 9-8 Subluxed lens. This lens with pseudoexfoliation is displaced inferiorly because zonular fibers at the superior edge of the lens are stretched, damaged, or broken. *Arrows* indicate the superior edge of the inferiorly displaced lens. Cataract surgery on a displaced lens requires meticulous preoperative planning to minimize surgical complications. *(Courtesy of Lisa Rosenberg, MD.)*

during surgery, the lens may tilt backward and out of the surgeon's reach. Thus, when iridodonesis or phacodonesis is detected preoperatively, it is helpful to confirm lens position with the patient supine during preoperative examination.

Zonular status may be determined by direct visualization of the lens equator through a widely dilated pupil or by use of a goniolens to visualize zonular fibers behind the dilated pupil. In the preoperative examination, if zonular disruption encompasses over 120°, the surgeon may consider removal of the cataract using 1 of 2 techniques: extracapsular cataract extraction (ECCE) or intracapsular cataract extraction (ICCE) (see the appendix).

Zonular incompetence becomes apparent intraoperatively with phacodonesis, decentration of the capsular bag, and sometimes vitreous prolapse into the anterior chamber. If phacodonesis prevents the use of a CCC or if zonular disruption exceeds 120°, the surgeon may convert from phacoemulsification to ECCE or ICCE. Otherwise, phacoemulsification can proceed safely with application of the same measures recommended in the Advanced Cataract section, earlier in this chapter. Reducing the flow rate diminishes turbulence and fluctuation in anterior chamber depth, lowering the risk of vitreous prolapse through the area of zonular absence. A larger capsulorrhexis allows easier separation of lens components within the capsular bag. Thorough hydrodissection and hydrodelineation of the nucleus facilitate smooth rotation during phacoemulsification. Viscodissection helps separate cortical attachments that may impede rotation. Excessive mechanical maneuvers in the nucleus, cortical aspiration, or inadvertent aspiration of the anterior capsule edge contributes to further zonular compromise. Viscodissection of cortical remnants and IOL insertion prior to complete cortical removal are maneuvers that help maintain capsular integrity. Tangential, rather than radial, removal of cortex from the bag minimizes zonular stress.

If capsular support is insufficient for safe phacoemulsification, capsular hooks or a CTR or CTR segments can be used (Videos 9-4, 9-5). Capsular hooks (Fig 9-9) support the anterior capsule edge in the area of weakened zonular fibers. They are placed through

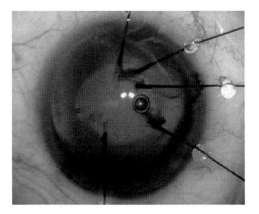

Figure 9-9 Hooks are placed around the anterior capsule edge to stabilize the capsular bag during phacoemulsification in this eye with a subluxed lens. Trypan blue solution is used to aid visualization of the capsular edge. *(Courtesy of Lisa Rosenberg, MD.)*

paracentesis incisions, and adjustment of tension on each hook recenters the capsule for phacoemulsification. CTRs provide support by exerting centrifugal force against the capsule equator to areas of absent or weakened zonular fibers.

 VIDEO 9-4 Insertion of capsular tension ring. *Courtesy of David F. Chang, MD.*

Because radial tension may further extend the capsular defect, placement of either capsular hooks or a CTR should be avoided if the anterior capsule is torn radially or if the capsulorrhexis is interrupted. The ring can be used in patients with posterior capsule defects as long as the anterior rhexis remains continuous. With a CTR in position, the surgeon can proceed to nuclear and cortical removal more safely and place the chosen IOL in the capsular bag ("in-the-bag" IOL). Insufficient zonular support can also be managed with a modified CTR or CTR segment sutured to the scleral wall. In the setting of severe instability, working in conjunction with a vitreoretinal surgeon to employ a pars plana approach may be advisable.

 VIDEO 9-5 Capsule hooks and capsular tension ring. *Courtesy of David F. Chang, MD.*

If zonular support is insufficient to use a 1-piece IOL in the capsular bag, the surgeon can choose from the following options:

- a 3-piece IOL with the haptics placed in the location of zonular weakness
- a 3-piece IOL placed in the ciliary sulcus (with or without optic capture)
- a transscleral-fixated or iris-fixated posterior chamber IOL
- an anterior chamber IOL

Premium IOLs, such as multifocal and toric lenses, should be avoided in eyes with capsular decentration or significant potential for decentration.

Crandall AS, Slade DS. Placement of endocapsular IOLs in eyes with zonular compromise. *Focal Points: Clinical Modules for Ophthalmologists.* San Francisco: American Academy of Ophthalmology; 2014, module 7.

Pseudoexfoliation Syndrome

Eyes with pseudoexfoliation are characterized by poor pupillary dilation and weakened zonular fibers. These findings increase the likelihood of intraoperative complications such as lens dislocation, capsular rupture, and vitreous loss. The techniques suggested for safe cataract surgery in these eyes are the same as those for advanced cataract and zonular dehiscence (discussed earlier in this chapter). Progressive capsular contraction, or capsular phimosis, is common in eyes with pseudoexfoliation. Possible dislocation of the implant into the vitreous is of concern. The surgeon should carefully consider the style of and placement for the chosen lens implant. Capsular contraction is less likely with a 3-piece lens placed inside the capsular bag. If capsular phimosis occurs, an Nd:YAG laser may be used to create radial incisions in the anterior capsule to release tension on the zonular fibers and maintain central lens position.

Cataract in Aniridia

The lens capsule in patients with aniridia is thinner and thus inherently more fragile than that in patients with normal lenses, which makes creation of a capsulorrhexis more challenging. Ideally, the edge of a well-centered capsulorrhexis should overlap the optic edge by 1 mm. Corneal haze and neovascularization in these eyes are common because of stem cell deficiency; capsular staining may aid visualization through the cornea during creation of an adequately sized capsular opening. Use of a high-viscosity OVD also optimizes visualization while stabilizing the capsular surface. The surgeon should avoid working inside the capsular bag to eliminate potential tension on the capsular rim. Low infusion helps reduce turbulence and capsular fluctuation. The capsule in aniridic eyes acts as a pseudo-iris when it opacifies.

Conditions Associated With Extremes in Axial Length

High Myopia

When the surgeon introduces the phaco tip into the anterior chamber of a highly myopic eye, the chamber may deepen dramatically, making lens manipulation difficult. To avoid extensive deepening of the anterior chamber, the surgeon is advised to lower the irrigation bottle and increase the flow rate before entering the eye with the phaco tip. Placing a second instrument between the iris and the anterior capsule prior to turning on infusion may prevent excess deepening. Despite this maneuver, these eyes are susceptible to lens–iris diaphragm retropulsion syndrome (LIDRS), wherein 360° of iridocapsular contact occurs, causing reverse pupillary block, pupillary dilation, and pain. A defect or laxity in the zonular fibers predisposes myopic eyes to LIDRS. Manual separation of the iris from the anterior capsule rim using a sideport instrument corrects the situation (see Chapter 8).

Preoperative IOL power calculation for myopic eyes indicates whether a special-order IOL such as a plano-power or minus-power implant is required. Whenever possible, the patient should receive an IOL because the lens implant serves as a barrier to the movement of the vitreous base and associated traction on the retina. Because myopic eyes are at increased risk of retinal detachment postoperatively, acrylic lens implants are favored when there is a strong possibility that the patient will later undergo vitreoretinal surgery. During vitreoretinal surgery, in the setting of an open posterior capsule, silicone IOLs develop condensation that compromises the retinal surgeon's view into the eye. Silicone lenses have also been observed to migrate through the capsular opening into the vitreous.

Cionni RJ, Barros MG, Osher RH. Management of lens-iris diaphragm retropulsion syndrome during phacoemulsification. *J Cataract Refract Surg.* 2004;30(5):953–956.

Nahra Saad D, Castilla Cespedes M, Martinez Palmer A, Pazos Lopez M. Phacoemulsification and lens-iris diaphragm retropulsion syndrome. *Ophthalmic Surg Lasers Imaging.* 2005; 36(6):512–513.

High Hyperopia and Nanophthalmos

The eye of a cataract patient with high hyperopia (axial length <22 mm) often has a shallow anterior chamber and is prone to uveal prolapse, iris damage, and excessive corneal endothelial trauma during cataract surgery. Anterior chamber deepening and intraocular tissue protection are achieved by using a high-viscosity OVD, a low aspiration rate, or elevation of the irrigation bottle prior to insertion of the phaco tip. Mannitol can be administered preoperatively to dehydrate the vitreous volume in a patient with no systemic contraindications to use of this medication. Iris prolapse is avoided by using an anterior corneal incision entry and by taking care not to overfill the eye with OVD. If all of these measures fail to provide sufficient anterior chamber volume for cataract removal, a small amount of liquid vitreous can be removed using a 25-gauge needle or vitrectomy handpiece through a pars plana puncture.

Nanophthalmos is a rare condition in which the eye is extremely short (axial length <20.5 mm) and the ratio of lens volume to eye volume is larger than normal. These eyes have shallow anterior chambers, narrow angles, and thickened sclerae, with little room for the surgeon to maneuver. Small-incision bimanual surgery is an alternative technique to consider. Intraoperative or postoperative uveal effusion is a unique hazard in nanophthalmic eyes. Maintaining positive pressure in the anterior chamber and limiting the length of the procedure aid in preventing intraoperative uveal effusion. Scleral windows should be considered as a prophylactic measure to treat uveal effusion. A sutured wound prevents hypotony from contributing to this complication postoperatively.

Hypotony

A shortened axial length with choroidal thickening is often accompanied by chronic hypotony and posterior scleral flattening. Hypotony makes biometry technically challenging and precise calculation of IOL power less predictable. To the extent possible, the clinician should determine the cause of hypotony and undertake specific treatment before cataract surgery. If the cataract obscures examination of the posterior segment, B-scan ultrasonography is helpful in revealing posterior segment pathology. A cyclodialysis cleft or retinal detachment requires a more extensive procedure combined with cataract surgery. Severe hypotony or pre-phthisis is a poor prognostic indicator for improvement in vision after cataract extraction.

Glaucoma and Cataract

Assessment

When cataract surgery is being considered in a patient with glaucoma, assessment of the patient's glaucoma control is incorporated into the surgical plan. It is challenging to predict the visual outcome in an eye with both cataract and glaucoma because both conditions may contribute to blurred vision, and the patient's visual symptoms may not be directly attributable to one condition or the other exclusively. An advanced visual field defect may limit visual improvement after cataract surgery. In contrast, an advanced cataract may exaggerate a mild visual field abnormality (Fig 9-10). Surgical options include cataract surgery alone, combined cataract and glaucoma surgery, and staged procedures of glaucoma surgery (trabeculectomy or tube shunt) followed by cataract surgery at a later time. Uncomplicated phacoemulsification alone may serve to lower the long-term IOP by 10%–34% in some eyes. Novel glaucoma procedures, collectively termed microinvasive glaucoma surgery (MIGS), such as canaloplasty, endoscopic cyclophotocoagulation (ECP), trabecular microbypass (iStent, Glaukos Corp, Laguna Hills, CA), and ab interno trabeculotomy (Trabectome, NeoMedix Inc, Tustin, CA) are amenable to combination with cataract extraction to further reduce IOP in a blebless, conjunctiva-sparing manner. Further randomized trials may determine the efficacy of these procedures compared with trabeculectomy, with one another, and with phacoemulsification alone. Small-incision cataract surgery with a clear corneal approach minimizes conjunctival damage, an essential consideration if filtering surgery is required in the future. In addition, a small incision at a temporal or superotemporal location makes cataract surgery in an eye with a

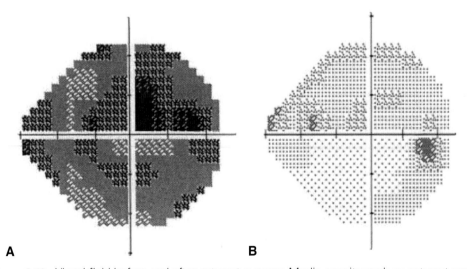

A   **B**

Figure 9-10 Visual field before and after cataract surgery. Media opacity such as cataract can impair the visual field. **A,** An abnormal Humphrey visual field in a glaucoma patient with a dense cataract. **B,** Improved Humphrey visual field following cataract removal and lens implantation. *(Courtesy of Lisa Rosenberg, MD.)*

functioning filtering bleb much easier, and it is also less likely to compromise IOP control by an existing functioning bleb. Issues that influence surgical approach include preoperative and desired postoperative IOP level, degree of damage to the optic nerve and visual field, number of medications required to control IOP, patient adherence, side effects of medication, and impact on quality of life. For a comprehensive discussion of surgical decision making in the glaucomatous eye as well as combined cataract and glaucoma surgery, see BCSC Section 10, *Glaucoma*.

Most of the surgical challenges in patients with both glaucoma and cataract are not unique to these eyes. For instance, zonular compromise and phacodonesis may complicate capsulorrhexis creation and lens removal in an eye with traumatic or pseudoexfoliation glaucoma. Uveitic glaucoma and miotic therapy may limit pupillary dilation and increase the risk of postoperative macular edema. Postoperative IOP elevation from retained OVD or inflammation occurs more commonly, and pressure rises to a higher level in glaucomatous eyes with reduced outflow through the trabecular meshwork. Management of these operative challenges is discussed in detail elsewhere in this chapter.

The use of topical prostaglandin medication has been associated with postoperative cystoid macular edema (CME), although proven cases are few. Because the occurrence of clinically significant postoperative CME after uncomplicated phacoemulsification is rare, it is difficult to attribute macular edema in the early postoperative period to the use of prostaglandin medication. In such cases, discontinuation of the prostaglandin is advisable to determine whether this medication is contributing to the edema.

Henderson BA, Kim JY, Ament CS, Ferrufino-Ponce ZK, Grabowska A, Cremers SL. Clinical pseudophakic cystoid macular edema. Risk factors for development and duration after treatment. *J Cataract Refract Surg.* 2007;33(9):1550–1558.

Cataract Surgery in an Eye With a Functioning Filter

Small-incision cataract surgery in the glaucomatous eye provides the surgeon with options that do not interfere with previous filtering surgery. With a temporal corneal incision, the surgeon avoids the superior conjunctiva and site of filtering surgery. If conversion to an extracapsular technique is indicated (eg, in the setting of extreme phacodonesis and zonular instability or capsular rupture with vitreous present in the anterior chamber), the surgeon may choose to extend the clear corneal incision to permit delivery of the crystalline lens. Alternatively, closure of the temporal incision and creation of a larger corneoscleral incision superiorly minimize astigmatism but may also compromise an existing filter. Aggressive control of postoperative inflammation is critical to ensure continued bleb function.

Francis BA, Singh K, Lin SC, et al. Novel glaucoma procedures: a report by the American Academy of Ophthalmology. *Ophthalmology.* 2011;118(7):1466–1480.

Shingleton BJ, O'Donoghue MW, Hall PE. Results of phacoemulsification in eyes with preexisting glaucoma filters. *J Cataract Refract Surg.* 2003;29(6):1093–1096.

Verges C, Cazal J, Lavin C. Surgical strategies in patients with cataract and glaucoma. *Curr Opin Ophthalmol.* 2005;16(1):44–52.

Uveitis

Chronic or recurring uveitis, as well as the corticosteroid therapy used to treat it, contributes to cataract formation. Decreased vision due to cataract must be differentiated from coexisting macular edema or posterior segment pathology. Fluorescein angiography or optical coherence tomography should be used preoperatively to identify CME. Complications can be minimized when inflammation has been controlled for several months before surgery and is treated aggressively after surgery. Topical and oral corticosteroids are the mainstay of therapy, and topical NSAIDs and cytotoxic agents may be used to supplement treatment.

Uveitic eyes dilate poorly and require expansion and lysis of iridolenticular adhesions, as discussed previously for small pupils. A pupillary membrane must be incised and stripped to avoid interference with the capsulorrhexis. Overly vigorous pupil stretching and manipulation lead to iris bleeding and fibrinous inflammation postoperatively. Meticulous cleanup of cortical material helps prevent exuberant postoperative inflammation.

Insertion of a silicone lens implant is discouraged because inflammatory precipitates may collect on the lens surface (Fig 9-11). Acrylic posterior chamber IOLs placed in the capsular bag are well tolerated and preferred in uveitic eyes. When complications arise and a lens cannot be inserted into the capsular bag, it may be advisable to omit placing a lens in the ciliary sulcus or implanting an anterior chamber lens. Other options may include leaving the patient aphakic or using a scleral-fixated lens. In types of uveitis associated with membrane formation, repeated Nd:YAG procedures may be necessary to clear the lens surface. (See also BCSC Section 9, *Intraocular Inflammation and Uveitis*.)

Abela-Formanek C, Amon M, Kahraman G, Schauersberger J, Dunavoelgyi R. Biocompatibility of hydrophilic acrylic, hydrophobic acrylic, and silicone intraocular lenses in eyes with uveitis having cataract surgery: Long-term follow-up. *J Cataract Refract Surg.* 2011; 37(1):104–112.

Kawaguchi T, Mochizuki M, Miyata K, Miyata N. Phacoemulsification cataract extraction and intraocular lens implantation in patients with uveitis. *J Cataract Refract Surg.* 2007; 33(2):305–309.

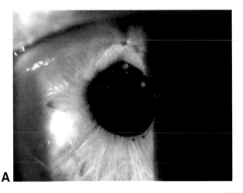 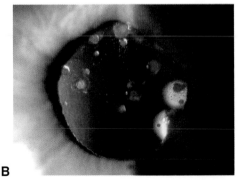

A **B**

Figure 9-11 Low-power **(A)** and high-power **(B)** views of a silicone intraocular lens with keratic precipitates. *(Courtesy of Steven Vold, MD; photography by Matthew Poe.)*

Retinal Conditions

Retinal Disease

Review of ocular records of the patient with retinal disease may reveal the visual acuity before the onset of cataract. Macular function tests, such as the macular photostress test or the potential acuity test (see Chapter 6), may help predict the visual outcome in patients with retinal disease. The clinician must interpret test results with caution because poor or equivocal performance on such tests does not rule out all benefit from cataract removal, whereas favorable results may be misleading. Optical coherence tomography and fluorescein angiography can detect the presence of diabetic or hypertensive retinopathy, degenerative changes, macular distortion, and leakage of fluid into the foveal area. Proper management of patient expectations is essential and especially prudent when eyes have vision-threatening retinal disease.

If diabetic macular edema is present and the view of the retina is adequate, the clinician may consider preoperative focal laser treatment or intravitreal injections of steroids or anti-vascular endothelial growth factor (anti-VEGF) medications. Ideally, cataract surgery should be delayed until the macular edema has resolved; this may take several months. The clinician may also consider perioperative administration of topical NSAIDs, as studies have shown that this may decrease the incidence of postoperative CME and that NSAIDs are beneficial in preventing macular edema in patients with diabetes mellitus.

If the patient is known to have peripheral vitreoretinopathy, a retina specialist should examine the patient before surgery to determine whether pretreatment with laser or cryotherapy would help reduce the risk of retinal tears or detachment. After prophylactic treatment, a period of at least 4 weeks should elapse before elective cataract surgery. (See also BCSC Section 12, *Retina and Vitreous.*)

If the view of the retina is restricted by a small pupil preoperatively, cataract surgery provides an opportunity to enlarge the pupil using stretch maneuvers, iris hooks, expansion devices, or multiple sphincterotomies. In addition, a generous anterior capsulotomy and complete cortical cleanup will enhance the view of the retinal periphery after surgery.

Whenever safely possible, the patient should receive a posterior chamber IOL. A silicone IOL should be avoided in a patient for whom vitrectomy is anticipated because, as mentioned earlier in this chapter, condensation on the posterior surface of the implant limits visibility during pars plana vitrectomy.

Colin J. The role of NSAIDs in the management of postoperative ophthalmic inflammation. *Drugs.* 2007;67(9):1291–1308.

Eriksson U, Alm A, Bjärnhall G, Granstam E, Matsson AW. Macular edema and visual outcome following cataract surgery in patients with diabetic retinopathy and controls. *Graefes Arch Clin Exp Ophthalmol.* 2011;249(3):349–359.

Hong T, Mitchell P, de Loryn T, Rochtchina E, Cugati S, Wang JJ. Development and progression of diabetic retinopathy 12 months after phacoemulsification cataract surgery. *Ophthalmology.* 2009;116(8):1510–1514.

Shah AS, Chen SH. Cataract surgery and diabetes. *Curr Opin Ophthalmol.* 2010;21(1):4–9.

Cataract Following Pars Plana Vitrectomy

Nuclear cataract formation is common after pars plana vitrectomy, especially in patients older than 50 years. Posterior subcapsular opacification is typical after the use of silicone oil during retinal surgery. In the absence of a vitreous cushion, the posterior capsule becomes more mobile; thus, the surgeon must pay careful attention to fluctuations in anterior chamber depth, avoiding surge upon breaking of vacuum when a piece of lens is aspirated (see Chapter 7). Lowering the irrigation bottle and fluid-flow rate prior to placing the phaco tip inside the eye is helpful. This maneuver is also recommended when zonular integrity is altered as a result of prior retinal surgery or preexisting ocular disease. The surgeon should beware of overfilling the anterior chamber with OVD in an effort to avoid further zonular stretch and breakage. Extra caution is also necessary to avoid losing pieces of the lens during hydrodissection when an inadvertent capsular break may have occurred during retinal surgery. A large capsulorrhexis allows prolapse of the nucleus during hydrodissection for an iris-plane phaco chop. If the surgeon selects an extracapsular surgical technique instead of phacoemulsification, the absence of vitreous reduces posterior pressure to aid lens expression. Alternatively, after capsulorrhexis and hydrodissection of the nucleus from its cortical attachments, the nucleus can be removed using a lens loop or irrigating vectis.

Cataract With Intraocular Silicone Oil

Cataract in an eye with silicone oil is usually very soft. The surgeon should avoid pressurizing the eye with excessive OVD or the high infusion pressure of balanced salt solution. During cataract surgery, silicone oil can migrate through a break in the zonular fibers if the anterior chamber is overfilled with OVD. The clinician should use low-flow irrigation or decrease the aspiration rate during surgery to minimize pressure on the zonular fibers and the risk of silicone oil migration into the anterior chamber. Droplets of silicone oil that were not apparent in the anterior chamber during surgery might become visible postoperatively. A few droplets are usually not toxic to the cornea. Silicone lens implants are contraindicated in these eyes because silicone oil adheres to the implant surface. The surgeon should create an inferior iridotomy if a patent one is not already present. (See Chapter 6 for a discussion of IOL calculations in eyes with silicone oil.)

Ocular Trauma

Ocular Assessment

When a patient presents with a history of ocular trauma sufficient to cause a dense cataract, the surgeon should suspect damage to other anterior segment structures. Damage to the corneal endothelium, zonular fibers, and anterior chamber angle all require an adjustment in surgical technique. Gonioscopy is essential when planning IOL placement. The surgeon must be hypervigilant when evaluating ocular findings and determining the potential for visual recovery (discussed in Chapter 6). Cataract may occur acutely after substantial trauma (see Chapter 5). A slowly progressive cataract after ocular trauma can be monitored while intraocular inflammation and other comorbidities are treated. The following sections discuss conditions related to and processes affected by the traumatized eye.

Visualization During Surgery

Corneal laceration and edema may impair the view into the eye such that phacoemulsification cannot be performed safely. Instead, an extracapsular approach may be advisable. Hemorrhage during surgery may further reduce visualization of the anterior segment. Use of OVDs and injection of intracameral air help occlude vessels and marginalize bleeding. If visualization remains inadequate, the surgeon should close the wound and pursue surgery later.

Inflammation

Acute and chronic inflammation are common in traumatized eyes. When uveitis is severe, it may mimic infectious endophthalmitis. Fibrin membranes on the iris lead to synechiae formation, pupil seclusion, and miosis. The surgeon should use pupil-enlarging maneuvers, as described previously in the section Small Pupil. In the setting of inflammation, a peripheral iridotomy is important for prevention of pupillary block glaucoma. Inflamed uveal tissue bleeds upon the slightest manipulation. OVDs should be used liberally to protect corneal endothelium and to improve the view into the anterior segment. Postoperative IOP elevation is typical and exacerbated by the use of OVD. Control of inflammation warrants cycloplegia as well as intensive topical and possibly oral corticosteroid therapy.

Retained Foreign Matter

A foreign body in the anterior chamber may be easier to see when the patient is seated upright at the slit lamp rather than positioned supine under the operating microscope. Irrigating solutions may dislodge a foreign body from its preoperative location. When an intraocular foreign body is suspected to be located in the posterior segment, indirect ophthalmoscopy is an excellent method to use if ocular media are sufficiently clear. When the view is obscured by cataract or hemorrhage, a computed tomography scan, x-ray, or ultrasonogram can help the clinician determine the presence and location of the foreign body. When a metallic foreign body is suspected, magnetic resonance imaging is contraindicated because the magnetic field could dislodge the foreign body. A dense cataract may be removed by either a pars plana or an anterior approach, followed by pars plana vitrectomy and removal of the foreign body.

Cataract in an Eye With Damage to Other Ocular Tissues

Iris trauma commonly coexists with traumatic cataract (Fig 9-12). Sphincter ruptures cause irregular pupil size and shape. The surgeon can repair iridodialysis at the time of cataract removal by suturing the iris root to the scleral spur. Though not apparent on slit-lamp examination, corneal endothelial damage can be significant and may not manifest until after surgery, when severe corneal edema occurs. Preoperative specular microscopy

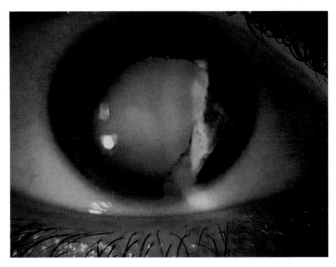

Figure 9-12 Traumatic cataract and iridodialysis secondary to a paintball injury. *(Courtesy of Mark H. Blecher, MD.)*

can be helpful in determining the status of the corneal endothelium and its ability to withstand cataract surgery. Trauma sufficient to cause iris tears and cataract also warrants careful inspection for zonular damage and posterior segment insult. Surgical planning to manage these findings intraoperatively is discussed in earlier sections of this chapter. If a retinal detachment is present, cataract removal may be necessary to allow adequate visualization for subsequent surgical repair.

Removal of Traumatic Cataract

A traumatic cataract may leak lens protein into the aqueous and vitreous, inciting uveitis and glaucoma. If cortical material is identified in the anterior chamber or if a mature cataract interferes with the diagnosis and treatment of injuries in the posterior segment, the cataract should be removed promptly. Rupture of the capsule causes rapid hydration of the lens cortex, leading to formation of a milky-white cataract. This type of cataract is usually soft and can be aspirated through the large port of the irrigating/aspirating handpiece. The surgeon should beware of preexisting capsule rupture that may not be visible on preoperative examination. Hydrodissection should be performed slowly to minimize the possibility of extending a capsular break and causing the lens to fall into the posterior segment.

If a hard nuclear cataract was present before the trauma, the surgeon should employ techniques for cataract removal (described in the section Zonular Dehiscence With Lens Subluxation or Dislocation, earlier in this chapter). An OVD can be used to provide a tamponade to anterior vitreous movement in areas of zonular incompetence. If vitreous has migrated into the anterior chamber, the surgeon must perform an anterior vitrectomy before removing the lens in order to avoid vitreous manipulation and retinal traction.

When the nucleus is markedly subluxed and vitreous fills a substantial part of the anterior chamber, the surgeon should consider a pars plana lensectomy, in collaboration with a retinal surgeon (see BCSC Section 12, *Retina and Vitreous*).

Vision Rehabilitation

Primary implantation of a posterior chamber lens after ocular trauma is recommended when intraocular inflammation and hemorrhage are minimal and the view of anterior segment structures is good. An anterior chamber IOL or transsclerally fixated posterior chamber lens may be necessary in case there is inadequate capsular support for a posterior chamber IOL. In rare situations, the surgeon may decide against placing an IOL primarily and instead insert an IOL as a secondary procedure later, after sufficient evaluation of the anterior segment and anterior angle anatomy. Scarring resulting from a corneal laceration changes the contour of the cornea, and inaccurate keratometry and biometry measurements can result in erroneous IOL power selection, increasing the risk of postoperative anisometropia. A rigid contact lens may be required to mask irregular astigmatism resulting from a corneal scar.

IOL Selection After Trauma

The clinician should tailor selection of a lens implant to the patient's ocular anatomy and to the desired postoperative outcome. As mentioned earlier, silicone lens implants should be avoided in patients with a history of uveitis; inflammatory debris is more likely to collect on the surface of this type of optic (see Fig 9-11) and impair vision than it is on hydrophobic acrylic IOLs. Acrylic lenses are preferred in these cases and in eyes that are more likely to undergo vitreoretinal surgery in the future. In eyes that have more than 4 clock-hours of inadequate zonular support but have an intact anterior capsule, a 3-piece posterior chamber lens may be placed in the ciliary sulcus. Alternatively, if there is no capsular support, a 3-piece lens may be sewn to the scleral wall. Finally, the design of current anterior chamber lenses is sufficiently flexible for the open-angle glaucomatous eye to tolerate. Ultimately, the choice of IOL is determined by the surgeon's experience with lens options and implantation methods.

Hannush SB. Sutured posterior chamber intraocular lenses. *Focal Points: Clinical Modules for Ophthalmologists.* San Francisco: American Academy of Ophthalmology; 2006, module 9.

Wagoner MD, Cox TA, Ariyasu RG, Jacobs DS, Karp CL; American Academy of Ophthalmology. Intraocular lens implantation in the absence of capsular support: a report by the American Academy of Ophthalmology. *Ophthalmology.* 2003;110(4):840–859.

Surgical Procedures for Extracapsular and Intracapsular Cataract Extraction

For an in-depth discussion of patient evaluation, preparation, and informed consent, see Chapter 6. For a discussion of anesthesia, antimicrobial prophylaxis, ophthalmic viscosurgical devices, types of intraocular lenses, and other topics relevant to cataract surgery, see Chapter 7.

Key Developments in Cataract Extraction

By 1600, anatomists had correctly identified the position of the crystalline lens (see the Introduction, Fig I-3), and the current definition of cataract, opacification of the lens, had been established. The initial method of extracapsular cataract extraction (ECCE), developed by Daviel (1696–1762), represented a substantial improvement over the much older couching technique. In ECCE, the lens is removed through an opening in the anterior capsule, and the capsular bag is left in place. Because of the large incision size used in ECCE, early ECCE was complicated by problems with wound healing, vitreous and uveal prolapse, and infection. In addition, lens remnant–induced inflammation and capsular opacification were common, and secondary discission of pupillary membranes was often necessary.

Intracapsular cataract extraction (ICCE), the removal of the lens with its capsule intact, was first performed in 1753 by Sharp (1709–1778). Various instruments were developed to grasp and extract the lens, including toothless forceps and suction cup–like devices called erysiphakes. Twentieth-century advances in ICCE included chemical dissolution of zonular fibers with α-chymotrypsin, reported by Barraquer in 1957, and use of the cryoprobe, introduced by Kelman in 1962. ICCE remained the most widely used method for cataract surgery in the United States until the late 1970s, when ECCE, and later phacoemulsification, predominated. The development of the binocular operating microscope, irrigation/aspiration (I/A) systems, ophthalmic viscosurgical devices (OVDs), and intraocular lenses (IOLs) reduced the complications associated with earlier versions of ECCE and helped it become a predominant procedure once again.

Extracapsular Cataract Extraction

Patient Preparation

After informed consent is obtained, the operative site is marked, and the pupil is maximally dilated. A "time-out" is performed to ensure that the surgical team is prepared for the correct surgical procedure on the correct patient, with the correct implant (see Chapter 7).

After the anesthesia has been administered and the eye is prepared and draped in sterile fashion, an eyelid speculum is placed.

Incision

A fornix-based conjunctival flap is made superiorly, followed by cauterization of the scleral bed. The initial incision usually consists of a limbal groove, fashioned with a round-tipped steel blade, sharp microknife, or diamond knife. Some surgeons prefer a slightly more posterior incision with anterior dissection, creating a scleral flap or tunnel. Nucleus expression requires a limbal chord length of 8–12 mm, smaller than the incision required for ICCE. A stab incision is made under the flap into the anterior chamber in preparation for anterior capsulotomy, and the cystotome is inserted to begin the procedure. The anterior chamber depth can be stabilized with OVDs, air bubble, or continuous fluid irrigation.

Anterior Capsulotomy

An anterior capsulotomy allows the surgeon to remove the cataract with the capsular bag intact and to ultimately stabilize the IOL, once implanted, within the capsular bag. The surgeon initiates a continuous curvilinear capsulorrhexis (CCC) by making a puncture or small tear in the anterior capsule using a cystotome needle or capsulorrhexis forceps with special tips for grasping and tearing. The edge of this tear is then grasped with the cystotome tip or with forceps and pulled around smoothly, removing a circular portion of the anterior capsule (see Chapter 7). The CCC used for ECCE needs to be larger (>6 mm) than the CCC created for routine phacoemulsification (approximately 5 mm) to allow for safe expression of an intact nucleus. Expression of a large or dense nucleus may require relaxing incisions in the CCC in order to avoid uncontrolled traumatic tears in the capsulorrhexis, which can lead to rupture of the posterior capsule. Alternatively, a cystotome needle may be used to make a series of connected punctures or small tears in a circular pattern (*can-opener capsulotomy;* Fig A-1). After the capsulotomy is completed, the initial limbal or scleral incision is widened to allow safe passage of the nucleus through the incision.

Nucleus Removal

Manual expression of the nucleus involves pressing on the inferior limbus to tip the superior pole of the nucleus up and out of the capsular bag. Applying additional counterpressure on the globe by using an instrument to indent the sclera posterior to the limbus, 180° away from the incision, expresses the nucleus from the anterior chamber. The surgeon removes the nucleus by loosening and elevating it from the capsule with the use of a hook

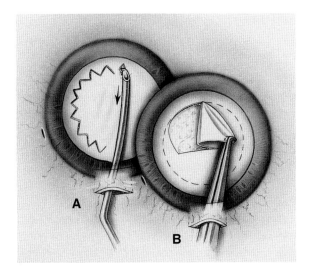

Figure A-1 Anterior capsulotomy techniques. **A,** In a can-opener incision, punctures are made peripherally and pulled centrally so that the torn edges connect. Each puncture site has the potential for a radial tear if stressed. **B,** In a capsulorrhexis, tearing is begun within the area to be excised and finished from the outside in. When stress lines in the free flap appear between forceps and the tear site, best control is maintained by regrasping the flap near the tear site. "Positive vitreous pressure" makes the tear travel peripherally; filling the anterior chamber with an ophthalmic viscosurgical device will counteract the posterior vitreous pressure and make it easier to complete the capsulorrhexis tear. *(Reproduced from Johnson SH. Phacoemulsification. Focal Points: Clinical Modules for Ophthalmologists. San Francisco: American Academy of Ophthalmology; 1994, module 6. Illustration by Christine Gralapp.)*

or irrigating cannula and then supporting it on a lens loop, spoon, or vectis that will subsequently be used to slide or irrigate the nucleus out of the chamber.

The incision is partially sutured to allow deepening of the anterior chamber with irrigation. Using the I/A equipment, the surgeon then aspirates the lens cortex under direct visualization in the pupillary space.

IOL Insertion

Prior to IOL insertion, the anterior chamber is usually filled with an OVD. A posterior chamber IOL may be inserted into the ciliary sulcus or into the capsular bag. Sulcus fixation typically requires an IOL with a larger overall diameter (at least 13 mm) and a large-diameter optic (at least 6 mm), which is more forgiving in case of postoperative decentration.

To insert the IOL into the capsular bag, an OVD is injected into the bag, with care taken to separate the anterior capsule flap completely from the posterior capsule. Direct visualization of haptic placement in the capsular bag during IOL insertion is critical.

Closure

The ECCE incision is typically closed with multiple interrupted sutures of 10-0 nylon or 1 running suture. Proper suture tension helps reduce postoperative astigmatism: loose sutures induce corneal flattening, whereas tight sutures cause corneal steepening in the axis of the suture.

Postoperative Course

Visual acuity on the first postoperative day should be consistent with the refractive state of the eye, the clarity of the ocular media, and the visual potential of the retina and optic nerve. Mild eyelid edema and erythema may be present. The cornea may also be mildly edematous. The anterior chamber should have normal depth, and a mild to moderate cellular reaction is typical. The posterior capsule should be clear, and the implant should be well positioned and stable. The red reflex should be bright and clear. Elevation in intraocular pressure (IOP) may be associated with retained OVD. Topical antibiotics, nonsteroidal anti-inflammatory drugs (NSAIDs), and corticosteroid eyedrops are generally prescribed postoperatively.

The postoperative course should be characterized by steady improvement in vision and comfort as the inflammatory reaction subsides. The refraction is typically stable by the fourth to sixth postoperative week, and spectacles may then be prescribed. If a significant amount of postoperative astigmatism is present in the axis of tight sutures, the clinician may selectively remove the sutures, as guided by wound stability, keratometry readings, or corneal topography measurements.

Manual Small-Incision Cataract Surgery

Manual small-incision cataract surgery (MSICS) is a variation of ECCE first described by Blumenthal in 1994. MSICS utilizes surgical instruments similar to those employed in ECCE, as well as a binocular operating microscope, but it does not require access to other high-technology instrumentation, making it particularly useful in areas of the world in need of high-volume, low-cost cataract extraction.

The primary differences between ECCE and MSICS are that, in the latter, a smaller incision and mechanical fragmentation of the nucleus for delivery are used. The scleral incision is made 1.5–2.0 mm posterior to the limbus in the form of a straight or frown-shaped groove 6–7 mm in length. Using a crescent blade, the surgeon tunnels this incision forward 1.5 mm, into clear cornea. The tunnel is shaped like a trapezoid, such that the internal incision is wider than the external scleral incision. This construction allows for delivery of the nucleus, which can be divided into smaller segments prior to removal, while maintaining a self-sealing external incision. A small, or soft, nucleus may be expressed intact with a Simcoe cannula (Fig A-2), vectis, or lens loop. A large or dense nucleus may require bimanual fragmentation prior to delivery.

Aspiration of cortex is performed using the Simcoe cannula. A rigid 6-mm polymethyl methacrylate (PMMA) lens is then placed into the capsular bag. A properly constructed wound should be self-sealing. If necessary, the wound may be closed with 10-0 nylon sutures.

Studies have shown that, in comparison to ECCE, MSICS allows a higher surgical volume and faster visual recovery and it results in less postoperative astigmatism and better uncorrected visual acuity (also called uncorrected distance visual acuity). Visual

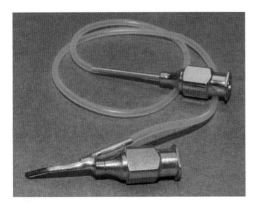

Figure A-2 Simcoe irrigating/aspirating cannula. *(Photograph by Carol Everhart Roper.)*

outcomes and complication rates for MSICS are similar to those for phacoemulsification performed in the developing world.

> Tabin GC, Feilmeier MR. Cataract surgery in the developing world. *Focal Points: Clinical Modules for Ophthalmologists.* San Francisco: American Academy of Ophthalmology; 2011, module 9.

Intracapsular Cataract Extraction

Patient Preparation

The preparation for planned ICCE is similar to that for ECCE. If retro-orbital anesthesia is used, preoperative orbital massage by digital pressure or compressive devices may be employed to decrease the pressure effect from the increased orbital volume produced by this anesthetic. Some surgeons use mannitol to decrease the orbital and vitreous volume. Mannitol should be used with caution in elderly patients and those with congestive heart failure, diabetes mellitus, or renal compromise.

Exposure of the Globe

After the skin and ocular surface have been prepared and the eye is draped, an eyelid speculum is placed. A bridle suture is usually required to hold the eye in a slight downward position. The surgeon can accomplish this step by placing a 6-0 silk suture beneath the superior rectus tendon or within sclera and securing the suture to the superior drape.

Incision

The surgeon creates either a fornix-based or a limbus-based conjunctival flap, and then uses cautery to achieve hemostasis. A scleral support ring may be necessary in young patients or in those with high myopia to avoid scleral collapse when the lens is extracted. In patients with deep-set eyes, the ring may be needed to improve exposure.

Incision placement varies according to surgeon preference and the patient's anatomy. More-anterior or corneal incisions may be of shorter chord length and result in less bleeding. However, closure of such incisions induces corneal steepening in the meridian of the incision. Incisions that are more posterior heal faster and, when covered by a conjunctival flap, are more comfortable to the patient. Posterior incisions induce less astigmatism and are less damaging to the corneal endothelium, but they cause more bleeding.

Sutures are preplaced across the incision and looped out of the way; their presence allows rapid closure of the eye in case of choroidal hemorrhage, Valsalva maneuver, or other causes of positive posterior pressure. An additional suture may be placed through the anterior lip of the incision only; this will allow the surgical assistant to elevate the cornea at the time of lens delivery, facilitating delivery.

Iridectomy and Lens Delivery

An iridectomy is performed at this point. If the eye has a small pupil, the surgeon may consider performing sector iridectomy, radial iridotomy, or multiple sphincterotomies or using iris hooks or pupil expanders.

α-Chymotrypsin, if available, can be injected via a cannula through the pupillary space into the posterior chamber. An iris retractor can be used to expose the superior surface of the lens. A cellulose sponge is employed to dry the anterior lens capsule. Next, the surgeon positions the cryoprobe, a hollow metal-tipped probe that is cooled by compressed nitrous oxide, on the lens surface. Once an ice ball has formed and the lens has adhered to the probe (Fig A-3), gentle to-and-fro maneuvers are used to deliver the lens. An iris retractor or cellulose sponge can be used to strip the vitreous from the posterior surface of the lens during delivery. Vitreous loss, combined with the larger incision of intracapsular surgery, contributes to posterior scleral collapse. Thus, the surgeon should anticipate the need for management of vitreous loss. The anterior vitrectomy apparatus that is part of the phacoemulsification machine can be used for controlled removal of vitreous. In addition, cellulose sponges may be used to engage vitreous, which can then be cut with Vannas scissors; this process should be repeated until all externalized vitreous has been removed.

Next, a lens implant may be inserted, or the patient may be left aphakic. An anterior chamber lens can be inserted after instillation of acetylcholine or carbachol. Other lens implant options include posterior chamber lenses with iris or scleral fixation.

The surgeon then uses sutures to close the incision while an OVD or balanced salt solution is utilized to keep the anterior chamber formed. The conjunctival flap is secured.

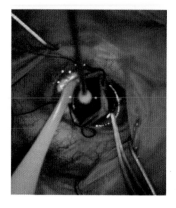

Figure A-3 Cryoextraction of cataract (intracapsular cataract extraction). The lens is being lifted out of the eye. *(Courtesy of Lisa F. Rosenberg, MD.)*

Subconjunctival or sub-Tenon injection of antibiotics or corticosteroids can be given at this point. A patch and shield should be applied.

Postoperative Course

The postoperative course is generally similar to that for ECCE. If the eye has been left aphakic, visual acuity can be estimated with a +10.00 to +12.00 D lens, or a +4.00 D lens can be used as a telescope. The surgeon should monitor the appearance of the cornea, the security of the wound, the depth of the anterior chamber, the degree of inflammatory reaction, and the IOP. Visualizing the posterior segment is important for evaluation of vitreous clarity and position and for detecting any retinal or optic nerve pathology.

It is not unusual to see mild eyelid edema and erythema. The upper eyelid may be moderately ptotic. The conjunctiva is often mildly hyperemic, and subconjunctival hemorrhage may be present. The cornea should be clear, but some superior corneal edema is often present from the bending of the cornea during lens extraction. This edema generally resolves during the first postoperative week. The anterior chamber should have normal depth with mild to moderate cellular reaction. The pupil should be round and the iridectomy, patent.

The postoperative course should be characterized by steady improvement in vision and comfort. Topical antibiotics, NSAIDs, and corticosteroids are typically used during the first postoperative weeks. The refraction generally becomes stable 6–12 weeks after intracapsular surgery, depending on the wound-closure technique employed. It usually takes longer to achieve a stable refraction after ICCE than after ECCE or other procedures, because of the larger incision required for ICCE.

Basic Texts

Lens and Cataract

Apple DJ, Auffarth GU, Peng Q, Visessook N. *Foldable Intraocular Lenses: Evolution, Clinicopathologic Correlations, and Complications.* Thorofare, NJ: Slack; 2000.

Bahadur GG, Sinskey RM. *Manual of Cataract Surgery.* 2nd ed. Boston: Butterworth-Heinemann; 1999.

Buratto L, Werner L, Zanini M, Apple DJ. *Phacoemulsification: Principles and Techniques.* 2nd ed. Thorofare, NJ: Slack; 2003.

Chang D. *Phaco Chop: Mastering Techniques, Optimizing Technology, and Avoiding Complications.* Thorofare, NJ: Slack; 2004.

Fine IH. *Clear Corneal Lens Surgery.* Thorofare, NJ: Slack; 1999.

Garg A, Fine IH, Alió JL, et al, eds. *Mastering the Techniques of Advanced Phaco Surgery.* New Delhi, India: Jaypee Brothers Medical Publishers; 2008.

Harding J. *Cataract: Biochemistry, Epidemiology, and Pharmacology.* New York: Chapman & Hall; 1991.

Henderson BA. *Essentials of Cataract Surgery.* 2nd ed. Thorofare, NJ: Slack; 2014.

Jaffe NS, Jaffe MS, Jaffe GF. *Cataract Surgery and Its Complications.* 6th ed. St Louis: Mosby; 1998.

Kohnen T, Koch DD, eds. *Essentials in Ophthalmology—Cataract and Refractive Surgery.* Berlin, Germany: Springer-Verlag; 2006.

Olsen RJ, Jin GJC, Ahmed IK, Crandall AS, Cionni RJ, Jones JJ. *Cataract Surgery from Routine to Complex: A Practical Guide.* Thorofare, NJ: Slack; 2011.

Pineda R, Espaillat A, Perez VL, Rowe S. *The Complicated Cataract: The Massachusetts Eye and Ear Infirmary Phacoemulsification Practice Handbook.* Thorofare, NJ: Slack; 2001.

Seibel BS. *Phacodynamics: Mastering the Tools and Techniques of Phacoemulsification Surgery.* 4th ed. Thorofare, NJ: Slack; 2004.

Steinert RF, ed. *Cataract Surgery.* 3rd ed. Philadelphia: Saunders; 2010.

Tasman W, Jaeger EA, eds. *Duane's Ophthalmology on DVD-ROM.* Philadelphia: Lippincott Williams & Wilkins; 2012.

Wilson ME Jr, Trivedi RH. *Pediatric Cataract Surgery: Techniques, Complications, and Management.* 2nd ed. Philadelphia: Lippincott Williams & Wilkins; 2014.

Related Academy Materials

The American Academy of Ophthalmology is dedicated to providing a wealth of high-quality clinical education resources for ophthalmologists.

Print Publications and Electronic Products

For a complete listing of Academy products related to topics covered in this BCSC Section, visit our online store at http://store.aao.org/clinical-education/topic/cataract -anterior-segment.html. Or call Customer Service at 866.561.8558 (toll free, US only) or +1 415.561.8540, Monday through Friday, between 8:00 AM and 5:00 PM (PST).

Online Resources

Visit the Ophthalmic News and Education (ONE®) Network at aao.org/onenetwork to find relevant videos, online courses, journal articles, practice guidelines, self-assessment quizzes, images and more. The ONE Network is a free Academy-member benefit.

Access free, trusted articles and content with the Academy's collaborative online encyclopedia, EyeWiki, at aao.org/eyewiki.

Requesting Continuing Medical Education Credit

The American Academy of Ophthalmology is accredited by the Accreditation Council for Continuing Medical Education (ACCME) to provide continuing medical education for physicians.

The American Academy of Ophthalmology designates this enduring material for a maximum of 10 *AMA PRA Category 1 Credits™*. Physicians should claim only the credit commensurate with the extent of their participation in the activity.

To claim *AMA PRA Category 1 Credits™* upon completion of this activity, learners must demonstrate appropriate knowledge and participation in the activity by taking the posttest for Section 11 and achieving a score of 80% or higher.

This Section of the BCSC has been approved by the American Board of Ophthalmology as a Maintenance of Certification Part II self-assessment and CME activity.

To take the posttest and request CME credit online:

1. Go to www.aao.org/cme-central and log in.
2. Click on "Claim CME Credit and View My CME Transcript" and then "Report AAO Credits."
3. Select the appropriate media type and then the Academy activity. You will be directed to the posttest.
4. Once you have passed the test with a score of 80% or higher, you will be directed to your transcript. *If you are not an Academy member, you will be able to print out a certificate of participation once you have passed the test.*

CME expiration date: June 1, 2019. *AMA PRA Category 1 Credits™* may be claimed only once between June 1, 2016, and the expiration date.

For assistance, contact the Academy's Customer Service department at 866-561-8558 (US only) or +1 415-561-8540 between 8:00 AM and 5:00 PM (PST), Monday through Friday, or send an e-mail to customer_service@aao.org.

Study Questions

Please note that these questions are not part of your CME reporting process. They are provided here for your own educational use and identification of any professional practice gaps. The required CME posttest is available online (see "Requesting CME Credit"). Following the questions are a blank answer sheet and answers with discussions. Although a concerted effort has been made to avoid ambiguity and redundancy in these questions, the authors recognize that differences of opinion may occur regarding the "best" answer. The discussions are provided to demonstrate the rationale used to derive the answer. They may also be helpful in confirming that your approach to the problem was correct or, if necessary, in fixing the principle in your memory.

1. What is the rate of cataract surgery in developed countries?
    a. up to 50 per million population per year
    b. up to 1000 per million population per year
    c. up to 10,000 per million population per year
    d. up to 50,000 per million population per year

2. What is a normal change in the human crystalline lens as it ages?
    a. It develops an increasingly curved shape, resulting in more refractive power.
    b. It becomes increasingly flat, resulting in less refractive power.
    c. There is an increase in the index of refraction as a result of the decreasing presence of insoluble protein particles.
    d. There is a decrease in the index of refraction as a result of the decreasing presence of insoluble protein particles.

3. How is metabolic waste removed from the crystalline lens?
    a. It is broken down by lysosomes.
    b. It is removed by the venous system of the lens.
    c. It is stored in the lens, not removed, contributing to the increase in lens size throughout life.
    d. It is removed via the aqueous humor.

4. Why are glutathione and vitamins E and C present in the anterior chamber?
    a. to adjust the pH and act as a buffer
    b. to protect the corneal endothelium
    c. to act as a free radical scavenger
    d. to induce DNA damage

5. On what presumption is the Helmholtz theory of accommodation based?

   a. Most of the change in lens shape occurs at the central anterior lens surface.

   b. The action of the anterior zonular fibers on the lens during accommodation results in flattening of the central anterior lens surface.

   c. The change in curvature of the posterior lens capsule contributes approximately 25% of the accommodative amplitude.

   d. As the ciliary muscle contracts, the zonular tension increases, resulting in bulging of the lens and increasing the dioptric power of the eye.

6. What change occurs in the lens in the presence of high levels of glucose?

   a. Glucose that is not phosphorylated to G6P enters the Krebs cycle.

   b. Hexokinase activity increases until all glucose is phosphorylated.

   c. Aldose reductase activity increases.

   d. Sorbitol is produced and then eliminated from the lens via diffusion through the capsule into the anterior chamber.

7. What process occurs in the crystalline lens during terminal differentiation?

   a. Lens epithelial cells elongate into lens fibers.

   b. The mass of cellular proteins is decreased.

   c. Glycolysis assumes a lesser role in metabolism.

   d. Cell organelles increase their metabolic activity.

8. What process results in formation of the Y-sutures seen in the adult lens?

   a. connection of the adult nucleus to the surrounding cortex

   b. scarring from the tunica vasculosa lentis

   c. elaboration of the adult nucleus around the fetal nucleus

   d. fusion of the embryonic cells within the fetal nucleus

9. A 30-year-old patient with Marfan syndrome presents with a new report of visual difficulty. Examination reveals early lens subluxation. What would be the best initial management strategy?

   a. planning for early lens extraction

   b. addition of prism to the patient's current prescription for glasses

   c. refraction with attention to presbyopic correction

   d. treatment with miotic eyedrops

10. What is a common symptom of cortical cataracts?

   a. better near vision than distance vision

   b. abrupt myopic shift

   c. glare under mesopic lighting conditions

   d. diminished color perception

11. What is the histologic change most commonly associated with posterior subcapsular cataracts (PSCs)?

    a. increased number of lamellar membrane whorls

    b. posterior migration of lens epithelial cells

    c. calcium deposition

    d. glycosaminoglycan deposits in the lens cell bodies

12. What type of cataract is associated with chalcosis?

    a. oil droplet cataract

    b. anterior subcapsular cataract

    c. PSC

    d. "sunflower" cataract

13. A patient presents with a mature lens and secondary glaucoma without evidence of pupillary block. What is the most likely diagnosis?

    a. phacomorphic glaucoma

    b. phacolytic glaucoma

    c. phacoantigenic uveitis

    d. lens particle glaucoma

14. If a patient has a dense, white cataract and the posterior pole is not visible, what test would be most helpful in determining whether cataract surgery is likely to improve vision?

    a. specular microscopy

    b. B-scan ultrasonography

    c. potential acuity pinhole test

    d. fluorescein angiography

15. A patient with nuclear sclerosis asks whether her cataract is "ripe" enough to be removed. What information would best allow the surgeon to answer appropriately?

    a. Snellen acuity

    b. glare test results documenting the level of decreased vision required for cataract surgery reimbursement under the patient's insurance plan

    c. the patient's confession that she does not feel comfortable driving at night because of glare but needs to continue to do so

    d. documentation of significantly decreased contrast sensitivity

16. Determining the axial length with an immersion technique or contact applanation is most appropriate in which setting?

    a. posterior chamber filled with silicone oil

    b. aphakic patient

    c. history of corneal refractive surgery

    d. dense vitreous hemorrhage

17. On the day of surgery, a patient arrives 30 minutes late to the surgery center. The order of cases is changed as a result, and another patient is taken to the operating room earlier than planned. What step would prevent the surgeon from placing an incorrect intraocular lens (IOL) implant?

   a. performing a "time-out" to confirm the patient's name and the operative eye

   b. having all lens implants for the day's cases available in the operating room before the start of surgery

   c. reviewing the patient's IOL calculations and ocular measurements immediately before the start of surgery

   d. designating one staff member to be responsible for the lens choice

18. A patient with a medical history significant for hypertension, diabetes mellitus, and coronary artery disease with cardiac stent placement is brought to the operating room for cataract surgery. Anesthetic is administered via a retrobulbar injection. Soon afterward, the orbit is taut, and the eye is noted to be proptotic, with significant ecchymosis of the eyelids and conjunctiva. The eye is extremely firm to palpation. What would be the most appropriate course of action?

   a. Perform ocular massage.

   b. Request that the anesthesiologist decrease intravenous sedation.

   c. Examine the fundus to assess whether globe penetration has occurred.

   d. Perform a lateral canthotomy and cantholysis.

19. An elderly patient is seen in the office, and slit-lamp examination reveals dense nuclear sclerotic cataracts and severe blepharitis. What would be the most appropriate course of action to prevent postoperative endophthalmitis?

   a. Plan to scrub the eyelids and lashes vigorously with 10% povidone-iodine soap on the day of surgery.

   b. Plan to use intravenous antibiotics in the irrigating solution.

   c. Plan for an extracapsular cataract extraction to minimize repeated manipulation of instruments in the eye and over the eyelashes.

   d. Recommend eyelid hygiene to the patient, and have the patient return for reevaluation before surgery.

20. While examining a patient for cataract surgery, the ophthalmologist notes that although the cornea is clear, there are significant cornea guttae. How would the ophthalmologist manage this patient intraoperatively?

   a. Increase the use of a cohesive ophthalmic viscosurgical device (OVD) during phacoemulsification.

   b. Increase the use of a dispersive OVD during phacoemulsification.

   c. Perform vigorous hydrodissection to prolapse the lens into the anterior chamber and minimize the amount of energy needed to create a groove in the nucleus.

   d. Prepare for possible penetrating keratoplasty by having corneal tissue available in the operating room.

21. What is the best initial treatment of a postoperative shallow anterior chamber caused by ciliary block glaucoma?
    a. cyclophotocoagulation
    b. cycloplegia and aqueous suppression
    c. miotics and peripheral iridotomy
    d. Nd:YAG laser posterior capsulotomy

22. What systemic medication is most likely to cause severe intraoperative floppy iris syndrome (IFIS)?
    a. alfuzosin
    b. doxazosin
    c. tamsulosin
    d. terazosin

23. What is the most characteristic finding on examination of a patient with blurred vision and toxic anterior segment syndrome (TASS)?
    a. hypopyon that presents 3–7 days postoperatively
    b. diffuse corneal edema that presents 1 day postoperatively
    c. elevated intraocular pressure with central corneal epithelial edema
    d. ocular pain with cells in the anterior vitreous

24. What type of IOL implant is most likely to cause negative dysphotopsia?
    a. anterior chamber IOL
    b. decentered multifocal IOL
    c. sulcus-fixated 1-piece acrylic IOL
    d. square-edge posterior chamber IOL in the capsular bag

25. What is an appropriate indication for combined keratoplasty and cataract extraction?
    a. nuclear cataract and irregular corneal astigmatism due to epithelial basement membrane dystrophy
    b. nuclear cataract and Fuchs endothelial dystrophy with vision worse in the morning
    c. recurrent herpes simplex keratitis with peripheral corneal scarring and moderate nuclear cataract
    d. brunescent cataract and cornea guttata with normal corneal thickness

26. What test is useful in the calculation of IOL power for a patient who has previously undergone laser in situ keratomileusis (LASIK)?
    a. corneal topography
    b. optical coherence tomography of the macula
    c. B-scan ultrasonography
    d. A-scan ultrasonography

27. A surgeon encounters IFIS after phacoemulsification has begun. What procedure would allow the surgeon to best manage the miotic pupil and floppy iris?

    a. insertion of 4 or 5 iris hooks through new corneal incisions

    b. insertion of a pupil expansion device (eg, Malyugin ring)

    c. insertion of a high-viscosity OVD and bimanual pupil stretching

    d. insertion of a capsular tension ring (CTR)

28. A patient has a white, intumescent cataract. In addition to the standard supplies and instruments for cataract surgery, what should the surgeon have ready for use in this patient?

    a. Malyugin ring

    b. CTR

    c. lens chopper

    d. trypan blue dye

29. During phacoemulsification, the surgeon realizes that zonular dialysis of 3 clock-hours (90°) is present. How should the surgeon proceed?

    a. Increase the bottle height and flow rate to maintain adequate anterior chamber depth.

    b. Close the corneal incision, and convert to an extracapsular cataract extraction with a superior corneoscleral incision.

    c. Proceed with phacoemulsification, and place an anterior chamber IOL.

    d. Place a CTR, complete phacoemulsification, and insert a posterior chamber IOL.

30. What procedure is best suited for cataract extraction in an eye with controlled uveitis and a small pupil?

    a. pupil stretching and lysis of any posterior synechiae, followed by phacoemulsification and placement of an acrylic IOL

    b. Malyugin ring insertion, followed by phacoemulsification and placement of a silicone IOL

    c. insertion of iris hooks, followed by phacoemulsification without IOL insertion

    d. extracapsular cataract extraction

Answer Sheet for Section 11 Study Questions

Question	Answer	Question	Answer
1	a b c d	16	a b c d
2	a b c d	17	a b c d
3	a b c d	18	a b c d
4	a b c d	19	a b c d
5	a b c d	20	a b c d
6	a b c d	21	a b c d
7	a b c d	22	a b c d
8	a b c d	23	a b c d
9	a b c d	24	a b c d
10	a b c d	25	a b c d
11	a b c d	26	a b c d
12	a b c d	27	a b c d
13	a b c d	28	a b c d
14	a b c d	29	a b c d
15	a b c d	30	a b c d

Answers

1. **c.** The rate of cataract surgery varies widely: in developed countries, it is up to 10,000 per million population per year, while in parts of the developing world, the rate may be as low as 50 surgeries per million. The World Health Organization has set a goal of 3000 surgeries per million population annually to adequately address the worldwide need for cataract extraction.

2. **a.** With age, the human lens develops an increasingly curved shape, which results in more refractive power. This change may be accompanied by—and in some cases offset by—a decrease in the index of refraction of the lens, probably resulting from an increase in water-insoluble proteins. As a result, either a myopic or hyperopic shift in refraction may occur.

3. **d.** After fetal development, the lens has no blood supply or organelles and depends on the aqueous humor for removal of metabolic waste. Changes in lens size occur throughout life as the lens epithelial cells at the equator continue to divide.

4. **c.** Glutathione and vitamins E and C are powerful free radical scavengers. They have no effect on the pH or the corneal endothelium. They actually protect DNA from being damaged by free radicals.

5. **a.** The Helmholtz theory of accommodation, developed in the mid-1800s, remains widely accepted. It is based on the presumption that, when a distance target is viewed, the eye's ciliary muscle is relaxed, causing the zonular fibers to flatten the central anterior surface of the lens. Conversely, when the eye attempts to focus on a near object, the ciliary muscle contracts, relaxing the tension on the zonular fibers. The central anterior surface of the lens is allowed to bulge, resulting in an increase in dioptric power. Despite the fact that the central posterior capsule is the thinnest part of the capsule, there is no change in curvature of the posterior aspect of the lens with contraction or relaxation of the ciliary muscle.

6. **c.** The hexokinase reaction is the rate-limiting step in glucose phosphorylation. When glucose concentration increases in the lens, the sorbitol pathway is activated; aldose reductase is the key enzyme in this pathway. Sorbitol is retained in the lens because of poor permeability, promoting lens opacification.

7. **a.** Terminal differentiation involves elongation of the lens epithelial cells into lens fibers. This change is associated with a tremendous increase in the mass of cellular proteins in the fiber cell membrane. The cells lose organelles, including nuclei, mitochondria, and ribosomes. The loss of cell organelles is optically advantageous; however, the cells then become more dependent on glycolysis for energy production and less active metabolically.

8. **d.** Y-sutures are formed when the ends of the secondary lens fibers of the fetal nucleus meet and interdigitate with the ends of fibers arising on the opposite side of the lens. An erect Y-suture appears anteriorly; an inverted Y-suture, posteriorly. In a clear or mildly cataractous adult lens, the Y-sutures can be seen in the center of the nucleus. The junction of the adult nucleus and the surrounding cortex is generally not visible but may be appreciated once the nucleus develops sclerosis; there is no morphologic distinction between the cortex and the nucleus. The tunica vasculosa lentis, a capillary network on the posterior surface of the lens capsule, regresses at approximately 9 weeks of gestation. A remnant may persist as a small opacity (Mittendorf dot).

9. **c.** Careful refraction improves vision in many patients with Marfan syndrome. Presbyopic correction may be required, even in young patients with this syndrome, as the subluxated lens lacks accommodative power because of the abnormal function of the zonular fibers. The position of the subluxated lens may remain stable over time, and lens surgery in patients with Marfan syndrome carries a high risk of complications; thus, lens extraction should be deferred until more conservative management is unsuccessful in achieving adequate vision. Prism correction is not indicated, because the diplopia that occurs with lens subluxation is most often monocular.

10. **c.** Glare is a common symptom of cortical cataracts. Near-vision preference occurs most commonly in patients with nuclear cataracts, as does a myopic shift. In patients with advanced nuclear cataracts, impaired color perception is common.

11. **b.** Posterior migration of lens epithelial cells and their enlargement are the typical histologic changes associated with posterior subcapsular cataracts (PSCs). Lamellar membrane whorls are seen on electron microscopy of nuclear cataracts. Calcium deposition is seen in hypermature cataracts. Glycosaminoglycan deposition is not a feature of cataracts.

12. **d.** Chalcosis occurs when an intraocular foreign body deposits copper in the Descemet membrane, anterior lens capsule, or other intraocular basement membranes. The term "sunflower" cataract refers to a petal-shaped deposition of yellow or brown pigment in the lens capsule that radiates from the anterior axial pole of the lens to the equator. Oil droplet cataracts can occur in galactosemia and posterior lenticonus, and the term is used to describe some dense nuclear cataracts. The "oil droplet" appearance of dense nuclear cataracts in galactosemia is due to a great difference between the density of the central nucleus and that of the surrounding cortex. The oil droplet appearance noted on red reflex examination in cases of posterior lenticonus is due to a bulge in the posterior capsule. In all of these cases, the best way to view the oil droplet is with retinoscopy or with direct ophthalmoscopy using a wide-angle view.

13. **b.** Phacolytic glaucoma occurs when denatured lens protein leaks through an intact but permeable capsule. The trabecular meshwork becomes clogged with the lens proteins and engorged macrophages. In phacomorphic glaucoma, the mature lens causes pupillary block and secondary angle closure. In phacoantigenic uveitis, leaking of lens protein produces a granulomatous inflammatory reaction. Lens particle glaucoma is associated with a penetrating lens injury or surgery.

14. **b.** B-scan ultrasonography is indicated to screen for retinal detachment, posterior staphyloma, occult tumors, or other posterior pathology that could affect the visual outcome. The potential acuity pinhole test and fluorescein angiography would not be possible with such a dense cataract. Specular microscopy would be indicated only if signs of corneal endothelial dysfunction were present.

15. **c.** In most cases, cataract surgery is an elective procedure. In determining whether surgery is the most appropriate option, the ophthalmologist must assess not only the clinical findings, but also the impact of vision changes on the patient's daily activities and lifestyle. Questionnaires for measuring visual function may be useful tools for evaluation and documentation.

16. **d.** To obtain accurate measurements, optical biometers require adequate clarity of the cornea, aqueous, lens, and vitreous. In the setting of significant corneal scarring, PSC, or vitreous hemorrhage, biometry may not be obtainable, and an immersion technique

or contact applanation would be more appropriate. Adjustments need to be made to biometry calculations when there are alterations in the average velocity through the ocular media, such as in the setting of aphakia or silicone oil in the posterior chamber. However, accurate measurements can still be achieved if these factors are taken into account.

17. **c.** Improper selection of an intraocular lens (IOL) is a preventable cause of a "refractive surprise." All information related to calculations for the patient's IOL should be available to the surgeon in the operating room. Before the procedure begins, the entire surgical team should participate in a "time-out" to confirm the patient's identity, the operative eye, the procedure, and the IOL to be implanted.

18. **d.** Possible complications of retrobulbar anesthesia include the following: retrobulbar hemorrhage; globe penetration; optic nerve trauma; extraocular muscle toxicity; intravenous injection with cardiac arrhythmia; and inadvertent intradural injection with associated seizures, respiratory arrest, and brainstem anesthesia.

    In this case, there was an increased risk of retrobulbar hemorrhage due to anticoagulation. The goal of treatment is to lower the intraocular pressure (IOP) as quickly as possible. Cataract surgery should not be performed, because the risk of iris prolapse through the wound and expulsive choroidal hemorrhage is increased.

19. **d.** The prevention of endophthalmitis is a much-debated topic. On the day of surgery, the use of 5% povidone-iodine solution in the fornix has been shown to decrease bacterial colony counts. However, vigorous scrubbing of the eyelids and lashes is generally not recommended, as doing so may actually disseminate bacteria onto the ocular surface immediately prior to surgery. Systemic antibiotics do not adequately penetrate an intact globe. While minimizing repeated manipulation of instruments over the eyelashes and in the eye is recommended, making a large incision for an extracapsular extraction would not be advised. Appropriate eyelid hygiene preoperatively would be the recommended course of action in this case.

20. **b.** Protecting the corneal endothelium with a coating agent, or dispersive ophthalmic viscosurgical device (OVD), would be recommended for an eye with cornea guttae. A cohesive agent, while maintaining space, would be easily expelled from the eye during phacoemulsification. Prolapsing the lens into a supracapsular position for phacoemulsification would not necessarily be helpful, as the phaco tip would then be closer to the endothelium. Unless corneal edema is observed preoperatively, the surgeon would not plan for a keratoplasty until some months postoperatively.

21. **b.** Causes of a shallow anterior chamber postoperatively include wound leak, capsular block, pupillary block, suprachoroidal hemorrhage, and ciliary block. If the cause is known to be ciliary block glaucoma and the other conditions are ruled out, initial treatment with cycloplegia and aqueous suppressants may relieve the condition. A peripheral iridotomy, while effective for pupillary block, does not relieve ciliary block. If the initial medical treatment fails, surgical disruption of the vitreous face or a vitrectomy may be necessary at a later time to permanently restore the normal aqueous circulation and anterior chamber depth.

22. **c.** Tamsulosin is a selective α_{1a}-adrenergic antagonist, commonly prescribed to treat lower urinary tract symptoms associated with benign prostatic hypertrophy. Selective α_{1a}-adrenergic antagonists have a greater effect on the iris dilator muscle than do nonselective agents. Alfuzosin is a nonselective α-adrenergic antagonist used to treat prostatic hypertrophy

and is less likely to cause the same degree of intraoperative floppy iris syndrome (IFIS) as the selective α_{1a} medications. Doxazosin and terazosin are also nonselective α-adrenergic antagonists; they are used to treat hypertension or prostatic hypertrophy.

23. **b.** Toxic anterior segment syndrome (TASS) presents within hours of surgery with relatively painless diffuse corneal edema and blurred vision. Elevated IOP shortly after surgery may be due to retained OVDs and may cause decreased vision, pain, and a central epithelial edema ("bedewing"). Endophthalmitis typically presents 3–10 days after surgery with pain, decreased vision, and anterior chamber and anterior vitreous inflammation.

24. **d.** Negative dysphotopsia (ND) is caused by the shadow (penumbra) cast on the nasal retina as light rays entering the eye from the temporal periphery interact with the nasal edge of a well-centered IOL in the capsular bag. It is seen with all types of IOLs placed in the capsular bag but is most common with smaller, square-edge optic designs. ND does not occur with anterior chamber IOLs. A 1-piece acrylic IOL in the ciliary sulcus increases the risk of uveitis-glaucoma-hyphema syndrome but not ND. Decentered posterior chamber IOLs of all types are associated with positive dysphotopsias.

25. **b.** Fluctuating vision that is worse in the morning indicates significant corneal endothelial dysfunction, which is an indication for keratoplasty (penetrating or endothelial). Concurrent removal of a cataract is indicated if the cataract is visually significant or likely to progress rapidly. Epithelial basement membrane dystrophy may require corneal debridement, not keratoplasty. Peripheral corneal scarring is unlikely to be visually significant. A dense cataract with mild endothelial dystrophy should generally be treated with cataract surgery alone.

26. **a.** Corneal topography is useful to determine whether there is irregular astigmatism, as well as to help determine the true corneal power. While optical coherence tomography (OCT) of the anterior segment may provide useful measurements, such as anterior chamber depth and corneal thickness, macular OCT does not assist in the calculation of IOL power. Immersion A-scan ultrasonography may be used in place of optical biometry, but contact A-scan is not accurate enough for IOL calculation in patients who have undergone refractive surgery.

27. **a.** Iris hooks and pupil expansion devices are both very useful in dealing with IFIS. However, when the pupil becomes miotic during surgery, after creation of a continuous curvilinear capsulorrhexis (CCC), iris hooks are a safer choice. A possible complication of Malyugin ring insertion after CCC is that the ring may inadvertently catch the edge of the capsulorrhexis. Iris hooks can be used to dilate the iris in a more controlled manner in this situation. Bimanual pupil stretching is not likely to keep the pupil sufficiently dilated and does not address the excessive motility of the floppy iris.

28. **d.** The surgeon should always be prepared for likely complications by having alternative surgical plans ready and the appropriate instruments available in the operating room. Staining the capsule of a white cataract aids direct visualization and promotes creation of a controlled CCC. Trypan blue dye would certainly be advantageous for capsular staining. If a pupil is miotic or there is zonular weakness, the surgeon should be ready to use other devices as the situation dictates.

29. **d.** For a patient with 90° of zonular dialysis, management consists of continued phacoemulsification and capsular tension ring (CTR) placement. The timing of the CTR placement depends on the extent of the zonular compromise and the surgeon's preference. Placement of the CTR before completion of phacoemulsification stabilizes the capsule

for further lens manipulation and extraction but makes cortical aspiration more difficult. Thorough cortical aspiration is easier if CTR placement is delayed until just before IOL insertion. However, there is a risk of extending the zonular dialysis if phacoemulsification is performed without adequate capsule support.

The flow rate and bottle height should not be increased, as doing so could cause vitreous to prolapse through the dialysis and into the anterior chamber. OVD may be used as a tamponade against the forward movement of vitreous in the area of the dialysis. Unless the situation deteriorates further, neither conversion to extracapsular cataract extraction nor use of an anterior chamber IOL would be necessary.

30. **a.** Uveitic eyes dilate poorly and require pupil expansion. This may be achieved in a variety of ways, including bimanual stretching, iris hooks, or pupil expansion devices. In an eye with controlled uveitis, an IOL should be placed. An acrylic IOL is well tolerated and preferred over a silicone IOL because of the risk of inflammatory precipitates collecting on the silicone IOL surface postoperatively.

Index

(*f* = figure; *t* = table)

A constant, in IOL power determination/power prediction formulas, 85

A-scan ultrasonography, for axial length measurement, in IOL power determination/selection, 82–83, 83*f*, 85, 87

Ab externo/ab interno approaches, for IOL dislocation repair, 145, 147*f*

Aberrometry, wavefront, intraoperative, in IOL power determination/selection
  astigmatism and, 124
  after refractive surgery, 86

Accommodating intraocular lenses, 122, 122*f*
  complications of, 151

Accommodation, 22–23, 23*t*
  aging affecting, 23
  amplitude of, 23
  changes with, 22–23, 23*t*
  Helmholtz hypothesis (capsular theory) of, 22

Accommodative intraocular lenses. *See* Accommodating intraocular lenses

Acid, ocular injuries caused by, cataract and, 59

ACIOL. *See* Intraocular lenses (IOLs), anterior chamber

Acne rosacea, cataract surgery in patient with, 172–173

Acrylic, for IOLs, 120. *See also* Foldable intraocular lens
  glistenings and, 151
  ocular trauma and, 193
  opacification and, 151
  uveitis and, 140, 188

Active transport/secretion, in lens
  epithelium as site of, 21
  pump–leak theory and, 21, 22*f*

Activities of Daily Vision Scale (ADVS), 71

Acyclovir, for herpes simplex virus infections, before cataract surgery, 175

ADVS (Activities of Daily Vision Scale), 71

Aerobic glycolysis, in lens glucose/carbohydrate metabolism, 18

Affinity constant (K_m), sorbitol in cataract development and, 19

Age/aging
  accommodative response/presbyopia and, 23
  cataracts related to, 5, 43–48. *See also* Age-related cataracts
  lens changes associated with, 11, 43–48
  lens proteins affected by, 17

Age-related cataracts, 5, 43–48. *See also specific type*
  cortical, 45–46, 46*f*, 47*f*, 48*f*, 49*f*, 50*f*
  in diabetes mellitus, 60
  epidemiology of, 5
  genetic contributions to, 41–42
  indications for surgery and, 72
  nuclear, 43–45, 45*f*
  nutritional deficiency and, 7, 63–64
  posterior subcapsular, 46–48, 51*f*

Age-Related Eye Disease Study (AREDS), 7, 63

AK. *See* Astigmatic keratotomy

AL. *See* Axial length

Alcohol, use/abuse of, cataract formation and, 63–64

Aldose reductase
  in cataract formation, 19
  in lens glucose/carbohydrate metabolism, 18*f*, 19

Aldose reductase inhibitors, cataract prevention/management and, 72

Alfuzosin, intraoperative floppy iris syndrome and, 74, 136, 137*t*

Alkalis (alkaline solutions), ocular injuries caused by, cataract and, 59

Alpha (α)-blockers, intraoperative floppy iris syndrome and, 74, 136–137, 137*t*

Alpha (α)-chymotrypsin, for ICCE, 195, 200

Alpha (α)-crystallins, 15, 15–16, 15*f*

Alport disease/syndrome, lenticonus in, 30

American Academy of Ophthalmology (AAO), Initiative in Vision Rehabilitation (patient handout/website), 71

American Society of Cataract and Refractive Surgery (ASCRS), on IOL power calculation, 85

Amikacin, for endophthalmitis, after cataract surgery, 163

Amiodarone, lens changes caused by, 53

Amniotic membrane transplantation/graft, for corneal edema after cataract surgery, 129

Amplitude, of accommodation, 23

Anaerobic glycolysis, in lens glucose/carbohydrate metabolism, 17, 17–19, 18*f*

Anesthesia, for cataract surgery, 91–92, 91*f*, 92*f*, 93*f*
  retrobulbar hemorrhage and, 158, 171

Angiographic cystoid macular edema, after cataract surgery, 163–164, 164*f*

Angle-closure glaucoma
  after cataract surgery, 136
    ciliary block/malignant glaucoma (aqueous misdirection) and, 139
  microspherophakia and, 33
  phacomorphic, 67, 68*f*

Aniridia, 33
  cataract and, 33, 34*f*
  surgery for, 184

Anisometropia
  asymmetric lens-induced myopia causing, 70
  second-eye cataract surgery for, 73

Ankyloblepharon, cataract surgery in patient with, 173

Ankylosing spondylitis, cataract surgery in patient with, 171, 171*f*

Anomalies, congenital. *See specific type and* Congenital anomalies

Anterior capsule fibrosis and phimosis, 153–154
  Nd:YAG laser capsulotomy for, 154, 154–157, 154*f*, 156*f*. *See also* Nd:YAG laser therapy, capsulotomy

Anterior capsule opacification, cataract surgery and, 152, 153

Anterior capsulotomy. *See* Capsulotomy, anterior

Anterior chamber
    flat or shallow, cataract surgery and, 134–136
        intraoperative complications and, 134–135
        posterior fluid misdirection syndrome and, 134–135
        postoperative complications and, 135–136
        preoperative considerations/IOL power
            determination and, 79, 84, 86–87
    gonioscopy/evaluation of, before cataract surgery, 79
    phacoemulsification in, 112
    vitreous prolapse in, 143–144
Anterior chamber intraocular lenses. See Intraocular
    lenses
Anterior lenticonus/lentiglobus, 30
Anterior polar cataracts, 35–36
Anterior pole, 9, 10f, 11f, 12f
Anterior pupillary membrane, 29, 29f
Anterior segment
    disorders of
        cataract and, 68
        cataract surgery complications causing, 132–144,
            137t. See also specific type
    trauma to, 190
Anterior segment dysgenesis syndrome, Peters anomaly
    and, 31–32
Antibiotics
    for endophthalmitis, after cataract surgery, 162, 162–163
    prophylactic, cataract surgery and, 93–95, 94f
        corneal melting and, 132
Anticholinesterase agents. See Cholinesterase/
    acetylcholinesterase inhibitors
Anticoagulant therapy, cataract surgery and, 74, 157,
    171–172, 172t
Antiglaucoma agents, cataracts and, 52
Anti-inflammatory agents, for cystoid macular edema,
    after cataract surgery, 164
Antimicrobial prophylaxis, for cataract surgery, 93–95, 94f
    corneal melting and, 132
Antioxidants, cataract prevention and, 7, 20, 72
Antiplatelet therapy, cataract surgery and, 157, 171–172,
    172t
Antipsychotic drugs, intraoperative floppy iris syndrome
    and, 136, 137t
Anti-VEGF agents
    for cystoid macular edema, 165
    for diabetic macular edema, 189
Aphakia
    congenital, 30
    after ICCE, 201
    IOLs for, 118–122
Aphakic (pseudophakic) bullous keratopathy, after
    cataract surgery, 129, 129f
    IOL design and, 149
Applanation ultrasonography, for axial length
    measurement, in IOL power determination/
    selection, 83
AquaLase liquefaction device, 125
Aquaporin 0 (major intrinsic protein/MIP), 16, 20–21
Aquaporins (water channels), 16, 20–21
Aqueous misdirection (malignant/ciliary block
    glaucoma), cataract surgery and, 139
Arachnodactyly, in Marfan syndrome, 40, 40f
AREDS (Age-Related Eye Disease Study), 7, 63
Arterial retrobulbar hemorrhage, cataract surgery and, 158

Arthritis
    cataract surgery in patient with, 171
    rheumatoid, cataract surgery in patient with, corneal
        melting/keratolysis and, 132
ASCRS (American Society of Cataract and Refractive
    Surgery), on IOL power calculation, 85
Aspiration
    in ECCE, 197
    in manual small-incision cataract surgery, 198, 199f
    in phacoemulsification, 102, 115
    pumps for, 103–104, 103f, 104f
Astigmatic keratotomy (AK), cataract surgery and, 123
Astigmatism
    in cataract patient, 174
        corneal topography before surgery and, 84, 174
        modification during surgery and, 123–124
        toric IOLs for, 124
    after cataract surgery, 131–132
        keratorefractive/refractive surgery and, 176, 177f
        manual small-incision surgery and, 198
    limbal relaxing incisions for, 123–124
Atkinson nerve block, for cataract surgery, 92, 93f
Atopic dermatitis, cataracts associated with, 66
Atropine, accommodation affected by, 23
Axes
    optic, 9, 10f
    visual, Nd:YAG laser capsulotomy location and, 155
Axial length (AL), 84–85
    extremes in, cataract surgery in patient with, 184–185
    in IOL power determination, 82–83, 83f, 85
        hypotony and, 185
        optical measurement of, 82, 85
        ultrasound measurement of, 82–83, 83f, 85, 87
        unexpected refractive results after surgery and,
            150, 176

B-scan ultrasonography, before cataract surgery, 81
Balanced salt solution (BSS), in phacoemulsification,
    110, 118
Barbados Eye Study, 6
Barrett formula, for IOL power determination/selection, 85
Basement membrane dystrophies, epithelial, cataract
    surgery in patient with, 174–175, 174f
BCVA. See Best-corrected visual acuity
Beaded filaments, 16
Beaver Dam Eye Study, 6
Behavioral/psychiatric disorders, cataract surgery in
    patient with, 169–170
Benign prostatic hypertrophy, α-blockers for, intraopera-
    tive floppy iris syndrome and, 74, 136–137, 137t
Best-corrected visual acuity (BCVA/corrected distance
    visual acuity), after cataract surgery, 126
    manual small-incision surgery and, 198–199
    multifocal IOLs and, 121–122
Beta (β)-crystallins, 16
Betagamma (β,γ)-crystallins, 15, 15f, 16
Biconvex design, for IOLs, 120
Biometry, before cataract surgery, 82, 82–83, 83f
    hypotony and, 185
    IOL power determination/selection and, 82–83,
        83f, 84–85, 87
Biomicroscopy, slit-lamp. See Slit-lamp biomicroscopy/
    examination

Bladder (Wedl) cells, 48, 152
Bleeding disorders, cataract surgery in patient with, 171–172
Blepharitis, cataract surgery in patient with, 172–173
Blindness, cataract causing, 5
Blood, cornea stained by, hyphema after cataract surgery and, 159
Blue-blocking intraocular lenses, 120
Blue-dot (cerulean) cataract, 37, 38f
Blunt trauma, lens injury/cataract caused by, 53–55, 54f
BMP. See Bone morphogenetic protein
Bone morphogenetic protein (BMP), lens placode formation and, 25
Brown-McLean syndrome, 128t, 130
Brunescent cataract, 44
    lens proteins in, 17
    surgery for, 180
        hydrodelineation in, 110, 180
BSS. See Balanced salt solution
Buerger disease (thromboangiitis obliterans), cataract caused by, 68
Bullous keratopathy, after cataract surgery, 129, 129f
    IOL design and, 149
Burns, thermal, cataract surgery incision, 131
Burst-mode phacoemulsification, 101

Calcium deposits, on IOLs, 151
Can-opener capsulotomy
    for ECCE, 196
    for phacoemulsification, 109–110
Canaloplasty, cataract surgery and, 186
Capsular block syndrome (CBS), 148–149
Capsular cataracts, 38
Capsular fibrosis, 153–154
    IOL decentration/dislocation and, 145
    Nd:YAG laser capsulotomy for, 154, 154–157, 154f, 156f. See also Nd:YAG laser therapy, capsulotomy
Capsular hooks, 182–183, 183f
Capsular/capsule opacification, 152–157, 184
    IOLs and, 153
    Nd:YAG laser capsulotomy for, 152, 153, 154, 154–157, 154f, 156f. See also Nd:YAG laser therapy, capsulotomy
Capsular phimosis, 153–154
    Nd:YAG laser capsulotomy for, 154, 154–157, 154f, 156f. See also Nd:YAG laser therapy, capsulotomy
    in pseudoexfoliation/exfoliation syndrome, 184
Capsular rupture, cataract surgery and, 142–143, 180–181
Capsular tension rings (CTRs), for zonular incompetence, 180, 181f, 183
Capsule, lens. See Lens capsule
Capsule staining, for cataract surgery, 178–179, 179f
Capsulorrhexis
    advanced cataract and, 180
    continuous curvilinear (CCC), 108–110, 109f
        capsule staining for, 178–179, 179f
        for ECCE, 196
        for phacoemulsification, 108–110, 109f
    for ECCE, 196, 197f
    for phacoemulsification, 108–110, 109f
        in zonular dehiscence with lens subluxation/ dislocation, 182

Capsulotomy
    anterior
        for ECCE, 196, 197f
        for phacoemulsification, 109–110
    can-opener, 109–110, 196, 197f
    Nd:YAG laser, 154–157, 154f, 156f
        for anterior capsule fibrosis and phimosis, 154, 154–157, 154f, 156f
        for capsular block syndrome, 149
        for capsule opacification, 152, 153, 154, 154–157, 154f, 156f
        complications of, 156–157
        contraindications to, 155
        indications for, 154–155
        lens particle glaucoma and, 67
        procedure for, 155–156, 156f
        retinal detachment and, 157, 166
Carbohydrates, metabolism of, in lens, 17–19, 18f
Carbonic anhydrase inhibitors (CAIs), for cystoid macular edema, after cataract surgery, 165
Catalase, in lens, 20
Cataract
    advanced, surgery for, 180
    age-related, 5, 43–48. See also Age-related cataracts
        epidemiology of, 5
        genetic contributions to, 41–42
    alcohol use/abuse and, 63–64
    astigmatism caused by, 123
    atopic dermatitis and, 66
    brunescent, 44
        lens proteins in, 17
        surgery for, 180
            hydrodelineation in, 110, 180
    capsular, 38
    cerulean, 37, 38f
    chemical injuries causing, 59
    in children, 34–39, 35t, 36f, 37f, 38f, 39f
        genetic contributions to, 41–42
    complete (total), 38
    congenital, 34–39, 35t, 36f, 37f, 38f, 39f
        aniridia and, 33, 34f
        bilateral, 35t
        genetic/hereditary factors in, 41–42
        unilateral, 35t
    contrast sensitivity affected by, 70
    contusion, 54, 54f
    coronary, 37
    cortical, 45–46, 46f, 47f, 48f, 49f, 50f
        characteristics and effects of, 45, 70t
        genetic contributions to, 41
        race and, 6
        uveitis and, 64–66, 64f
    corticosteroids causing, 51–52, 64, 188
    degenerative ocular disorders and, 68
    diabetic, 60–61, 60f
        "sugar," aldose reductase in development of, 19
        surgery for, 170
            preoperative evaluation and, 80–81
    drug-induced, 51–53, 52f
    electrical injury causing, 59, 59f
    epidemiology of, 5–7
    evaluation of, 69–88, 70t
    fundus evaluation in patient with, 80–81

in galactosemia, 61, 61*f*
glassblower's, 57
glaucoma and, 186–187, 186*f*
    management of, 186–187
    preoperative evaluation/care and, 186–187, 186*f*
history in, 69–71, 70*t*
    surgery evaluation and, 74–76
hypermature, 46, 49*f*
    phacolytic glaucoma and, 67
hypocalcemic, 61–62
incidence/prevalence of, 5, 6
infantile, 34–39, 35*t*, 36*f*, 37*f*, 38*f*, 39*f*. *See also*
    Cataract, congenital
intralenticular foreign body causing, 57
intumescent, 46
    surgery for, 179–180
ischemia causing, 68
after keratoplasty, 176
lamellar (zonular), 34–35, 36*f*
lens proteins and, 17
management of, 71–88. *See also* Cataract surgery
    in glaucoma, 186–187, 186*f*
    low-vision aids in, 71
    nonsurgical, 71–72
    pharmacologic, 72
mature, 46, 48*f*
    phacolytic glaucoma and, 67
membranous, 38, 39*f*
metabolic, 60–62, 60*f*, 61*f*, 62*f*
morgagnian, 46, 50*f*
in myotonic dystrophy, 62, 62*f*
nuclear, 43–45, 45*f*
    characteristics and effects of, 43, 44, 70, 70*t*
    in children/congenital, 38, 39*f*
    genetic contributions to, 42
    hyperbaric oxygen therapy and, 20, 65
    race and, 6
    vitrectomy and, 55, 190
nutritional disease and, 7, 63–64
oil droplet, 44, 61, 61*f*
oxidative damage and, 19–20
pediatric, 34–39, 35*t*, 36*f*, 37*f*, 38*f*, 39*f*. *See also*
    Cataract, congenital
perforating/penetrating injuries causing, 55, 55*f*, 56*f*
persistent fetal vasculature and, 42
phacolytic glaucoma and, 67
phacomorphic glaucoma and, 67, 68*f*
polar, 35–36, 37*f*
    surgery for, 180–181
        hydrodissection/nucleus rotation and, 111, 181
posterior lenticonus/lentiglobus and, 30
postvitrectomy, 55, 190
in pseudoexfoliation syndrome, 65
race and, 6
radiation-induced, 57–58
after refractive surgery, 176–177, 177*f*
risk factors for development of, 6–7
rosette, 54, 54*f*
rubella, 38–39
in siderosis bulbi, 58–59, 58*f*
silicone oil use and, 83, 120, 190
smoking/tobacco use and, 6–7, 63–64
"snowflake," 60, 60*f*

statin use and, 53
steroid-induced, 51–52, 64, 188
subcapsular, posterior, 46–48, 51*f*
    characteristics and effects of, 47, 70*t*
    corticosteroids causing, 51–52
    ischemia causing, 68
    in myotonic dystrophy, 62
    race and, 6
    silicone oil use and, 190
    uveitis and, 64
    vitrectomy and, 55, 190
subtypes of, distribution of, 6
"sugar," aldose reductase in development of, 19
"sunflower," in chalcosis/Wilson disease, 59, 62
sutural (stellate), 37, 37*f*
tetanic, 61–62
total (complete), 38
traumatic, 53–59, 54*f*, 55*f*, 56*f*, 59*f*, 190–193, 192*f*
    surgery for, 192
uveitis and, 64–65, 64*f*, 139–140
visual acuity and, 69–70, 70*t*
    postoperative outcome and, 126
    preoperative evaluation and, 75–76
vitrectomy and, 55, 190
in Wilson disease, 62
zonular (lamellar), 34–35, 36*f*
Cataract surgery, 89–126. *See also specific procedure and*
    Phacoemulsification
in acne rosacea, 172–173
α-blocker use and, 74
anesthesia for, 91–92, 91*f*, 92*f*, 93*f*
anterior capsule fibrosis and phimosis and, 153–154
anterior segment complications of, 132–144, 137*t*
anticoagulant use and, 74, 157, 171–172, 172*t*
antimicrobial prophylaxis for, 93–95, 94*f*
    corneal melting and, 132
astigmatism and
    induced, 131–132
    modification of preexisting, 123–124
    toric IOLs for, 124
axial length extremes and, 184–185
biometry before, 82, 82–83, 83*f*
    hypotony affecting, 185
    IOL power determination/selection and, 82–83,
        83*f*, 84–85, 87
in bleeding diathesis, 171–172
in blepharitis, 172–173
Brown-McLean syndrome after, 128*t*, 130
bullous keratopathy after, 129, 129*f*
    IOL design and, 149
capsular block syndrome and, 148–149
capsular opacification and contraction and, 152–157,
    184
    Nd:YAG laser capsulotomy for, 152, 153, 154,
        154–157, 154*f*, 156*f*. *See also* Nd:YAG laser
        therapy, capsulotomy
capsular rupture and, 142–143
capsule staining and, 178–179, 179*f*
capsulorrhexis in, 108–110, 109*f*
    capsule staining for, 178–179, 179*f*
choroidal hemorrhage and. *See* Cataract surgery,
    suprachoroidal hemorrhage/effusion and
ciliary block (malignant) glaucoma and, 139

in claustrophobia, 169
clear corneal incision for, 106–107, 106f
communication with patient and, 169–170, 170
complications of, 127–167. See also specific type
   anterior segment, 132–144, 137t
   antimicrobial prophylaxis in prevention of, 93–95, 94f
   capsular opacification and contraction and, 152–157
   corneal, 128–132, 128t, 129f
   endophthalmitis, 127, 140, 160–163, 161f
   hemorrhage, 157–160
   intraoperative, 127
   IOL implantation and, 144–152, 144f, 146f, 147f, 148f
   retinal, 163–167, 164f
conjunctival evaluation before, 78
corneal complications and, 128–132, 128t, 129f
corneal conditions and, 174–177, 174f, 177f
corneal edema and, 128–130, 128t
corneal evaluation before, 78–79
   pachymetry, 84
   topography, 84, 86, 174
corneal melting/keratolysis after, 132
   in patient with dry eye, 132
cyclodialysis and, 139
cystoid macular edema and, 163–165, 164f, 187
   in glaucoma, 164, 187
   after Nd:YAG capsulotomy, 157
   vitreous prolapse and, 143–144
in dementia/mental disability, 169–170
Descemet membrane detachment and, 131
in diabetes mellitus, 170
   preoperative evaluation and, 80–81
elevated intraocular pressure after, 75, 128t, 129, 136. See also Elevated intraocular pressure
endophthalmitis after, 127, 140, 160–163, 161f
   prevention of, 93–95, 94f, 161–162
endothelial keratoplasty and, 175, 175–176
epithelial/fibrous ingrowth and, 128t, 132–133
external eye examination before, 77–78
external ocular abnormalities and, 172–174
extracapsular cataract extraction (ECCE), 90, 90f, 196–198, 197f. See also Extracapsular cataract extraction
femtosecond laser, 125–126
filtering bleb (inadvertent) after, 130–131
filtering surgery and, cataract surgery following, 187
flat or shallow anterior chamber and, 134–136
   intraoperative complications and, 134–135
   posterior fluid misdirection syndrome and, 134–135
   postoperative complications and, 135–136
   preoperative considerations/IOL power determination and, 79, 84, 86–87
fluid-based phacolysis, 125
Fuchs heterochromic uveitis and, 64–65
fundus evaluation before, 80–81
glaucoma and, 186–187, 186f
   filtering surgery before, 187
   preoperative evaluation and, 186–187, 186f
globe exposure for, 105, 105f, 199
hemorrhage and, 157–160
high hyperopia and, 185
high myopia and, 184–185

historical overview/key developments in, 89–91, 89f, 90f, 195
hyphema after, 149, 158–159
in hypotony, 185
hypotony/flat anterior chamber after, 135
   suprachoroidal effusion/hemorrhage and, 159, 160
incisions for. See also Incisions, for cataract surgery
   complications related to, 130–131, 134
   for ECCE, 196
   for ICCE, 199–200
   leaking, 118, 130–131
      flat anterior chamber and, 135
   for phacoemulsification
      clear corneal, 106–107, 106f
      scleral tunnel, 107–108, 107f
indications for, 72–74
informed consent for, 87–88
intracapsular cataract extraction (ICCE), 90, 199–201, 200f. See also Intracapsular cataract extraction
intraoperative floppy iris syndrome and, 74, 178
IOLs and, 115–117, 118–122. See also Intraocular lenses
   complications of, 144–152, 144f, 146f, 147f, 148f
iridodialysis and, 138
iris trauma and
   in patient with preexisting iris trauma, 191, 192f
   as surgical complication, 138
in keratoconjunctivitis sicca, 173
keratoplasty and, 175, 175–176
   with IOL insertion (triple procedure), 175
key developments in, 195
laser photolysis, 125
lens anatomy alterations and, 179–184, 181f, 182f, 183f
lens–iris diaphragm retropulsion syndrome and, 138, 184
lens visualization and, 177–179, 178f, 179f
   trauma affecting, 191
limbal relaxing incisions and, 123–124
macular function evaluation before, 82
   retinal disease and, 189
malignant glaucoma (aqueous misdirection/ciliary block glaucoma) and, 139
manual small-incision, 198, 199f
measurements taken before, 82–84, 83f
medical status and, 72, 170–171
in mucous membrane pemphigoid, 173
in nanophthalmos, 185
in neurocognitive/neurodevelopmental disorders, 169–170
nucleus removal in
   in ECCE, 196–197
   in ICCE, 200, 200f
   in phacoemulsification, 111, 112–114, 113f. See also Phacoemulsification
ophthalmic viscosurgical devices (viscoelastic agents) in, 95–97. See also Ophthalmic viscosurgical devices
outcomes of, 126
   improving, 87
paracentesis for, 105
in patient with communication obstacles, 169–170, 170
patient preparation for, 87–88

phacoemulsification, 98–118. *See also*
Phacoemulsification
posterior capsule opacification and, 152–153
Nd:YAG laser capsulotomy for, 152, 153, 154–157,
154*f*, 156*f*. *See also* Nd:YAG laser therapy,
capsulotomy
posterior capsule rupture and, 142–143
posterior fluid misdirection syndrome and, 134–135
postoperative care and
after ECCE, 198
after ICCE, 201
potential acuity estimation before, 81–82
preoperative evaluation/preparation for, 74–76, 87–88
in pseudoexfoliation/exfoliation syndrome, 79, 184
pseudophakic/aphakic bullous keratopathy after, 129,
129*f*
IOL design and, 149
psychosocial considerations in, 72, 76, 169–170
pupil expansion and, 177–178, 178*f*
in uveitis, 191
pupillary capture and, 148, 148*f*
IOL decentration and, 145
rate of, 5–6
red reflex and, 178–179, 179*f*
refraction before, 76
refractive errors after, 86
after refractive surgery, 176–177, 177*f*
IOL power calculation and, 85–87, 176, 177*f*
with refractive surgery, 123–124. *See also* Cataract
surgery, astigmatism and
retained foreign matter and, 191
retained lens material and, 140–141
retinal complications and, 163–167, 164*f*
retinal detachment after, 127
family history as risk factor and, 75
Nd:YAG laser capsulotomy and, 157, 166
in retinal disease, 189
retinal light toxicity and, 166
retrobulbar hemorrhage and, 158, 171
same-day bilateral, 73
scleral tunnel incisions for
ECCE and, 196
phacoemulsification and, 107–108, 107*f*
second-eye, 73
slit-lamp examination before, 78–80
small pupil and, 177–178, 178*f*
specular microscopy before, 84
suprachoroidal hemorrhage/effusion and, 159, 171
delayed, 160
expulsive, 159–160
flat anterior chamber and, 134
systemic conditions and, 170–172, 171*f*
toxic anterior segment syndrome and, 129, 133–134
after trauma, 190–193, 192*f*
in triple procedure, 175
uveitis after, 139–140
in uveitis patient, 64–65, 75, 140
visual function evaluation before, 71, 72, 76–77
visual function evaluation after, 126
vitreal complications/vitreous abnormalities and
with ICCE, 200
posterior detachment, 166
prolapse, 142, 143–144
vitreocorneal adherence, 130

wound closure for
complications associated with, 130–131
after ECCE, 197–198
after ICCE, 200–201
postoperative endophthalmitis and, 161
wound dehiscence/rupture and, 131
zonular abnormalities and, 179–184
iris coloboma/corectopia and, 180
nucleus rotation and, 111
zonular dehiscence with lens subluxation or
dislocation and, 181–183, 182*f*, 183*f*
zonular anatomy alterations and, 179–184
Cation balance, in lens, maintenance of, 21, 22*f*
Cavitation, 99
CBS. *See* Capsular block syndrome
CCC. *See* Continuous curvilinear capsulorrhexis
CDC (Centers for Disease Control), cataract
epidemiology and, 5
Ceftazidime, for endophthalmitis, after cataract surgery,
162
Cefuroxime, intracameral, during cataract surgery, 94, 162
Centers for Disease Control (CDC), cataract
epidemiology and, 5
Central nervous system (CNS), disorders of, cataract
surgery in patient with, 169–170
Cerulean cataract, 37, 38*f*
Chalcosis, 59
Chatter, 99, 100
Chemical injury (burns)
during cataract surgery, corneal edema and, 128*t*
cataracts caused by, 59
Children, cataract in, 34–39, 35*t*, 36*f*, 37*f*, 38*f*, 39*f*. *See
also* Cataract, pediatric
Chloride, in lens, 21
Chlorpromazine
intraoperative floppy iris syndrome and, 136, 137*t*
lens changes caused by, 52
Cholinesterase/acetylcholinesterase inhibitors
(anticholinesterase agents), cataracts caused by, 52
Chondroitin sulfate, as viscoelastic, 95
Chopping techniques, in phacoemulsification, 114
Choroidal hemorrhage/suprachoroidal hemorrhage,
cataract surgery and, 159, 171
delayed, 160
expulsive, 159–160
flat or shallow anterior chamber and, 134
Chromophores, ultraviolet-absorbing, IOLs with, 120
Chronic obstructive pulmonary disease (COPD),
cataract surgery in patient with, 170
Chymotrypsin (α-chymotrypsin), for ICCE, 195, 200
Cigarette smoking, cataract development and, 6–7,
63–64
Ciliary block, after cataract surgery, flat or shallow
anterior chamber and, 135
Ciliary block glaucoma (malignant glaucoma/aqueous
misdirection), cataract surgery and, 139
Ciliary muscle, in accommodation, 22–23, 23*t*
Clarity, optical, of ophthalmic viscosurgical device, 97
Claustrophobia, cataract surgery in patient with, 169
Clear corneal incision, for cataract surgery, 106–107, 106*f*
in glaucoma, 186
after radial keratotomy, 177
Closed-loop intraocular lenses, pseudophakic bullous
keratopathy and, 149

Closed-loop speculum, for globe exposure, in cataract surgery, 105f
CME. See Cystoid macular edema
CNS. See Central nervous system
Coagulation, disorders of, cataract surgery in patient with, 171–172
Coatability, of ophthalmic viscosurgical device, 97
Cohesive ophthalmic viscosurgical devices/viscoelastics, 96
Collagen, in lens capsule, 11
Colobomas
    iris, cataract surgery in patient with, 180
    lens, 30–31, 31f
Color vision, defects in, cataract and, 44, 70
Communication, between clinician and patient, cataract surgery and, 169–170, 170
Complete cataract, 38
Confrontation testing, before cataract surgery, 82
Congenital anomalies. See also specific type
    of lens, 30–39, 30f, 31f, 32f, 33f, 34f, 35t, 36f, 37f, 38f, 39f
Congenital aphakia, 30. See also Aphakia
Congenital cataract, 34–39, 35t, 36f, 37f, 38f, 39f. See also specific type and Cataract, congenital
    genetic/hereditary factors in, 41–42
Congenital rubella syndrome, cataracts and, 38–39
Conjunctiva, examination of, before cataract surgery, 78
Conjunctival flaps
    for ECCE, 196
    for ICCE, 199
    leak causing inadvertent filtering bleb and, 130–131
    for postoperative corneal edema, 129–130
Connective tissue disorders, cataract surgery in patient with, 170–171, 171f
Consent, informed, for cataract surgery, 87–88
Contact applanation, for axial length measurement, in IOL power determination/selection, 83
Continuous curvilinear capsulorrhexis (CCC), 108–110, 109f
    capsule staining for, 178–179, 179f
    for ECCE, 196
    for phacoemulsification, 108–110, 109f
Contrast sensitivity, cataracts and, 70, 77
Contrast sensitivity testing, 77
Contusion cataract, 54, 54f
Contusion injury, lens damage caused by, 53–55, 54f
Copper
    foreign body of, 59
    "sunflower" cataract and, 59
    in Wilson disease/chalcosis, 59, 62
Corectopia, cataract surgery in patient with, 180
Cornea
    blood staining of, hyphema after cataract surgery and, 159
    deposits in, copper/Wilson disease causing, 59, 62
    disorders of
        as cataract surgery complication, 128–132, 128t, 129f
        cataract surgery in patient with, 174–177, 174f, 177f, 191–192
    edema of
        after cataract surgery, 128–130, 128t
            ECCE, 198
            ICCE, 201
            persistent, with vitreocorneal adherence, 130
        cataract surgery in patient with, 191–192

epithelium of, defects/persistent defects of, after cataract surgery, 132, 173
examination of, before cataract surgery, 78–79, 84
guttae/guttata
    Brown-McLean syndrome and, 130
    cataract surgery and, 79
melting of (keratolysis), cataract surgery and, 132
    in patient with dry eye, 132
opacification of, in Peters anomaly, 31
thickness/rigidity of, measurement of, before cataract surgery, 78–79
topography of
    cataract surgery and, 84, 86, 174
    IOL power determination/selection and, after refractive surgery, 86
transplantation of
    cataract/cataract surgery and, 56, 175, 176
    for corneal edema after cataract surgery, 129
    in triple procedure, 175
Corneal dystrophies, cataract/cataract surgery in patient with, 84, 174–175, 174f
Corneal incision, clear, for cataract surgery, 106–107, 106f
    in glaucoma, 186
Corneal melting (keratolysis), cataract surgery and, 132
    in patient with dry eye, 132
Coronary cataract, 37
Corrected distance visual acuity (best-corrected visual acuity), after cataract surgery, 126
    manual small-incision surgery and, 198–199
    multifocal IOLs and, 121–122
Cortex, lens, 10f, 12f, 13
Cortical cataracts, 45–46, 46f, 47f, 48f, 49f, 50f
    characteristics and effects of, 45, 70t
    genetic contributions to, 41
    race and, 6
    uveitis and, 64–65, 64f
Cortical spokes, 46, 47f
Corticosteroids (steroids)
    cataracts caused by, 51–52, 64, 188
    for cystoid macular edema, after cataract surgery, 165
Couching, 89, 89f
Cough, cataract surgery in patient with, 170
Coupling, astigmatic keratotomy and, 123
Cover tests, before cataract surgery, 77–78
Cranial nerve III (oculomotor nerve), in accommodation, 23
Cryoprobe, for lens extraction, 195
    in ICCE, 200
Crystallins, 15–16, 15f
    α, 15, 15–16, 15f
    β, 16
    β,γ, 15, 15f, 16
    γ, 16
CTRs. See Capsular tension rings
Cuneiform opacities, 46, 47f
Cyclodialysis, after cataract surgery, 139
Cycloplegia/cycloplegics, 23
Cystoid macular edema (CME), postoperative, cataract surgery and, 163–165, 164f, 187
    in glaucoma, 164, 187
    after Nd:YAG capsulotomy, 157
    vitreous prolapse and, 143–144
Cystotome, for ECCE, 196
Cytoskeletal (urea-soluble) lens proteins, 15f, 16–17

Deafness (hearing loss), cataract surgery in patient with, 170

Decentration/dislocation (IOL), 127, 144–147, 144f, 146f, 147f

Degenerations, cataracts associated with, 68

Delayed suprachoroidal hemorrhage, after cataract surgery, 160

Dementia, cataract surgery in patient with, 169–170

Dermatitis, atopic, cataracts associated with, 66

Descemet membrane, detachment of, after cataract surgery, 131

Descemet stripping endothelial keratoplasty, cataract formation and, 56

Developmental defects. See also specific type and Congenital anomalies
of lens, 39–42, 40f

Diabetes mellitus, cataracts associated with, 19, 60–61, 60f
"sugar," aldose reductase in development of, 19
surgery for, 170
preoperative evaluation and, 80–81

Diabetic macular edema, cataract surgery and, 80, 189

Diabetic retinopathy, cataract surgery, 80–81, 189

Diaphragm pump, for phacoemulsification aspiration, 103, 104f

Diffusion, glucose transport into lens and, 17

Diplopia, monocular, in cataracts, 43–44, 45, 47, 70–71

Dislocated lens, 40. See also Ectopia lentis
cataract surgery in patient with, 181–183, 182f, 183f
traumatic, 40, 54–55, 54f

Dislocation/decentration (IOL), 127, 144–147, 144f, 146f, 147f

Dispersive ophthalmic viscosurgical devices/viscoelastics, 96

"Divide and conquer nucleofractis," 112–114, 113f

Doxazosin, intraoperative floppy iris syndrome and, 74, 136–137, 137t

Drugs, lens changes caused by, 51–53, 52f

Dry eye, cataract surgery in patient with, 173
corneal melting/keratolysis and, 132

Dulcitol (galactitol), in cataract formation, 61

Duty cycle, in phacoemulsification, 100

Dysphotopsias, IOLs and, 150–151

Dystrophies, corneal, cataract/cataract surgery in patient with, 84, 174–175, 174f

ECCE. See Extracapsular cataract extraction

Echothiophate, cataract and, 52

Ectoderm, in lens development, 25, 26f

Ectopia lentis, 39–41, 40f
cataract surgery in patient with, 181–183, 182f, 183f
et pupillae, 42
in homocystinuria, 41
in hyperlysinemia, 41
isolated/simple, 40
in Marfan syndrome, 40–41, 40f
traumatic, 40

Edema, corneal. See Cornea, edema of

Effusion, suprachoroidal, cataract surgery and, 159
flat or shallow anterior chamber and, 134

EK. See Endothelial keratoplasty

Electrical injury, lens damage/cataracts caused by, 59, 59f

Electrolytes, in lens, maintenance of balance of, 21, 22f

Elevated intraocular pressure
cataract surgery and, 75, 128t, 129, 136
corneal edema and, 129
ECCE, 198
epithelial ingrowth and, 133
expulsive suprachoroidal hemorrhage and, 159, 160
flat or shallow anterior chamber and, 134, 135–136
in glaucoma, 67, 75, 187
postoperative hyphema and, 159
retained lens material and, 141
retrobulbar hemorrhage and, 158
stromal/epithelial corneal edema and, 129
in glaucoma
cataract surgery and, 75
phacolytic glaucoma, 67
Nd:YAG laser capsulotomy and, 156
phacoemulsification lowering, 186

Elliptical phacoemulsification, 101

Elschnig pearls, 152

Emanation theory of vision, 3

Embryonic lens nucleus, 13, 27f
opacification of (congenital nuclear cataract), 38, 39f

Emulsification. See also Phacoemulsification
locations of, 111–112

Endophthalmitis
phacoanaphylactic (phacoantigenic uveitis), 66
postoperative, 127, 140, 160–163, 161f
acute, 162
chronic (delayed-onset), 162, 163
prevention of, 93–95, 94f, 161–162

Endophthalmitis Study Group of the European Society of Cataract and Refractive Surgeons (ESCRS), on postoperative endophthalmitis, 94, 162

Endophthalmitis Vitrectomy Study (EVS), 161, 162

Endothelial dystrophies, cataract surgery in patient with, 175

Endothelial keratoplasty (EK)
cataract surgery and, 175, 175–176
in triple procedure, 175
for corneal edema after cataract surgery, 129

Energy, phaco, 99. See also Power

Enophthalmos, cataract surgery in patient with, 77

Enterococcus, postoperative endophthalmitis caused by, 161

EPHA2 gene, in age-related cataracts, 41–42

Epicapsular star, 31, 32f

Epimerase deficiency, galactosemia/cataract formation and, 61

Epinephrine, for intraoperative floppy iris syndrome, 138

Epithelial defects, corneal/persistent corneal, after cataract surgery, 132, 173

Epithelial dystrophies, basement membrane, cataract surgery in patient with, 174–175, 174f

Epithelial edema, after cataract surgery, 128–130, 128t

Epithelial ingrowth (downgrowth), cataract surgery and, 128t, 132–133

Epithelium, lens, 10f, 12–13, 12f
active transport and, 21
development of, 27, 27f
opacification of (capsular cataract), 38

Equator (lens), 9, 10f, 12f

Erysiphakes, 195

ESCRS (Endophthalmitis Study Group of the European Society of Cataract and Refractive Surgeons), on postoperative endophthalmitis, 94, 162
Essential/progressive iris atrophy, cataract and, 68
EVS (Endophthalmitis Vitrectomy Study), 161, 162
Exfoliation. *See also* Exfoliation/pseudoexfoliation syndrome
  true, infrared radiation/heat causing, 57
Exfoliation/pseudoexfoliation syndrome, 65–66, 65*f*
  cataract surgery in patient with, 79, 184
  IOL decentration/dislocation and, 144
  postoperative hyphema and, 158
  zonular incompetence and, 65–66, 181, 182*f*, 184
Exposure keratitis, cataract surgery in patient with, 174
Expulsive choroidal/suprachoroidal hemorrhage, cataract surgery and, 159–160
External (outer) eye
  cataract surgery in patient with abnormalities of, 172–174
  examination of, before cataract surgery, 77–78
Extracapsular cataract extraction (ECCE), 90, 90*f*, 196–198, 197*f*. *See also* Cataract surgery
  for advanced cataract, 180
  anterior capsulotomy in, 196, 197*f*
  complications of, 135–136, 195, 198
    intraoperative complications and, 134–135
    posterior fluid misdirection syndrome and, 134–135
    postoperative complications and, 135–136
  historical overview/key developments in, 90, 90*f*, 119, 195
  incisions for, 196
  IOLs for, 197
  lens particle glaucoma and, 67
  manual small-incision cataract surgery and, 198, 199*f*
  nucleus removal in, 196–197
  ocular trauma affecting visualization and, 191
  patient preparation for, 196
  posterior capsule opacification and, 152–153
    Nd:YAG laser capsulotomy for, 152, 153, 154–157, 154*f*, 156*f*. *See also* Nd:YAG laser therapy, capsulotomy
  postoperative course and, 198
  retained lens fragments after, 141
  retinal detachment and, 166
  suture-induced astigmatism after, 132
  wound closure and, 197–198
  in zonular dehiscence with lens subluxation or dislocation, 182
Extracapsular IOL dislocation, 144, 144*f*, 145
Eye
  anatomy of, early conceptions of, 3, 3*f*, 4*f*
  axial length of
    extremes of, cataract surgery in patient with, 184–185
    in IOL power determination, 82–83, 83*f*, 85
      hypotony affecting, 185
      unexpected refractive results after surgery and, 150, 176
Eye marking, before phacoemulsification, 104
Eyedrops (topical medications)
  anesthetic, for cataract surgery, 92
  antibiotic, after cataract surgery, 95
    corneal melting and, 132

Eyelid disorders, cataract surgery in patient with, 174
Eyelid speculum, for globe exposure, in cataract surgery, 105, 105*f*

Facial nerve block, for cataract surgery, 92, 93*f*
Facilitated diffusion, glucose transport into lens and, 17
Feiz and Mannis formula, for IOL power determination/selection, 86
Femtosecond laser, for cataract extraction, 125–126
Fetal lens nucleus, 13, 27*f*, 28, 28–29, 28*f*
  opacification of (congenital nuclear cataract), 38, 39*f*
Fetal vasculature, persistent. *See* Persistent fetal vasculature
Fibrillin, defects in, in Marfan syndrome, 40
Fibrous ingrowth (downgrowth), corneal edema after cataract surgery and, 128*t*, 133
Filensin, 16
Filtering bleb
  cataract surgery in eye with, 187
  inadvertent, after cataract surgery, 130–131
Filtering procedures, cataract surgery after, 186, 187
Flaps, conjunctival
  for ECCE, 196
  for ICCE, 199
  leak causing inadvertent filtering bleb and, 130–131
  for postoperative corneal edema, 129–130
Flat anterior chamber. *See* Anterior chamber, flat or shallow
Flexible-loop anterior chamber intraocular lenses, 119, 120*f*
Floppy iris syndrome, intraoperative, 74, 136–138, 137*t*
  pupil expansion devices for, 178
Flow rate, in phacoemulsification, 102
  vacuum rise time and, 102
Fluid-based phacolysis, 125
Fluidics, terminology used in, 102–103
Fluorescein angiography (FA), in cataract surgery evaluation, 82, 188, 189
Foldable intraocular lenses, 116, 120, 120*f*, 121*f*
  insertion of, 116
Followability, in phacoemulsification, 102
Foot-pedal controls, phaco machine, 99
Foreign bodies
  intralenticular, 57
  intraocular, retained
    cataract surgery and, 191
    siderosis and, 58–59, 58*f*
Fornices, sterilization of, during cataract surgery, 94
FOXC1 gene, in Peters anomaly, 32
Free radicals, lens damage and, 19–20
Frequency, in phacoemulsification, 99
Fuchs corneal dystrophy, IOL implantation and, 149
Fuchs heterochromic uveitis, cataracts/cataract surgery in, 64–65, 64*f*
Fundus, evaluation of, before cataract surgery, 80–81

G6P. *See* Glucose-6-phosphate
Galactitol (dulcitol), in cataract formation, 61
Galactokinase, defective/deficiency of, galactosemia/cataract formation and, 61
Galactose, in cataract formation, 61
Galactose 1-phosphate uridyltransferase (Gal-1-PUT), galactosemia caused by defects in, 61

Galactosemia, 61
Gamma (γ)-crystallins, 16
Gap junctions, in lens, 20
General anesthesia. *See also* Anesthesia
    for cataract surgery, 92
        in arthritis, 171
        in claustrophobia, 169
        in patient unable to communicate, 170
Genetic/hereditary factors, in age-related cataracts,
    41–42
Geometric optics, IOLs and, 120, 121*f*
Germinative zone, 12, 12*f*
Glare
    cataracts and, 45, 47, 70, 70*t*, 77
    with IOLs, 144, 150–152
Glare testing, in cataract evaluation, 77
Glassblower's cataract, 57
Glaucoma
    cataracts and, 52, 56, 186–187, 186*f*
        management of, 186–187, 186*f*
        preoperative evaluation/care and, 75
    ciliary block, cataract surgery and, 139
    IOL implantation and, 149
    lens-induced, 67–68, 68*f*
    lens particle, 67
    microspherophakia and, 33
    phacolytic, 67
    phacomorphic, 67, 68*f*
Glaucoma surgery
    cataract development after, 56
    cataract surgery and, 186–187, 187
Glaukomflecken, 68
Glistenings, IOL, 151
Globe
    exposure of
        for ICCE, 199
        for phacoemulsification, 105, 105*f*
    stabilization of, for clear corneal incision, 106
Glucose
    in cataract formation, 19, 60. *See also* Diabetes mellitus
    metabolism of, in lens, 17–19, 18*f*
Glucose-6-phosphate (G6P), in lens glucose/
    carbohydrate metabolism, 17, 18*f*
Glutathione, in lens, oxidative changes and, 17, 20
Glutathione peroxidase, in lens, 20
Glycolysis, in lens glucose/carbohydrate metabolism, 17,
    17–19, 18*f*
"Golden ring" sign, 110
Gonioscopy
    before cataract surgery, 79
    in lens particle glaucoma, 67
    in trauma evaluation, 190
Gundersen flap, 129

Haigis formula, for IOL power determination/
    selection, 85
Handpiece, phaco, 98, 98*f*
Haptic, of IOL, insertion of lens and, 116, 117, 119, 119*f*
Hearing loss (deafness), cataract surgery in patient with,
    170
HEDS (Herpetic Eye Disease Study), 175
Helmholtz hypothesis (capsular theory) of
    accommodation, 22

Hemorrhages. cataract surgery and, 157–160
    patient receiving anticoagulation therapy and, 74,
        157, 171–172
    retrobulbar, 158, 171
    suprachoroidal/choroidal, 159, 171
        delayed, 160
        expulsive, 159–160
        flat anterior chamber and, 134
Hemostasis, disorders of, cataract surgery in patient
    with, 171–172
Hepatolenticular degeneration (Wilson disease), 62
Herpes simplex virus (HSV), ocular infection/
    inflammation caused by, cataract surgery and, 175
Herpetic Eye Disease Study (HEDS), 175
Heterochromia iridis, in siderosis bulbi, 58*f*
Hexokinase, in lens glucose/carbohydrate metabolism,
    17, 18*f*, 19
Hexose monophosphate (HMP) shunt, in lens glucose/
    carbohydrate metabolism, 17, 18*f*, 19
High hyperopia, cataract surgery in patient with, 185
High myopia, cataract surgery in patient with, 184–185
Historical methods, for IOL power calculation after
    refractive surgery, 86–87
History, in cataract, 69–71, 70*t*
    evaluation for surgery and, 74–76
HMG-CoA (3-hydroxy-3-methylglutaryl coenzyme-A)
    reductase inhibitors, cataracts and, 53
HMP shunt. *See* Hexose monophosphate shunt
Hoffer Q formula, for IOL power determination/
    selection, 85, 86
Holladay formulas, for IOL power determination/
    selection, 85, 87
Homocystinuria, 41
Horizontal phaco chop technique, 114
HPMC. *See* Hydroxypropyl methylcellulose
Hyaloid artery/system, tunica vasculosa lentis
    development and, 29, 29*f*
Hyaluronate/sodium hyaluronate, as viscoelastic, 95
Hydrodelineation, in phacoemulsification, 110
    for advanced cataract, 180
    for posterior polar cataract, 181
    for zonular dehiscence with lens subluxation or
        dislocation, 182
Hydrodissection, in phacoemulsification, 110
    for advanced cataract, 180
    for posterior polar cataract, 111, 181
    for traumatic cataract, 192
    for zonular dehiscence with lens subluxation or
        dislocation, 182
Hydrogel polymers, for IOLs, capsular opacification
    and, 153
3-Hydroxy-3-methylglutaryl coenzyme-A (HMG-CoA)
    reductase inhibitors, cataracts and, 53
Hydroxypropyl methylcellulose (HPMC), as
    viscoelastic, 95
Hyperbaric oxygen therapy, oxidative lens damage/
    cataracts and, 20, 65
Hyperlysinemia, 41
Hypermature cataract, 46, 49*f*
    phacolytic glaucoma and, 67
Hyperopia
    after cataract surgery, prior refractive surgery and, 177
    cataract surgery in patient with, 185

Hyphema, after cataract surgery, 149, 158–159
Hypocalcemia, cataracts associated with, 61–62
Hypopyon, after cataract surgery, 140
Hypotony
   cataract/cataract surgery in patient with, 68, 185
   during/after surgery
      flat anterior chamber and, 135
      suprachoroidal effusion/hemorrhage and, 159, 160

IA. *See* Irrigation/aspiration
IAPB (International Agency for the Prevention of
   Blindness), 6
ICCE. *See* Intracapsular cataract extraction
IFIS. *See* Intraoperative floppy iris syndrome
Immersion ultrasonography, for axial length
   measurement, in IOL power determination/
   selection, 83, 83*f*
Incision leaks, after cataract surgery, 118, 130–131
   flat anterior chamber and, 135
Incisions, for cataract surgery
   clear corneal, 106–107, 106*f*
   closure of
      complications associated with, 130–131
      after ECCE, 197–198
      postoperative endophthalmitis and, 161
   complications associated with, 130–131
      flat or shallow anterior chamber, 134
   dehiscence/rupture of, 131
   for ECCE, 196
      wound closure and, 197–198
   for ICCE, 199–200
   induced astigmatism and, 131–132
   for manual small-incision surgery, 198
   modification of preexisting astigmatism and, 123–124
   for phacoemulsification
      clear corneal, 106–107, 106*f*
      scleral tunnel, 107–108, 107*f*
   postoperative leaking and, 118, 130–131
      flat anterior chamber and, 135
   scleral tunnel
      for ECCE, 196
      for phacoemulsification, 107–108, 107*f*
   self-sealing, beveled/biplanar, clear corneal incisions
      and, 106–107, 106*f*
   thermal wounds of, 131
Index of refraction. *See* Refractive index
Infantile cataract, 34–39, 35*t*, 36*f*, 37*f*, 38*f*, 39*f*. *See also*
   Cataract, congenital
Inflammation (ocular), cataracts/cataract surgery and,
   64–66, 64*f*, 139–140, 170–171
   postoperative, 139–140
      retained lens material and, 141
   trauma and, 191
Informed consent, for cataract surgery, 87–88
Infrared (IR) radiation, lens affected by, 57
Instrumentation. *See* Ophthalmic instrumentation;
   Surgical instruments
Interlenticular opacifications, IOL, 151
International Agency for the Prevention of Blindness
   (IAPB), 6
Intracameral injections during cataract surgery
   cefuroxime, 94, 162
   lidocaine, 92, 137

Intracapsular cataract extraction (ICCE), 90, 199–201,
   200*f*. *See also* Cataract surgery
   globe exposure for, 199
   historical overview/key developments in, 90, 119,
      120*f*, 195
   incision for, 199–200
   IOLs for, 200
   iridectomy/lens delivery in, 200, 200*f*
   patient preparation for, 199
   postoperative course for, 201
   postoperative flat or shallow anterior chamber and,
      135
   retinal detachment and, 166
   suture-induced astigmatism after, 131–132
   wound closure and, 200–201
   in zonular dehiscence with lens subluxation or
      dislocation, 182
Intracapsular IOL dislocation, 144, 144*f*, 145
Intralenticular foreign bodies, 57
Intraocular foreign bodies, retained
   cataract surgery and, 191
   siderosis and, 58–59, 58*f*
Intraocular lenses (IOLs), 115–117, 118–122. *See also*
   Cataract surgery
   accommodating, 122, 122*f*
      complications of, 151
   anterior chamber (ACIOLs), 117, 119, 120*f*
      after capsular rupture, 142–143
      closed-loop, pseudophakic bullous keratopathy
         and, 149
      complications of, 146
      flexible-loop, 119, 120*f*
      history of development of, 119, 120*f*
      after ICCE, 200
      insertion of, 117
   blue-blocking, 120
   capsular block syndrome and, 148–149
   capsular opacification and, 153
   after capsular rupture, 142–143
   closed-loop, pseudophakic bullous keratopathy and,
      149
   complications of, 144–152, 144*f*, 146*f*, 147*f*, 148*f*
      induced-astigmatism, 132
   corneal disease and, 128*t*
   cystoid macular edema and, 165
   decentration and dislocation of, 127, 144–147, 144*f*,
      146*f*, 147*f*
      laser capsulotomy and, 156
   design modifications and, 119–122, 120*f*, 121*f*, 122*f*
   flexible-loop, 119, 120*f*
   foldable, 116, 120, 120*f*, 121*f*
      insertion of, 116
   glare and, 144, 150–152
   history of, 118–119, 118*f*
   hyphema after cataract surgery and, 159
   insertion of, 115–117
      anterior chamber, 117
      after capsular rupture, 142–143
      complications of, 144–152, 144*f*, 146*f*, 147*f*, 148*f*
      after ECCE, 197
      after ICCE, 200
      posterior chamber, 116–117
      procedures after, 117–118

iris-fixated, 119, 119*f*
  after ICCE, 200
  insertion of, 116–117, 119*f*
  after keratoplasty, 176
  pseudophakic bullous keratopathy and, 149
after keratoplasty, 176
with keratoplasty and cataract surgery (triple procedure), 175
laser capsulotomy affecting, 155–156, 156
for manual small-incision cataract surgery, 198
multifocal, 121–122, 121*f*
  complications of, 151
  contraindication to, capsular decentration and, 183
  dry eye therapy before use of, 173
in myopia, 184–185
after ocular trauma, 193
opacification of, 151
posterior chamber (PCIOLs), 116–117, 118*f*, 119–122, 119*f*, 120*f*, 121*f*
  after capsular rupture, 143
  decentration of, 145
  after ECCE, 197
  history of development of, 118–119, 119*f*
  insertion of, 116–117
  after keratoplasty, 176
  after ocular trauma, 193
  pupillary capture of, 148, 148*f*
  in retinal disease, 189
  scleral/iris-fixated (sutured), 116–117, 119, 119*f*
    after ICCE, 200
    after keratoplasty, 176
    uveitis and, 188
  uveitis and, 188
power determination for, 84–87
  biometry in, 82–83, 83*f*, 84–85, 87
    hypotony affecting, 185
  formulas for, 84, 85–87
  historical methods for, 86–87
  improving outcomes of surgery and, 87
  incorrect, 85
  in myopia, 184
  preventing errors in, 87
  refraction and, 76
  refractive surgery and, 85–87, 176, 177*f*
  triple procedure and, 175
  unexpected refractive results after surgery and, 86, 149–150
pseudoaccommodating, 122
  complications of, 151
pseudophakic bullous keratopathy and, 149
pupil evaluation and, 78
pupillary capture of, 148, 148*f*
in retinal disease, 189
silicone oil use and, 83, 120, 190
toric, 124
  complications of, 151
  contraindication to, capsular decentration and, 183
  dry eye therapy before use of, 173
traumatic cataract and, 193
with UV-absorbing chromophores, 120
in uveitis, 188
  postoperative inflammation and, 140

uveitis-glaucoma-hyphema (UGH) syndrome and, 149
  decentration and, 145
Intraocular pressure
  decreased, after cataract surgery, flat anterior chamber and, 135
  elevated/increased. *See* Elevated intraocular pressure
Intraocular surgery. *See* Ocular (intraocular) surgery
Intraoperative floppy iris syndrome (IFIS), 74, 136–138, 137*t*
  pupil expansion devices for, 178
Intravitreal injection
  cataract formation and, 56
  corticosteroid
    after cataract surgery, 163
    for cystoid macular edema, 165
  for endophthalmitis, postoperative, 162
Intumescent cortical cataract, 46
  surgery for, 179–180
IOLs. *See* Intraocular lenses
Ionizing radiation, cataracts caused by, 57
IR radiation. *See* Infrared radiation
Iridectomy
  for anterior chamber IOL insertion, 117, 136
  in ICCE, 200
Iridodialysis
  during cataract surgery, 138
  cataract surgery in patient with, 191
Iridodonesis, cataract surgery and, 79, 181–182
Iris
  absence of/rudimentary (aniridia), 33
    cataract and, 33, 34*f*
      surgery for, 184
  atrophy of, cataract and, 68
  coloboma of, cataract surgery in patient with, 180
  evaluation of, before cataract surgery, 79
  heterochromia of (heterochromia iridis), in siderosis bulbi, 58*f*
  traumatic damage to
    during cataract surgery, 138
    cataract surgery in patient with, 191
Iris-clip intraocular lenses, pseudophakic bullous keratopathy and, 149
Iris-fixated posterior chamber intraocular lenses, 116–117, 119, 119*f*
  after ICCE, 200
  after keratoplasty, 176
  pseudophakic bullous keratopathy and, 149
Iris hooks
  for pupil expansion, 177, 178*f*
  for zonular incompetence, 180
Iris plane, phacoemulsification at, 112
Iris sphincter, damage to, cataract surgery in patient with, 191
Iris suture fixation, peripheral, for IOL decentration, 145, 146*f*
Iron, foreign body of, siderosis caused by, 58–59, 58*f*
Irregular astigmatism, keratorefractive/refractive surgery and, cataract surgery outcome and, 176, 177*f*
Irrigation
  in ECCE, 197
  in phacoemulsification, 101–102, 115
    posterior fluid misdirection and, 134–135
    toxic solutions exposure and, corneal edema caused by, 129, 133–134

Irrigation/aspiration (IA). *See also* Aspiration; Irrigation
  in ECCE, 197
  in manual small-incision cataract surgery, 198
  in phacoemulsification, 115
    posterior fluid misdirection and, 134–135
Irvine-Gass syndrome, 163–165, 164f. *See also* Cystoid
  macular edema
Ischemia, cataracts caused by, 68

K_m (Michaelis/affinity constant), sorbitol in cataract
  development and, 19
Kayser-Fleischer ring, 62
Kelman phaco tip, 101
Keratectomy, photorefractive (PRK). *See* Photorefractive
  keratectomy
Keratitis, exposure, cataract surgery in patient
  with, 174
Keratoconjunctivitis sicca, cataract surgery in patient
  with, 173
  corneal melting/keratolysis and, 132
Keratolysis (corneal melting), cataract surgery and, 132
  in patient with dry eye, 132
Keratometry, in IOL power determination/selection,
  84, 174
  corneal irregularities and, 174
  refractive surgery and, 86
  unexpected refractive results after surgery and, 150
Keratopathy, bullous, after cataract surgery, 129, 129f
  IOL design and, 149
Keratoplasty
  cataract formation after, 176
  cataract surgery and IOL implantation combined
    with (triple procedure), 175
  for corneal edema after cataract surgery, 129
  endothelial (EK)
    cataract surgery and, 175, 175–176
    for corneal edema after cataract surgery, 129
    in triple procedure, 175
  penetrating (PKP)
    cataract/cataract surgery and, 56, 175, 176
    for corneal edema after cataract surgery, 129
    in triple procedure, 175
Keratorefractive surgery, cataract/cataract surgery and,
  123–124, 176–177, 177f
  IOL power calculation and, 85–87, 176, 177f
  preoperative evaluation/planning and, 76, 79
Keratotomy
  astigmatic (AK), cataract surgery and, 123
  radial (RK)
    cataract surgery after, 79, 177
    IOL power calculation and, 86
    hyperopic shift and, 177
Ketorolac
  for cystoid macular edema, after cataract surgery,
    165
  for intraoperative floppy iris syndrome, 138
K_m (Michaelis/affinity constant), sorbitol in cataract
  development and, 19
Kuglen hook, for pupil expansion, 177

Labetalol, intraoperative floppy iris syndrome and, 137,
  137t
Lamellae, zonular, 11
Lamellar (zonular) cataracts, 34–35, 36f

Laser capsulotomy (Nd:YAG), 154–157, 154f, 156f
  for anterior capsule fibrosis and phimosis, 154,
    154–157, 154f, 156f
  for capsular block syndrome, 149
  for capsule opacification, 152, 153, 154, 154–157,
    154f, 156f
  complications of, 156–157
  contraindications to, 155
  indications for, 154–155
  lens particle glaucoma and, 67
  procedure for, 155–156, 156f
  retinal detachment and, 157, 166
Laser in situ keratomileusis. *See* LASIK
Laser photolysis, 125
Laser pupilloplasty
  for cataracts, 71–72
  for IOL decentration/dislocation, 145
LASIK (laser in situ keratomileusis), cataract surgery
  after, 177
  IOL power calculation and, 86
Lens (crystalline)
  age-related changes in, 43–48. *See also* Age-related
    cataracts
  alcohol use/abuse and, 63–64
  anatomy of, 9–13, 9f, 10f, 11f, 12f
    altered, cataract surgery and, 179–184, 181f, 182f,
      183f
    early conceptions of, 3, 3f, 4f
  biochemistry and metabolism of, 11, 14–23
  capsule of. *See* Lens capsule
  carbohydrate metabolism in, 17–19, 18f
  changing shape of. *See* Accommodation
  chemical injuries affecting, 59
  colobomas of, 30–31, 31f
  coloration change in, 43, 44f
  congenital anomalies and abnormalities of, 30–39,
    30f, 31f, 32f, 33f, 34f, 35t, 36f, 37f, 38f, 39f
  cortex of, 10f, 12f, 13
  degenerative ocular disorders and, 68
  development/embryology of, 25–42
    congenital anomalies and abnormalities and,
      30–39, 30f, 31f, 32f, 33f, 34f, 35t, 36f, 37f, 38f, 39f
    developmental defects and, 39–42, 40f
    normal, 25–29, 26–27f, 28f, 29f
  diabetes mellitus affecting, 60–61, 60f
  dislocated, 39–40. *See also* Ectopia lentis
    cataract surgery in patient with, 181–183, 182f,
      183f
    traumatic, 40, 54–55, 54f
  disorders of, 43–68. *See also specific disorder and*
    Cataract
  drug-induced changes in, 51–53, 52f
  electrical injury of, 59, 59f
  epithelium of, 10f, 12–13
    active transport and, 21
    development of, 27, 27f
    opacification of (capsular cataract), 38
  evaluation of, before cataract surgery, 79–80
  foreign body in, 57
  free radicals affecting, 19–20
  glaucoma and, 67–68, 68f
  in homocystinuria, 41
  hyperbaric oxygen therapy associated with changes
    in, 20, 65

in hyperlysinemia, 41
ischemic damage to, 68
luxed/luxated, 40. *See also* Ectopia lentis
    cataract surgery in patient with, 181–183, 182*f*, 183*f*
    traumatic, 40, 54–55, 54*f*
in Marfan syndrome, 40–41, 40*f*
metabolic diseases affecting, 60–62, 60*f*, 61*f*, 62*f*
molecular biology of, 15–17, 15*f*
nucleus of, 10*f*, 12*f*, 13
    congenital cataract of, 38, 39*f*
    embryonic, 13, 27*f*
        opacification of (congenital nuclear cataract),
            38, 39*f*
    fetal, 13, 27*f*, 28, 28–29, 28*f*
        opacification of (congenital nuclear cataract),
            38, 39*f*
    opacification of. *See* Nuclear cataract
    removal/disassembly of
        in ECCE, 196–197
        in ICCE, 200–201, 200*f*
        in manual small-incision cataract surgery, 198,
           199*f*
        in phacoemulsification, 111, 112–114, 113*f*
        rotation of, in phacoemulsification, 111
nutritional diseases affecting, 63–64
oxidative damage to, 19–20
perforating and penetrating injury of, 55, 55*f*, 56*f*
    glaucoma and, 67
physiology of, 20–23
pseudoexfoliation/exfoliation syndrome and, 65–66,
    65*f*
radiation affecting, 57–58
removal of. *See* Cataract surgery; Phacoemulsification
retained, cataract surgery and, 140–141
size of, 11
smoking/tobacco use and, 63–64
subluxed/subluxated, 39–40, 40*f*. *See also* Ectopia
    lentis
    cataract surgery in patient with, 181–183, 182*f*,
        183*f*
    traumatic, 40, 54–55, 54*f*
sutures of, 13
    development of, 27*f*, 28–29
    opacification of (sutural/stellate cataract), 37, 37*f*
transport functions in, 21, 22*f*
traumatic damage to, 53–59, 54*f*, 55*f*, 56*f*, 58*f*, 59*f*
    phacoantigenic uveitis and, 66, 191
    surgery and, 190–193, 192*f*
uveitis and, 64–65, 64*f*, 66. *See also* Phacoantigenic
    (lens-associated) uveitis
water and cation balance in, maintenance of, 21, 22*f*
zonular fibers/zonules of, 9, 10*f*, 12
    absent/abnormal, cataract surgery and, 179–184
        iris coloboma/corectopia and, 180
        nucleus rotation and, 111
    development of, 29
    evaluation of, before cataract surgery, 80
    in pseudoexfoliation/exfoliation syndrome, 65–66,
        181, 182*f*, 184
Lens capsule, 10*f*, 11, 11*f*, 12*f*
    development of, 27, 27*f*
    exfoliation of, infrared radiation/heat causing, 57
    rupture of, cataract surgery and, 142–143
    staining, in cataract surgery, 178–179, 179*f*

Lens crystallins, 15–16, 15*f*. *See also* Crystallins
Lens fibers
    accommodation and, 22
    development of, 12–13, 12*f*
        primary fibers, 26–27, 27*f*
        secondary fibers, 27–28, 27*f*
            microspherophakia and, 33
        zonular (zonules of Zinn), 9, 10*f*, 12
            absent/abnormal, cataract surgery and, 179–184
                iris coloboma/corectopia and, 180
                nucleus rotation and, 111
            development of, 29
            evaluation of, before cataract surgery, 80
            in pseudoexfoliation/exfoliation syndrome, 65–66,
                181, 182*f*, 184
Lens-induced glaucoma, 67–68, 68*f*
Lens–iris diaphragm retropulsion syndrome (LIDRS),
    138, 184
Lens particle glaucoma, 67
Lens pit, 25, 26*f*
Lens placode, 25, 26*f*
Lens proteins, 15–17, 15*f*
    aging affecting, 17
    crystallins, 15–16, 15*f*. *See also* Crystallins
    cytoskeletal and membrane, 15*f*, 16–17
    in phacoantigenic uveitis/endophthalmitis, 66, 191
    in phacolytic glaucoma, 67
    traumatic cataract and, 66, 192
    urea-insoluble (membrane structural), 15*f*, 16–17
    urea-soluble (cytoskeletal), 15*f*, 16–17
    water-insoluble, 15, 15*f*
        age affecting, 17
    water-soluble, 15, 15*f*. *See also* Crystallins
        conversion of to water-insoluble, 17
Lens vesicle, formation of, 25, 26*f*
Lenticonus/lentiglobus, 30, 30*f*
    anterior, 30
    posterior, 30, 30*f*
Lenticular myopia (myopic shift), 43, 70
Lentiglobus. *See* Lenticonus/lentiglobus
Lester hooks, for pupil expansion, 177
Leukomas, in Peters anomaly, 31
Lidocaine
    for cataract surgery, 92
    for intraoperative floppy iris syndrome, 137
LIDRS. *See* Lens–iris diaphragm retropulsion
    syndrome
Lieberman speculum, for globe exposure, in cataract
    surgery, 105*f*
Light toxicity, retinal, cataract surgery and, 166
Limbal groove, for ECCE, 196
Limbal relaxing incisions (LRIs), cataract surgery and,
    123–124
Lipid peroxidation, in lens opacification, 19
Local anesthesia. *See* Anesthesia
Locus vacuus, 3, 3*f*
LogMAR, cystoid macular edema after cataract surgery
    and, 164
Low-vision aids, for cataract, 71
LRIs. *See* Limbal relaxing incisions
Lutein, cataract risk affected by, 7
Luxed/luxated lens, 40. *See also* Ectopia lentis
    cataract surgery in patient with, 181–183, 182*f*, 183*f*
    traumatic, 40, 54–55, 54*f*

Macular degeneration, cataract surgery in patient with, 80
Macular edema
    cystoid (CME), postoperative, cataract surgery and, 163–165, 164f, 187
        in glaucoma, 164, 187
            after Nd:YAG capsulotomy, 157
            vitreous prolapse and, 143–144
    diabetic, cataract surgery and, 80, 189
Macular function tests, before cataract surgery, 82
    retinal disease and, 189
Major intrinsic protein (MIP/aquaporin), 16, 20–21
Malignant glaucoma (aqueous misdirection/ciliary block glaucoma), cataract surgery and, 139
Malyugin ring, for pupil expansion, 178f
Manual small-incision cataract surgery (MSICS), 198, 199f
    in eye with functioning filter, 187
    in glaucoma, 186, 187
MAR (minimum angle of resolution), logarithm of (logMAR), cystoid macular edema after cataract surgery and, 164
Marcus Gunn pupil (relative afferent pupillary defect), cataract surgery on patient with, 78
Marfan syndrome, 40–41, 40f
Mature cataract, 46, 48f
    phacolytic glaucoma and, 67
Mazzocco foldable intraocular lens, 120, 120f
McCannel sutures/technique, for IOL decentration, 145
Medical history, cataract surgery evaluation and, 72, 170–171
Meibomian gland dysfunction, cataract surgery and, 172–173
Membrane structural (urea-insoluble) lens proteins, 15f, 16–17
Membranous cataract, 38, 39f
Meridians, 9
Mesodermal dysgenesis, Peters anomaly and, 31–32
Metabolic disorders, cataracts and, 60–62, 60f, 61f, 62f
Metallosis, lens damage/cataracts caused by, 58–59, 58f
Methionine, in homocystinuria, 41
Methylcellulose
    hydroxypropyl (HPMC), as viscoelastic, 95
    as viscoelastic, 95
Michaelis constant (K_m), sorbitol in cataract development and, 19
Microinvasive glaucoma surgery (MIGS), cataract surgery and, 186
Microscope
    specular, examination before cataract surgery and, 84
    surgical/operating
        for manual small-incision cataract surgery, 198
        retinal light toxicity and, 166
Microspherophakia, 32–33, 33f
MIGS. See Microinvasive glaucoma surgery
Minimum angle of resolution (MAR), logarithm of (logMAR), cystoid macular edema after cataract surgery and, 164
Miotics, for glaucoma, cataract/cataract surgery and, 52
MIP. See Major intrinsic protein
Mittendorf dot, 29, 31, 32f
Monocular diplopia, in cataracts, 43–44, 45, 47, 70–71
Morgagnian cataract, 46, 50f
Morgagnian globules, 46
Motility examination. See Ocular motility, assessment of

MSICS. See Manual small-incision cataract surgery
Mucous membrane pemphigoid, cataract surgery in patient with, 173
Multifocal intraocular lenses, 121–122, 121f
    complications of, 151
    contraindication to, capsular decentration and, 183
    dry eye therapy before use of, 173
Multiplanar incisions, clear corneal, 106, 106f
Mydriasis, after cataract surgery, 138
Myopia
    cataract causing, 43, 70, 70t
    cataract surgery in patient with, 184–185
        retinal detachment and, 166
    lenticular (myopic shift), 43, 70
Myopic shift, in cataracts (lenticular myopia), 43, 70
Myotonic dystrophy, lens disorders/cataracts in, 62, 62f

Na^+,K^+-ATPase (sodium-potassium pump), in lens
    active transport, 21
    pump–leak theory and, 21, 22f
Nadbath-Ellis block, for cataract surgery, 93f
NADP, in lens glucose/carbohydrate metabolism, 18f, 19
NADPH, in lens glucose/carbohydrate metabolism, 18f, 19
Nanophthalmos, cataract surgery in patient with, 185
National Eye Institute Visual Function Questionnaire (NEI-VFQ), 71
Nd:YAG laser therapy
    capsulotomy, 154–157, 154f, 156f
        for anterior capsule fibrosis and phimosis, 154, 154–157, 154f, 156f
        for capsular block syndrome, 149
        for capsule opacification, 152, 153, 154, 154–157, 154f, 156f
        complications of, 156–157
        contraindications to, 155
        indications for, 154–155
        lens particle glaucoma and, 67
        procedure for, 155–156, 156f
        retinal detachment and, 157, 166
    photolysis, 125
    vitreolysis
        for cystoid macular edema, after cataract surgery, 165
        for vitreous prolapse in anterior chamber, 143
"Near clear" incision, for cataract surgery, 107
Near visual acuity, age-related loss of, 23
Negative dysphotopsias, IOLs and, 150–151
NEI-VFQ (National Eye Institute Visual Function Questionnaire), 71
Nerve block, facial, for cataract surgery, 92, 93f
Neurocognitive/neurodevelopmental disorders, cataract surgery in patient with, 169–170
Neurocristopathy, Peters anomaly and, 31–32
Neurologic disorders, cataract surgery in patient with, 169–170
Nonsteroidal anti-inflammatory drugs (NSAIDs)
    corneal melting after cataract surgery associated with, 132, 173
    for cystoid macular edema, after cataract surgery, 165
NSAIDs. See Nonsteroidal anti-inflammatory drugs
Nuclear cataracts, 43–45, 45f
    characteristics and effects of, 43, 44, 70, 70t
    congenital, 38, 39f
    genetic contributions to, 42

hyperbaric oxygen therapy and, 20, 65
race and, 6
vitrectomy and, 55, 190
Nuclear disassembly/removal, 111
techniques of, 112–114, 113f
chopping techniques, 114
phaco fracture, 112–114, 113f
Nuclear sclerosis, 43, 45f, 48f, 50f. See also Nuclear
cataracts
smoking and, 6–7
Nucleofractis, "divide and conquer," 112–114, 113f
Nucleus (lens). See Lens (crystalline), nucleus of
Nutritional deficiency, cataract formation and, 7, 63–64

O'Brien nerve block, for cataract surgery, 92, 93f
Occlusion, in phacoemulsification, 102
OCT. See Optical coherence tomography/biometry
Ocular history, in cataract, 69–71, 70t
evaluation for surgery and, 75–76
Ocular hypotension. See Hypotony
Ocular motility, assessment of, before cataract surgery,
77–78
Ocular (intraocular) surgery
cataract and, 55–57
lens particle glaucoma and, 67
Ocular trauma
assessment of, 190–191
cataract surgery after, 190–193, 192f
ectopia lentis caused by, 40
lens damage/cataracts caused by, 53–59, 54f, 55f, 56f,
58f, 59f, 190–193, 192f
glaucoma and, 67
phacoantigenic uveitis and, 66, 191
surgery for, 192
Oculomotor nerve. See Cranial nerve III
Oil droplet appearance/cataract, 44
in galactosemia, 61, 61f
in lenticonus/lentiglobus, 30
1-piece foldable intraocular lens, insertion of, 116
Opacities. See also Cataract
fundus evaluation with, 81
IOL, 151
Open-loop speculum, for globe exposure, in cataract
surgery, 105f
Operating/surgical microscope
for manual small-incision cataract surgery, 198
retinal light toxicity and, 166
Ophthalmic instrumentation, for cataract surgery,
retinal light toxicity and, 166
Ophthalmic viscosurgical devices (OVDs/viscoelastic
agents), 95–97
advanced cataract and, 180
aniridia and, 184
capsular block syndrome and, 148
capsular rupture during surgery and, 142–143
in ECCE, 197
elevated intraocular pressure and, 136
high hyperopia and, 185
in ICCE, 200
inflamed eye and, 191
intumescent cataract and, 179–180
IOL implantation and, 116, 117, 117–118
in keratoconjunctivitis sicca, dry eye therapy before
use of, 173

in phacoemulsification, 105, 109, 110, 112, 115, 116,
117–118
physical properties of, 96
posterior polar cataract and, 181
pupil expansion and, 178
selection of, 97
traumatic cataract and, 191, 192
uveitis and, 191
zonular dehiscence with lens subluxation or
dislocation and, 182
Ophthalmoscopy, before cataract surgery, 80–81
Optic axis, 9, 10f
Optic cup, development of, 25
Optic nerve (cranial nerve II), evaluation of, before
cataract surgery, 81
Optic vesicle, lens development and, 25, 26f
Optical clarity, of ophthalmic viscosurgical device, 97
Optical coherence tomography/biometry (OCT)
before cataract surgery, 82
in IOL power determination, 82, 84–85, 87
Optical (ocular) medium/media, opaque. See Cataract;
Opacities
OVDs. See Ophthalmic viscosurgical devices
Overrefraction, cataract surgery evaluation and, 76
Oxidative lens damage, 19–20
Oxygen therapy, hyperbaric, oxidative lens damage and,
20, 65

Pachymetry, before cataract surgery, 84
PAM (Potential Acuity Meter). See Potential acuity
estimation/Potential Acuity Meter
Pannus, cataract surgery in patient with, 79
Paracentesis, in phacoemulsification, 105
Parasympatholytic agents, accommodation affected by, 23
Parasympathomimetic agents, accommodation affected
by, 23
Pars plana vitrectomy
for capsular rupture during cataract surgery, 143
cataract/cataract surgery after, 55, 190
for IOL decentration/dislocation, 145
for postoperative endophthalmitis, 162
for retained lens fragments after phacoemulsification,
141
for retinal detachment, cataract surgery/IOL and, 166
Patient education, before cataract surgery, 87–88
PAX6 gene mutation
in aniridia, 33
in Peters anomaly, 32
PCIOL. See Intraocular lenses (IOLs), posterior chamber
PCO. See Posterior capsular/capsule opacification
Pemphigoid, mucous membrane, cataract surgery in
patient with, 173
Penetrating injuries, lens damage caused by, 55
glaucoma and, 67
Penetrating keratoplasty. See Keratoplasty, penetrating
Pentose phosphate pathway (hexose monophosphate
shunt), in lens glucose/carbohydrate metabolism,
17, 18f, 19
Perforating injuries, lens damage caused by, 55, 55f, 56f
Peribulbar anesthesia, for cataract surgery, 91
Peripheral iris suture fixation, for IOL decentration,
145, 146f
Peristaltic pump, for phacoemulsification aspiration,
103, 103f

Peroxidation, lipid, in lens opacification, 19
Persistent corneal epithelial defects, after cataract surgery, 132, 173
Persistent fetal vasculature (PFV/persistent hyperplastic primary vitreous), 42
Peters anomaly, 31–32
PFV. *See* Persistent fetal vasculature
Phaco chop technique, 114
Phaco fracture technique, 112–114, 113*f*
Phaco handpiece, 98, 98*f*
Phaco tip, 98*f*, 100, 101*f*
Phacoanaphylactic endophthalmitis, 66
Phacoantigenic uveitis, 66
Phacodonesis, cataract surgery and, 182
Phacodynamics, terminology used in, 102–103
Phacoemulsification, 90–91, 98–118. *See also* Cataract surgery
  for advanced cataract, 180
  anterior capsulotomy for, 109–110
  in anterior chamber, 112
  anticoagulant use and, 171–172, 172*t*
  aspiration system for, 102, 115
  burst-mode, 101
  capsular rupture during, 142–143
  capsule staining for, 178–179, 179*f*
  capsulorrhexis in, 108–110, 109*f*
  clear corneal incision for, 106–107, 106*f*
  cystoid macular edema after, 164, 187
  elliptical, 101
  eye marking/time-out before, 104–105
  flat or shallow anterior chamber and, 134–136
    intraoperative complications and, 134–135
    posterior fluid misdirection syndrome and, 134–135
    postoperative complications and, 135–136
  foldable IOLs for, 116, 120, 120*f*. *See also* Foldable intraocular lenses
  in glaucoma, 186
    after filtering surgery, 187
    intraocular pressure lowered by, 186
  globe exposure for, 105, 105*f*
  high myopia and, 184–185
  historical overview of, 90–91
  hydrodelineation in, 110
  hydrodissection in, 110
  incisions for
    clear corneal incisions, 106–107, 106*f*
    scleral tunnel incisions, 107–108, 107*f*
  instrumentation for, 98–99, 98*f*
  for intumescent cataract extraction, 179–180
  IOLs for, 115–117, 118–122
    procedures after insertion of, 117–118
  at iris plane, 112
  irrigation in, 101–102, 115
    posterior fluid misdirection and, 134–135
    toxic solutions exposure and, corneal edema caused by, 129, 133–134
  lens particle glaucoma and, 67
  locations of, 111–112
  nuclear rotation in, 111
  nucleus disassembly/removal in, 111
    locations for emulsification and, 111–112
    techniques of, 112–114, 113*f*
      chopping techniques, 114
      phaco fracture, 112–114, 113*f*

  ocular trauma affecting visualization and, 191
  paracentesis for, 105
  after pars plana vitrectomy, 190
  posterior capsule opacification and, 152–153
    Nd:YAG laser capsulotomy for, 152, 153, 154–157, 154*f*, 156*f*. *See also* Nd:YAG laser therapy, capsulotomy
  in posterior chamber, 111–112
  for posterior polar cataract, 180–181
    hydrodissection/nucleus rotation and, 111, 181
  power delivery and, 99
    advances in, 100–101, 100*f*
  procedure for, 104–118
  pulsed, 100
  retained lens fragments after, 141
  retinal detachment and, 127, 166–167
  scleral tunnel incisions for, 107–108, 107*f*
  supracapsular, 110
  suprachoroidal effusion/hemorrhage risk and, 171
  torsional, 101
  for traumatic cataract, 192
  in triple procedure, 175
  ultrasonic technology terminology and, 99–100
  after vitrectomy, 190
  in zonular dehiscence with lens subluxation or dislocation, 181–183, 182*f*, 183*f*
Phacolysis, fluid-based, 125
Phacolytic glaucoma, 67
Phacomorphic glaucoma, 67, 68*f*
Phakinin, 16
Phenothiazines, lens changes caused by, 52, 52*f*
Phenylephrine, for intraoperative floppy iris syndrome, 138
Phimosis, capsular, 153–154
  Nd:YAG laser capsulotomy for, 154, 154–157, 154*f*, 156*f*
  in pseudoexfoliation/exfoliation syndrome, 184
Phosphofructokinase, in lens glucose/carbohydrate metabolism, 17, 18*f*
Photolysis, laser, 125
Photorefractive keratectomy (PRK), cataract surgery after, 177
  IOL power calculation and, 86
Phototherapeutic keratectomy, for corneal/epithelial erosions, 129
Piezoelectric crystal, in phacoemulsification handpiece, 99, 100
Pigmentations/pigment deposits, lens
  aging and, 43, 44*f*
  blunt injury causing (Vossius ring), 53
  drugs causing, 52, 52*f*
Pilocarpine
  accommodation affected by, 23
  cataracts caused by, 52
Pits, lens, 25, 26*f*
PITX2 gene, in Peters anomaly, 32
PKP. *See* Keratoplasty, penetrating (PKP)
Placode, lens, 25, 26*f*
Pleomorphism, specular microscopy in evaluation of, before cataract surgery, 84
PMMA. *See* Polymethyl methacrylate
Polar cataracts, 35–36, 37*f*
  surgery for, 180–181
    hydrodissection/nucleus rotation and, 111, 181
Polymegethism, specular microscopy in evaluation of, before cataract surgery, 84

Polymethyl methacrylate (PMMA), IOLs made from, 116, 118, 119
  capsular opacification and, 153
  insertion of, 116
  for manual small-incision cataract surgery, 198
Polyol (sorbitol) pathway
  in cataract formation, 19
  in lens glucose/carbohydrate metabolism, 18f, 19
Polyopia, in cataracts, 70–71
Positive dysphotopsias, IOLs and, 150
"Positive vitreous pressure," flat or shallow anterior chamber and, 134
Posterior capsular/capsule opacification (PCO), cataract surgery and, 152–153
  Nd:YAG laser capsulotomy for, 152, 153, 154–157, 154f, 156f. See also Nd:YAG laser therapy
Posterior capsular rupture, cataract surgery and, 142–143
Posterior chamber, phacoemulsification in, 111–112
Posterior chamber intraocular lenses. See Intraocular lenses
Posterior fluid misdirection syndrome, 134–135
Posterior lenticonus/lentiglobus, 30, 30f
Posterior polar cataract, 36
  surgery for, 180–181
    hydrodissection/nucleus rotation and, 111, 181
Posterior pole, 9, 10f, 12f
Posterior pupillary membrane, 29f
  remnant of (Mittendorf dot), 29, 31, 32f
Posterior subcapsular cataract (PSC), 46–48, 51f
  characteristics and effects of, 47, 70t
  corticosteroids causing, 51–52
  ischemia causing, 68
  in myotonic dystrophy, 62
  race and, 6
  silicone oil use and, 190
  uveitis and, 64
  vitrectomy and, 55, 190
Posterior synechiae, in uveitis, lens changes/cataract and, 64
Posterior vitreous detachment (PVD), retinal detachment after cataract surgery and, 166
Postoperative care of cataract surgery patient
  antimicrobial prophylaxis, 95
  after ECCE, 198
  after ICCE, 201
Postoperative endophthalmitis, 127, 160–163, 161f
  prevention of, 93–95, 94f, 161–162
Postvitrectomy cataract, 55, 190
Potassium, in lens, 21
Potassium balance, in lens, pump–leak theory of maintenance of, 21, 22f
Potential acuity estimation/Potential Acuity Meter (PAM), in cataract surgery evaluation, 81–82
Power, in phacoemulsification, 100
  delivery of, 99
    advances in, 100–101, 100f
Power (optical), IOL, determination of, 84–87
  biometry in, 82–83, 83f, 84–85, 87
    hypotony affecting, 185
  formulas for, 84, 85–87
  historical methods for, 86–87
  improving outcomes of surgery and, 87
  incorrect, 85
  preventing errors in, 87

refraction and, 76
refractive surgery and, 85–87, 176, 177f
triple procedure and, 175
unexpected refractive results after surgery and, 86, 150
Power prediction formulas, for IOLs, 84, 85–87
Prazosin, intraoperative floppy iris syndrome and, 74, 136–137, 137t
Prednisolone, for cystoid macular edema, after cataract surgery, 165
"Premium" IOLs, 120–121
  contraindication to, capsular decentration and, 183
  dry eye therapy before use of, 173
Preoperative assessment/preparation for cataract surgery, 74–76, 87–88
  antimicrobial prophylaxis and, 93–94
  in diabetes mellitus, 80–81
  ECCE, 196
  ICCE, 199
  medical evaluation and, 170–171
  ocular trauma and, 190–191
Presbyopia, 23
Preussner formula, for IOL power determination/selection, 85
Primary aphakia, 30. See also Aphakia
Primary coloboma, 30–31. See also Coloboma
Primary lens fibers, development of, 26–27, 27f
Primary vitreous, persistent hyperplasia of. See Persistent fetal vasculature
PRK. See Photorefractive keratectomy
Proparacaine, for cataract surgery, 92
Propionibacterium acnes, uveitis/endophthalmitis after cataract surgery caused by, 140, 162
Prostaglandins, cystoid macular edema after cataract surgery and, 164, 187
PSC. See Posterior subcapsular cataract
Pseudoaccommodating intraocular lenses, 122
  complications of, 151
Pseudoexfoliation/exfoliation syndrome, 65–66, 65f
  cataract surgery in patient with, 79, 184
  IOL decentration/dislocation and, 144
  postoperative hyphema and, 158
  zonular incompetence and, 65–66, 181, 182f, 184
Pseudophakia, surgically induced, cataract surgery and, 166–167
Pseudophakic (aphakic) bullous keratopathy, after cataract surgery, 129, 129f
  IOL design and, 149
Pseudophakodonesis
  anterior capsule contraction and, 154
  IOL dislocation and, 145
Pseudoplasticity, of ophthalmic viscosurgical device, 96
Pulse (term), in phacoemulsification, 100
Pulsed phacoemulsification, 100
Pulseless disease (Takayasu arteritis), cataract caused by, 68
Pump–leak theory, 21, 22f
Pupil expansion devices, 177, 178f
  for intraoperative floppy iris syndrome, 178
  for traumatic inflammation, 191
Pupillary block
  after cataract surgery, flat or shallow anterior chamber and, 135–136
  microspherophakia causing, 33
  phacomorphic glaucoma and, 67, 68f

Pupillary capture, after cataract surgery, 148, 148f
 IOL decentration and, 145
Pupillary light reflex (pupillary response to light), in
 cataract surgery evaluation, 78
Pupillary membrane
 anterior, 29, 29f
 in cataract surgery, 188
 posterior, 29f
 remnant of (Mittendorf dot), 29, 31, 32f
Pupilloplasty
 for cataracts, 71–72
 for IOL decentration/dislocation, 145
Pupils
 displacement of (corectopia), cataract surgery in
  patient with, 180
 in ectopia lentis et pupillae, 42
 examination of, before cataract surgery, 78
 Marcus Gunn (relative afferent pupillary defect),
  cataract surgery on patient with, 78
 size of, cataract surgery and, 78, 177–178, 178f
  IOL selection and, 78
  trauma and, 191
  uveitis and, 188
PVD. See Posterior vitreous detachment
Pyridoxine (vitamin B_6), for homocystinuria, 41

Q formula, Hoffer, for IOL power determination/
 selection, 85

Race, cataract development and, 6
Radial keratotomy (RK)
 cataract surgery after, 79, 177
  IOL power calculation and, 86
 hyperopic shift and, 177
Radiation, cataracts caused by, 57–58
RAM. See Retinal Acuity Meter
RAPD. See Relative afferent pupillary defect
Red reflex
 in complete cataract, 38
 after ECCE, 198
 in lenticonus/lentiglobus, 30
 poor, cataract surgery and, 178–179, 179f
Refracting power, in IOL power determination, 84
Refraction, clinical, in cataract
 nonsurgical management and, 71
 before surgery/IOL power determination, 76
Refractive errors, unexpected, after cataract surgery, 86,
 149–150
Refractive index, of lens, 11
Refractive surgery, cataract/cataract surgery and,
 123–124, 176–177, 177f
 IOL power calculation and, 85–87, 176, 177f
 preoperative evaluation/planning and, 76, 79
Regression formulas, for IOL power determination/
 selection, 85–87
Relative afferent pupillary defect (RAPD/Marcus Gunn
 pupil), cataract surgery in patient with, 78
Relaxing incisions
 for anterior capsule contraction, 154f, 156
 limbal, cataract surgery and, 123–124
Resolution, minimum angle of (MAR), logarithm of
 (logMAR), cystoid macular edema after cataract
 surgery and, 164
Retained lens material, cataract surgery and, 140–141

Retina
 examination of, before cataract surgery, 80–81
 light injury of, during cataract surgery, 166
 oxidative lens damage during surgery on, 20
Retinal Acuity Meter (RAM), in cataract surgery
 evaluation, 81
Retinal detachment
 after cataract surgery, 127, 166–167
  family history as risk factor and, 75
  Nd:YAG laser capsulotomy and, 157, 166
 after Nd:YAG laser capsulotomy, 157, 166
 posterior vitreous detachment and, cataract surgery
  and, 166
Retinal disease
 after cataract surgery, 163–167, 164f
 cataract surgery in patient with, 189
Retinal ischemia, cataract surgery and, 80–81
Retinal light toxicity, cataract surgery and, 166
Retinal pigment epithelium (RPE), burns of, during
 cataract surgery, 166
Retinitis pigmentosa (RP), cataract/cataract surgery in
 patient with, 68
Retinoscopy, before cataract surgery, 80
Retrobulbar anesthesia, for cataract surgery, 91, 91f
 hemorrhage and, 158, 171
Retrobulbar hemorrhage, cataract surgery and, 158, 171
Rhegmatogenous retinal detachment. See Retinal
 detachment
Rheumatoid arthritis, cataract surgery in patient with,
 corneal melting/keratolysis and, 132
Riders, 35
Ridley intraocular lens, 118–119, 118f
Right to Sight, 6
Rise time, in phacoemulsification, 102, 103
RK. See Radial keratotomy
Rosacea, cataract surgery in patient with, 172–173
Rosette cataract, 54, 54f
RRD (rhegmatogenous retinal detachment). See Retinal
 detachment
Rubella, congenital, cataracts and, 38–39

Salisbury Eye Evaluation project, 6
Scleral buckling/buckle, for retinal detachment, after
 cataract surgery, 166–167
Scleral-fixated posterior chamber intraocular lenses
 after ICCE, 200
 insertion of, 116–117
 after keratoplasty, 176
 ocular trauma and, 193
 uveitis and, 188
Scleral support ring, for ICCE, 199
Scleral tunnel incisions, for cataract surgery, 107–108,
 107f
 after radial keratotomy, 177
Scleritis, cataract surgery in patient with, 170–171
Sclerosis, nuclear, 43, 45f, 48f, 50f
 smoking and, 6–7
Sclerotomy, for suprachoroidal hemorrhage, 160
Sculpting, in phacoemulsification, settings for, 111
"Second sight," 43, 70
Secondary aphakia, 30. See also Aphakia
Secondary coloboma, 31. See also Coloboma
Secondary lens fibers, development of, 27–28, 27f
 microspherophakia and, 33

Segment removal, in phacoemulsification, settings for, 111

Self-sealing incision, for cataract surgery, 118
   beveled/biplanar, clear corneal incision and, 106–107, 106*f*

Seventh nerve palsy, cataract surgery in patient with, 174

Shallow anterior chamber. *See* Anterior chamber, flat or shallow

Siderosis/siderosis bulbi, 58–59, 58*f*

Siepser slipknot technique, for IOL decentration, 145, 146*f*

Silicone foldable intraocular lenses, 120. *See also* Foldable intraocular lenses
   IOL opacification and, 151
   after ocular trauma, 193
   in uveitis, 188, 188*f*

Silicone oil, cataract/cataract surgery and, 83, 120, 190

Silodosin, intraoperative floppy iris syndrome and, 74, 136, 137*t*

Simcoe cannula, 198, 199*f*

Simple diffusion, glucose transport into lens and, 17*f*

Simvastatin, cataract risk and, 53

Sjögren syndrome, cataract surgery in patient with, corneal melting/keratolysis and, 132

Slit-lamp biomicroscopy/examination, before cataract surgery, 78–80
   limitations of, 80

Small-incision cataract surgery, 198, 199*f*
   in eye with functioning filter, 187
   in glaucoma, 186, 187

Smoking/smoking cessation, cataract development and, 6–7, 63–64

Snellen acuity. *See* Visual acuity

"Snowflake" cataract, 60, 60*f*

Social history, cataract surgery evaluation and, 72, 76

Sodium, in lens, 21

Sodium balance, in lens, pump–leak theory of maintenance of, 21, 22*f*

Sodium hyaluronate, as viscoelastic, 95

Sodium-potassium pump (Na$^+$,K$^+$-ATPase), in lens
   active transport, 21
   pump–leak theory and, 21, 22*f*

Soemmering ring, 152

Sorbitol/sorbitol pathway
   in cataract formation, 19, 60
   in lens glucose/carbohydrate metabolism, 18*f*, 19

Space maintenance, by ophthalmic viscosurgical device, 97

Specular microscopy, before cataract surgery, 84

Sphincter muscle (iris), damage to, cataract surgery in patient with, 191

Spondylitis, ankylosing (AS), cataract surgery in patient with, 171, 171*f*

SRK/T formula, for IOL power determination/ selection, 85

Staphylococcus
   aureus, postoperative endophthalmitis caused by, 140, 161
   epidermidis, uveitis/endophthalmitis after cataract surgery caused by, 140, 162

Statins, cataracts and, 53

Stellate (sutural) cataracts, 37, 37*f*

Steroids. *See* Corticosteroids

Stop and chop technique, in phacoemulsification, 114

Streptococcus, postoperative endophthalmitis caused by, 161

Stroke/stroke length (phacoemulsification), 99, 100

Stromal edema, after cataract surgery, 128–130, 128*t*

Subcapsular cataract, posterior, 46–48, 51*f*
   characteristics and effects of, 47, 70*t*
   corticosteroids causing, 51–52
   ischemia causing, 68
   in myotonic dystrophy, 62
   race and, 6
   silicone oil use and, 190
   uveitis and, 64
   vitrectomy and, 55, 190

Subluxation, IOL, 144–147, 144*f*, 146*f*, 147*f*. *See also* Decentration/dislocation

Subluxed/subluxated lens, 39–40, 40*f*. *See also* Ectopia lentis
   cataract surgery in patient with, 181–183, 182*f*, 183*f*
   traumatic, 40, 54–55, 54*f*

Sub-Tenon drug administration
   corticosteroid, in cystoid macular edema, after cataract surgery, 165
   lidocaine, for cataract surgery, 92, 92*f*

"Sugar" cataracts, aldose reductase in development of, 19

"Sunflower" cataract, in chalcosis/Wilson disease, 59, 62

Sunglasses, ultraviolet-absorbing lenses and, cataract prevention and, 58

Sunlight. *See* Ultraviolet light

Superoxide dismutase, in lens, 20

Supracapsular phacoemulsification, 110

Suprachoroidal effusion, cataract surgery and, 159
   flat or shallow anterior chamber and, 134

Suprachoroidal hemorrhage/choroidal hemorrhage, cataract surgery and, 159, 171
   delayed, 160
   expulsive, 159–160
   flat or shallow anterior chamber and, 134

Surface ectoderm, lens development and, 25, 26*f*

Surface tension, of ophthalmic viscosurgical device, 96

Surge, in phacoemulsification, 102

Surgical instruments, for phacoemulsification, 98–99, 98*f*

Sutural cataracts, 37, 37*f*

Sutures (lens), 13
   development of, 27*f*, 28–29, 28*f*
   opacification of (sutural/stellate cataract), 37, 37*f*

Sutures (surgical)
   for cataract surgery
      astigmatism and, 131–132
      posterior chamber IOL fixation and, 116–117, 119, 119*f*
   McCannel, for IOL decentration, 145

Swinging flashlight test, for relative afferent pupillary defect, before cataract surgery, 78

Symblepharon, cataract surgery in patient with, 173

Synechiae, posterior, in uveitis, lens changes/cataract and, 64

Takayasu arteritis (pulseless disease), cataract caused by, 68

Tamoxifen
   cataract risk and, 53
   maculopathy caused by, 53

Tamsulosin, intraoperative floppy iris syndrome and, 74, 136, 137, 137t

TASS. See Toxic Anterior Segment Syndrome

Tension rings, capsular, for zonular incompetence, 180, 181f, 183

Terazosin, intraoperative floppy iris syndrome and, 74, 136–137, 137t

Tetanic cataract, 61–62

Tetracaine, for cataract surgery, 92

TGF-β. See Transforming growth factor βs

Thermal injury (burns), cataract surgery incision, 131

Thioridazine, lens changes caused by, 52

3-piece foldable intraocular lens, insertion of, 116

Thromboangiitis obliterans (Buerger disease), cataract caused by, 68

Time-out
    before ECCE, 196
    before phacoemulsification, 104–105

Tobacco use, cataract development and, 6–7, 63–64

Topical anesthesia, for cataract surgery, 92

Topography, corneal, before cataract surgery, 84, 86, 174

Toric intraocular lenses, 124
    complications of, 151
    contraindication to, capsular decentration and, 183
    dry eye therapy before use of, 173

Torsional phacoemulsification, 101

Total cataract, 38

Toxic anterior segment syndrome (TASS), 129, 133–134

Toxic solutions, exposure to during cataract surgery, corneal edema caused by, 129, 133–134

Trabeculectomy, cataract risk and, 56

Transforming growth factor βs (TGF-βs), in pseudoexfoliation/exfoliation syndrome, 65

Transplantation, corneal
    cataract/cataract surgery and, 56, 175, 176
    in triple procedure, 175

Transport mechanisms, lens, 21, 22f

Trauma
    assessment of, 190–191
    cataract surgery after, 190–193, 192f
    ectopia lentis caused by, 40
    lens damage/cataracts caused by, 53–59, 54f, 55f, 56f, 58f, 59f, 190–193, 192f
        glaucoma and, 67
        phacoantigenic uveitis and, 66, 191
        surgery for, 192

Triple procedure, 175

Trypan blue dye, for capsule staining, 178–179, 179f

Tunica vasculosa lentis, 29, 29f
    remnant of
        epicapsular star, 31, 32f
        Mittendorf dot, 29, 31, 32f

Twin studies, in age-related cataract, 41–42

UDP galactose 4-epimerase deficiency, galactosemia/cataract formation and, 61

UGH syndrome. See Uveitis-glaucoma-hyphema (UGH) syndrome

Ultrasonic (term), 99

Ultrasonography/ultrasound
    before cataract surgery, 81, 82–83, 83f, 87
        hypotony and, 185
    in IOL power determination/selection, 82–83, 83f, 87

for phacoemulsification, 98
    terminology related to, 99–100

Ultraviolet-absorbing chromophores/filters, IOLs with, 120

Ultraviolet-absorbing lenses, cataract prevention and, 58

Ultraviolet (UV) light (ultraviolet radiation)
    eye disorders/injury associated with
        cataracts, 57–58
        pseudoexfoliation, 65–66, 65f
    lenses absorbing, cataract prevention and, 58

Urea-insoluble (membrane structural) lens proteins, 15f, 16–17

Urea-soluble (cytoskeletal) lens proteins, 15f, 16–17

UV light/radiation. See Ultraviolet light

Uveitis
    cataracts and, 64–65, 64f, 188
        after cataract surgery, 139–140
        surgery in patients with, 64–65, 75, 140, 170–171, 188, 188f
    Fuchs heterochromic, cataracts/cataract surgery in, 64–65, 64f
    phacoantigenic, 66

Uveitis-glaucoma-hyphema (UGH) syndrome, IOL implantation and, 149
    decentration and, 145

Vacuum (phacoemulsification), 98, 103

Vacuum rise time (phacoemulsification), 102, 103

van Lint nerve block, for cataract surgery, 92, 93f

Vancomycin, for postoperative endophthalmitis, 162

VDA (Visual Disability Assessment), 71

Venous retrobulbar hemorrhage, cataract surgery and, 158

Venturi pump, for phacoemulsification aspiration, 103, 104f

Vertical chopping techniques, in phacoemulsification, 114

Vesicle
    lens, formation of, 25, 26f
    optic, lens development and, 25, 26f

VF-14 (Visual Function Index), 71

Videokeratography, IOL power determination/selection after refractive surgery and, 86

Vimentin, 16

Viscodissection, 115. See also Ophthalmic viscosurgical devices
    for advanced cataract, 180
    in zonular dehiscence with lens subluxation or dislocation, 182

Viscoelastic agents. See Ophthalmic viscosurgical devices

Viscoelasticity, of ophthalmic viscosurgical device, 96

Viscomydriasis, 97

Viscosity, of ophthalmic viscosurgical device, 96

Viscosurgical devices, ophthalmic (viscoelastic agents). See Ophthalmic viscosurgical devices

VISION 2020, 6

Vision loss/impairment. See also Visual acuity
    cataract and, 5, 69–71, 70t
        indications for surgery and, 72–73

Vision rehabilitation, in cataracts, 71
    ocular trauma and, 193

Visual acuity
  in cataract, 69–70, 70*t*
    indications for surgery and, 72–73
    preoperative evaluation and, 75–76, 76
  after cataract surgery, 126
    cystoid macular edema and, 163, 164
    with ECCE, 198
    endophthalmitis and, 161, 162
    with ICCE, 201
    incorrect lens power and, 85
    with manual small-incision surgery, 198–199
    multifocal IOLs and, 121–122
Visual axis, Nd:YAG laser capsulotomy location and, 155
Visual Disability Assessment (VDA), 71
Visual field defects, in glaucoma, cataract/media opacities and, 186, 186*f*
Visual field testing, before cataract surgery, 82
Visual function, measuring, in cataract evaluation, 71
  before surgery, 71, 72, 76–77
  after surgery, 126
  indications for surgery and, 72
Visual Function Index (VF-14), 71
Visual loss/impairment. *See* Vision loss/impairment
Vitamin B₆ (pyridoxine), for homocystinuria, 41
Vitamins
  deficiencies of, cataracts caused by, 63
  supplementary, cataract prevention and, 7, 20
Vitrectomy
  for capsular rupture during cataract surgery, 142, 143
  cataract/cataract surgery after, 20, 55, 75, 190
  for IOL decentration/dislocation, 145
  oxidative lens damage and, 20
  pars plana. *See* Pars plana vitrectomy
  for postoperative cystoid macular edema, 165
  for postoperative endophthalmitis, 162
  for retained lens fragments after phacoemulsification, 141
  for retinal detachment, 166
  for vitreocorneal adherence/persistent corneal edema, 130
  for vitreous prolapse, 142, 143–144
Vitreocorneal adherence, after cataract surgery, 130
Vitreolysis, Nd:YAG laser
  for cystoid macular edema, after cataract surgery, 165
  for vitreous prolapse in anterior chamber, 143
Vitreoretinopathies, cataract surgery in patient with, 189
Vitreous
  biopsy of, for endophthalmitis after cataract surgery, 162
  cataract surgery complications and
    endophthalmitis, 161
    with ICCE, 200
    posterior vitreous detachment, 166
    prolapse, 142, 143–144
    vitreocorneal adherence, 130
  primary, persistent hyperplasia of. *See* Persistent fetal vasculature
Vitreous block. *See also* Ciliary block glaucoma
  after cataract surgery, 139

Vitreous detachment, posterior (PVD), retinal detachment after cataract surgery and, 166
Vitreous pressure, positive, flat or shallow anterior chamber and, 134
von Graefe knife, 90
Vossius ring, 53

WAGR syndrome, 33
Warfarin/warfarin derivatives, cataract surgery in patient taking, 171
Water and electrolyte balance, in lens, maintenance of, 21, 22*f*
Water channels (aquaporins), 16, 20–21
Water-insoluble lens proteins, 15, 15*f*
  aging affecting, 17
Water-soluble lens proteins, 15, 15*f*. *See also* Crystallins
  conversion of to water-insoluble, 17
Wavefront aberrometry, intraoperative, in IOL power determination/selection
  astigmatism and, 124
  after refractive surgery, 86
Wedl (bladder) cells, 48, 152
Weill-Marchesani syndrome, microspherophakia in, 33
WHO (World Health Organization), cataract epidemiology and, 5
Wilms tumor, aniridia and, 33
Wilson disease (hepatolenticular degeneration), 62
World Health Organization (WHO), cataract epidemiology and, 5
Wound closure, after cataract surgery
  complications associated with, 130–131
  after ECCE, 197–198
  after ICCE, 200–201
  postoperative endophthalmitis and, 161
Wound dehiscence/rupture, after cataract surgery, 131
Wound leaks, after cataract surgery, 118, 130–131
  flat anterior chamber and, 135

Y-sutures, lens, 13
  development of, 28, 28*f*
  opacification of (sutural/stellate cataract), 37, 37*f*

Z syndrome, 151
Zeaxanthin, cataract risk affected by, 7
Zinn, zonules of (zonular fibers). *See* Zonular fibers, lens
Zonular (lamellar) cataracts, 34–35, 36*f*
Zonular dehiscence, cataract surgery and, 181–183, 182*f*, 183*f*
  iris coloboma/corectopia and, 180
Zonular fibers, lens (zonules of Zinn), 9, 10*f*, 12
  absent/abnormal, cataract surgery and, 179–184
    iris coloboma/corectopia and, 180
    nucleus rotation and, 111
  development of, 29
  evaluation of, before cataract surgery, 80
  in pseudoexfoliation/exfoliation syndrome, 65–66, 181, 182*f*, 184
Zonular lamella, 11
Zonules, of Zinn (zonular fibers). *See* Zonular fibers, lens